Immunohistochemistry

Immunohistochemistry

A Technical Guide to Current Practices

Edited by

Trung Nguyen

Peter MacCallum Cancer Centre

CAMBRIDGE
UNIVERSITY PRESS

CAMBRIDGE
UNIVERSITY PRESS

University Printing House, Cambridge CB2 8BS, United Kingdom

One Liberty Plaza, 20th Floor, New York, NY 10006, USA

477 Williamstown Road, Port Melbourne, VIC 3207, Australia

314–321, 3rd Floor, Plot 3, Splendor Forum, Jasola District Centre, New Delhi – 110025, India

103 Penang Road, #05–06/07, Visioncrest Commercial, Singapore 238467

Cambridge University Press is part of the University of Cambridge.

It furthers the University's mission by disseminating knowledge in the pursuit of education, learning, and research at the highest international levels of excellence.

www.cambridge.org
Information on this title: www.cambridge.org/9781009107723
DOI: 10.1017/9781009106924

First published 2022

Printed in the United Kingdom by TJ Books Limited, Padstow Cornwall

A catalogue record for this publication is available from the British Library.

Library of Congress Cataloging-in-Publication Data
Names: Nguyen, Trung, 1976– editor.
Title: Immunohistochemistry : a technical guide to current practices / edited by Trung Nguyen.
Other titles: Immunohistochemistry (Nguyen)
Description: Cambridge, United Kingdom ; New York, NY : Cambridge University Press, 2022. | Includes bibliographical references and index.
Identifiers: LCCN 2021047523 (print) | LCCN 2021047524 (ebook) | ISBN 9781009107723 (paperback) | ISBN 9781009106924 (ebook)
Subjects: MESH: Immunohistochemistry
Classification: LCC RB46.6 (print) | LCC RB46.6 (ebook) | NLM QW 504.5 | DDC 616.07/56–dc23
LC record available at https://lccn.loc.gov/2021047523
LC ebook record available at https://lccn.loc.gov/2021047524

ISBN 978-1-009-10772-3 Paperback

A dedication to one and all,
For mum and dad, our salvation when we fall.
To those here and to those who have passed,
You are still with us; eternal love forever lasts.

Contents

List of Contributors viii
Preface ix

1 **Immunohistochemistry Fundamentals** 1
Enisa Hasic

2 **Immunohistochemistry Quality Assurance and Quality Control** 24
Bronwyn Christiansen and Hazel Chambers

3 **Automation and Robotics with the Leica Bond III** 67
Anthony F. Henwood

4 **Automation and Robotics with the Roche Ventana BenchMark ULTRA** 85
Ahida Batrouney

5 **Automation and Robotics with the Agilent Dako Omnis** 120
Andrew Dinan

6 **Immunohistochemistry for Research Applications** 160
Trung Nguyen

7 **Troubleshooting Immunohistochemistry** 183
David Gan

8 **Current Status of Immunohistochemistry** 210
Trung Nguyen

9 **Immunohistochemistry for Future Applications** 253
Candice J. Clarke

Index 266

Contributors

Ahida Batrouney. BAppSc
Senior Scientist – Immunohistochemistry, Anatomical Pathology
The Royal Melbourne Hospital, Australia

Hazel Chambers. BSc, MSc, FAIMS
Senior Scientist – Immunohistochemistry, Anatomical Pathology
Royal Children's Hospital, Australia

Bronwyn Christiansen. BAppSc, FAIMS
Principal Scientist – Anatomical Pathology
Royal Children's Hospital, Australia

Candice J. Clarke. BSc (Hons), MSc (MBT), MBA (Health Management)
Senior Medical Laboratory Scientist – Anatomical Pathology
New South Wales Health Pathology
Concord Repatriation General Hospital, Australia

Andrew Dinan. BSc (Hons)
Senior Scientist – Immunohistochemistry, Anatomical Pathology
The Alfred Hospital, Australia

David Gan. AssocDip Clinical Laboratory Techniques
IHC Supervisor – Anatomical Pathology
Princess Alexandra Hospital
Australia

Enisa Hasic. BSc
Hospital Scientist – Anatomical Pathology
Prince of Wales Hospital, Australia

Anthony F. Henwood. MSc, BAppSc, GradDipSysAnalys, CT(ASC), FFSc(RCPA)
Principal Scientist – Anatomical Pathology
The Children's Hospital at Westmead Australia
Adjunct Fellow – School of Medicine, University of Western Sydney, Australia
Visiting Lecturer – School of Life Sciences, University of Technology Sydney, Australia

Trung Nguyen. BAppSc, FAIMS
Principal Scientist – Anatomical Pathology
Peter MacCallum Cancer Centre, Australia

Preface

Immunohistochemistry (IHC) is a fascinating piece of technology. It has many facets and offers diverse perspectives, depending on how it is used. As a platform, it is employed in both diagnostic and research applications within medical science. Protein expression and morphological relationships within tissue structures are gained by visualizing antigen–antibody attractions at the cellular level. At its core, it is an analytical tool requiring complete understanding of all of its intricacies so that its full potential can be realized.

Alongside the humble haematoxylin and eosin (H&E) stain, IHC is a member of the 'golden trinity' of histology testing which includes the traditional special stains and the new frontier of molecular technologies (electron microscopy is a highly specialized technique and considered separate because of its unique fixation requirements). Special stains, IHC and molecular assays for the most part can be performed on formalin fixed paraffin embedded (FFPE) tissue blocks. For this reason, IHC has cemented itself as an invaluable part of a pathologist's toolkit. In addition, diagnostic histopathology has entered the 'molecular age', and this venture has implications for targeted therapies. Novel treatment regimens are tailored to specific tumour profiles. Certainly, the concept of personalized medicine is rapidly expanding, bringing with it the importance of IHC as an analytic tool.

Antibodies are fundamental to IHC. Unfortunately, not all are created equal. Some clones are functionally better because they are more robust and reliable. Finding a clone that consistently performs well for any given situation can be difficult. The inherent challenges are to explore and utilize these immunoglobulins for a wide range of clinical situations. The theory is simple: find an antibody to bind to an antigen in a tissue section and apply a label so that the reaction can be localized. The practicalities of this idea, however, are not so straightforward.

This book directs the reader to areas within IHC that are important to know, with ideas proven to work in real-world settings. Special emphasis is placed on lean and efficient principles. Both the theoretical and the practical are covered in chapters written by authors who are current practising medical scientists in diagnostic histology laboratories. These contributors have made all the mistakes, worked at the coalface of IHC and successfully troubleshooted their way out of many predicaments over the years. They are experts in this field of medical science and are willing to share their collective experiences with the readership.

Throughout the book, common themes emerge. Validation is the method of selecting suitable antibody clones, and the foundation to successful IHC is adherence to the principles of pre-analytic, analytic and post-analytic standardization. The contributors concentrate on the reasons IHC assays fail. Protocols can become quite technical or unnecessarily complicated, and there are numerous traps to avoid for the inexperienced investigator. In gaining a deeper understanding of the technology, it is hoped that the laboratory worker can consistently achieve a clean, crisp and optimized IHC stain.

Chapter 1 explores fundamental themes and serves as a basic introduction to IHC, highlighting pioneers of this technology throughout the years and looking at the different types of assays that have been used up to the current practice of polymer detection systems. Chapter 2 presents a discussion on the important aspect of quality matters and standardization requirements. Chapters 3, 4 and 5 examine current generation automation and robotic technologies for IHC. They are surveyed from a user's perspective in the form of three popular instruments advocated by Leica Biosystems, Ventana Medical Systems and Agilent Technologies. A personal perspective is offered in terms of design and user friendliness. Strategies to maximize workflow efficiencies are also included. Chapter 6 is dedicated to researchers wishing to utilize IHC for their projects. In particular, the various components of the assay are addressed in a chronological fashion so that the protocol can be tailored to a specific objective. Chapter 7 investigates when errors occur and offers troubleshooting guidance for 'sticky' situations through practical solutions and explanations. Chapter 8 is a treatise on the status of IHC in diagnostic applications. The current state of affairs is examined with examples taken from lung, breast, bowel and melanoma pathologies. Finally, the book concludes with a glimpse into the future and searches for the next 'big' thing associated with IHC technology.

This book has two main objectives. The first is to outline the current best practice for IHC analytical testing for those who are interested in the technology and for those who are at the laboratory bench. The second is to convey to the reader how the IHC technique has matured in the second decade of the twenty-first century. There is a need for such a resource because IHC technology evolves. It is prudent for the laboratory worker to keep up to date on current best practices and there is no greater resource than the professionals who are employing IHC technology daily in their working lives.

Chapter 1

Immunohistochemistry Fundamentals

Enisa Hasic

Overview

Demonstrating changes at the cellular level via morphology is the current gold standard in diagnostic histopathology. Most pertinent to tumour pathology, cells expressing observable antigenic proteins provide valuable information as to their lineage, disease status and operational conditions. Detecting these 'expressions' and evaluating them within a clinical context gives confidence to the clinician considering relevant therapies. Likewise, interpreting disease pathways and simulating models helps researchers address relevant hypotheses (de Matos et al. 2010).

Immunohistochemistry (IHC) is a technology employed to 'tag' specific sites within tissue and observe the reaction. The ability to do so renders IHC, a powerful tool in diagnostics and research applications. The discipline is made up of three elements: *immunology*, *histology* and *chemistry*. Employing antibodies to identify antigenic sites within tissue utilizes concepts from immunology. Establishing the technique upon the study of cells and tissues explains the histology reference. Principles of chemistry are used to visualize the reaction detected from a 'label' bound directly or indirectly to the antibodies, an idea explored further in what follows.

Immunohistochemistry originated in 1890 with the discovery of serum antibodies and their use to combat disease (Childs 2014). This chapter begins with a homage to the pioneering work of early investigators and their valuable contributions throughout the years. A revolution of imagination, ingenuity and curiosity from scientists and clinicians worldwide, buoyed by their successes in research but also undeterred by their failures, led to discoveries still impacting disease diagnoses and treatments today. This chapter endeavours to highlight individual contributors to this progressing technology.

Although IHC is built from a solid theoretical basis centred upon the antigen–antibody attraction, setbacks and uncertainties often arise within IHC practice. A basic rundown of IHC principles is offered and includes the relationship of the antigen and antibody complex within IHC assays. Variations adopted from the 'standard' IHC protocol are then explored and compared to current standard practices. Common terms such as 'immunocytochemistry', 'immunolabelling', 'immunofluorescence' and 'immunoperoxidase staining' are delved into. All share the same principles with IHC but can be differentiated with subtle modifications to the technique. A discussion as to the differences is provided in this chapter whilst the highlighting of important phrases and explanations gives context to the technique. A brief mention of manual techniques and automation systems along with specific examples of using IHC in real practice should serve as a good introduction to the discipline as well as to the book. By this chapter's end, it should be evident how IHC has come to be regarded as the diagnostic tool of choice in anatomical pathology.

Laying the Foundations

From IHC's humble beginnings to the present day, the story of IHC is one to be celebrated and disseminated. It is an account of a collective effort from inquisitive minds whose discoveries contributed not only to the development of IHC, but also to the impact it has made on disease investigation and drug development. The effects have been so huge that possibilities from this technology continue to be redefined. Most will attest that IHC has been a 'game changer' in diagnostic histopathology.

Seeking treatment for diphtheria in the 1890s, researchers made a pivotal discovery in the form of serum therapy which can be viewed as one of the foundations of IHC. To combat the 50,000 German fatalities from the disease each year, three eminent scientists collaborated on researching how to effectively treat patients with what we now know is a toxin originating from a bacterial infection. Dr Emil von Behring (Figure 1.1) at the Pharmacological Institute, University of Bonn, in association with Robert Koch and his colleague Shibasaburo Kitasato, found that rabbits, guinea pigs, rats and horses injected with attenuated forms of *Corynebacterium diphtheriae* produced 'antitoxins' (antibodies) in their sera that could then be used to treat patients. In 1891, the mortality rate from the disease reduced from more than 50% to 13%, a drop so important that in 1901, Dr von Behring received the first Nobel Prize in Physiology or Medicine for this important breakthrough and was instilled as the founder of serum therapy.

Although successful, this 'passive' serum treatment prevented diphtheria for only a short time. In 1901, while searching for a treatment that worked longer, Dr von Behring injected patients directly with attenuated bacteria or with mixtures of antiserum and attenuated bacteria so that patients produced their own antibodies. This discovery led to the first 'active' immunization strategy.

In 1891, a tetanus serum was introduced as a therapeutic agent against tetanus in animals valuable to agriculture. At the onset of the First World War, as many lives were lost not from the battlefield but from tetanus, the serum was injected into soldiers. For preventing the disease during battle and saving many lives, Dr von Behring was awarded the Prussian Iron Cross Medal as a 'Saviour of German Soldiers' (NobelPrize.org).

These two occasions directed investigators to the wonders of antibodies. Although antibodies were still mysterious in the early 1900s, researchers already knew their value in medicine. To define them and to establish a standard by which they could be measured, Dr von Behring worked with Professor Paul Ehrlich (Figure 1.2) at Robert Koch's Institute in collecting serum from large animals and working on the serum therapy protocol. By 1913, Dr von Behring had

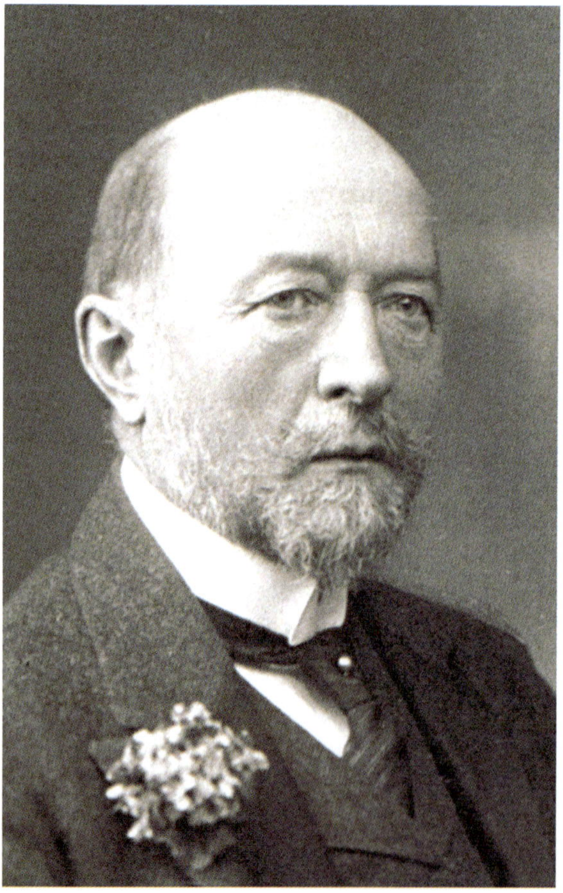

Figure 1.1 Dr Emil von Behring

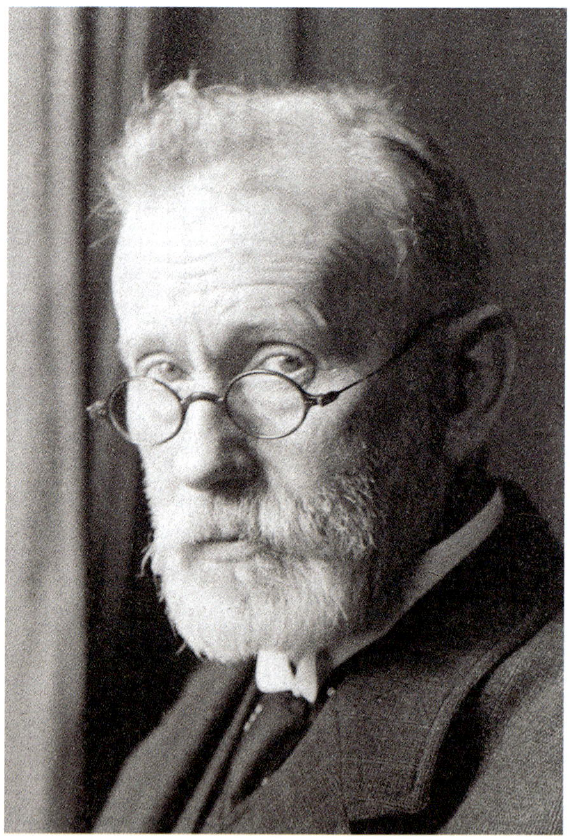

Figure 1.2 Professor Paul Ehrlich

produced his first active vaccine. Having attenuated both diphtheria antigen and antibody (mixing both active and passive therapy), the vaccine was aimed at both long-term protection against and short-term neutralization of the bacteria (Childs 2014).

Professor Paul Ehrlich was a pioneer in pathology renowned for his contributions in the fields of histochemistry, haematology and microbiology. Notable works include the theory and practice of staining animal tissues with aniline dyes, his research categorizing dyes into basic, acidic or neutral groups, and the classification of blood cell granules. In histology, Ehrlich is synonymous with a specific preparation of a working haematoxylin formulation bearing his name.

In 1896, Professor Ehrlich was appointed director of the Institute for the Control of Therapeutic Sera. Researching the characteristics and mechanisms of the antigen–antibody reaction, he found that the infective agent comprised two groups, the toxic region and the toxoid. The latter in his view was the group responsible for fuelling the production of antibodies. He noticed that heat enhanced the antigen–antibody reaction while cold restricted it, and that the binding was specific but could be broken with hydrochloric acid. For this groundbreaking work, Professor Ehrlich was awarded the Nobel Prize in Physiology or Medicine in 1908.

Basic Principles of Immunohistochemistry

The overall aim of IHC is to detect the presence, distribution and location of specific molecules (antigens) in cells and tissue. To make this possible, the three main concepts of *immunology*, *histology* and *chemistry* are required. Immunohistochemistry first employs antibodies to identify antigens and second affords the ability to visualize the reaction. Although less sensitive than Western blots or enzyme-linked immunosorbent assays (ELISA), IHC has the main advantage of enabling the investigator to observe and understand disease processes in a morphological context within an intact tissue environment.

Immunology Concepts

Antibodies, otherwise known as immunoglobulins, are serum proteins produced by B-cell lymphocytes that play an important role in an animal's defence system. They have the ability to bind with specific antigens that the body sees as foreign, thus initiating an immune response. The term 'antigen' is coined from two words: 'antibody' and 'generator' (Male and Roitt 1998). More precisely, it is the epitope on the antigen that the antibody recognizes. Multiple epitopes can be found in one antigen molecule.

Figure 1.3 represents an antibody with two light chains and two heavy chains arranged in a 'Y' shape. The light chain is connected to the heavy chain via a sulphide bond and the two heavy chains are joined together by a disulphide bridge. Note the distinct areas of the Fab and Fc regions. The binding site is at the Fab location and this is where the antibody latches onto the epitope. It is also called the variable region because this Fab site adapts to all of the variations an epitope can present to the animal. The Fc region belongs to a cascade of events that ultimately recruits phagocytes to destroy the pathogen. This body of knowledge came from the combined effort of astute workers, some of whom are now highlighted.

In 1897 at Vienna's Serotherapeutic Institute, Dr Rudolf Kraus demonstrated a method to detect antigen–antibody complexes. His precipitin reaction resulted from incubations of serum containing anti-cholera antibodies obtained from rabbits with soluble *Vibrio cholerae* bacterial infiltrates. He proved it again with serum containing anti-typhoid antibodies with *Salmonella enterica* serotype Typhi bacterial infiltrates. Each incubation resulted in the production of insoluble clumps of antigen–antibody complexes.

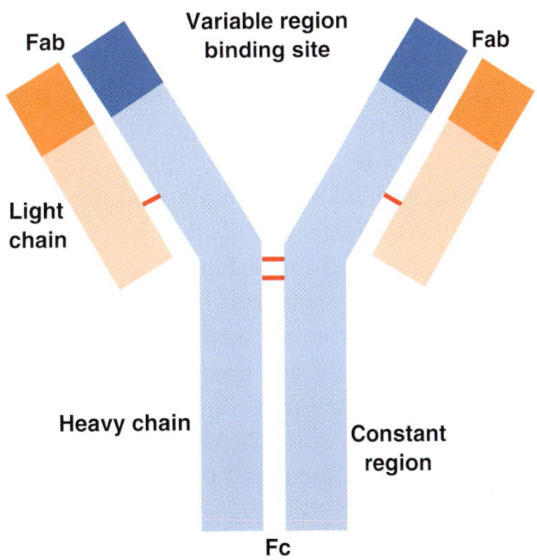

Figure 1.3 Schematic of an antibody

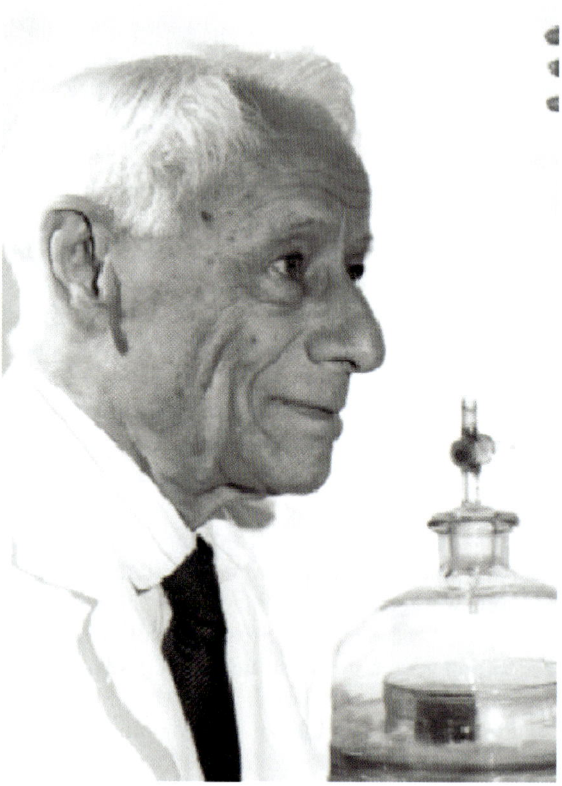

Figure 1.4 Dr Michael Heidelberger. Courtesy University archives, Rare Book & Manuscript Library, Columbia University Libraries

The precipitation reaction was of great interest to researchers, but it wasn't until 1920 that the next significant breakthrough was made. Figure 1.4 shows Dr Michael Heidelberger, a person highly regarded as one of the fathers of immunology and the founder of modern immunochemistry, a branch of biochemistry that examines the mammalian immune system on a molecular level. He established the first coloured antigen–antibody complex. Under the tutelage of Dr Oswald Avery, himself a notable figure in early DNA research, Dr Heidelberger identified the protein nature of antibodies and noted that the antigens he was working with were polysaccharides (Van Epps 2006). Further discoveries revealed antibody origin, function and specificity. These revelations assisted in understanding immune reaction chemistry and molecular mechanisms, which then led to more effective antisera for the treatment and prevention of bacterial infections.

Throughout his career, Dr Heidelberger received many awards in recognition for his work. He received 15 honorary degrees, 46 medals and 2 Albert Lasker awards in 1953 and 1978. For his work in developing quantitative analyses of antibodies, he was decorated with the Louis Pasteur Gold Medal in 1960. This prestigious honour is given by the Swedish Medical Society once every 10 years. Dr Heidelberger's other significant prizes include the Bronze Medal of the City of Paris (1964), the National Medal of Science (1967) and the Louisa Gross Horwitz Prize in 1977 (Stacey, 1994).

In the 1930s, Professor John Richardson Marrack was another researcher intrigued by the antigen–antibody complex and its crystal lattice-like formation. He believed the antibody as well as the antigen had more than one binding site and that the precipitating complex formed was the result of an antibody bridging with two multivalent antigen molecules. Working with diphtheria, he showed the toxin–antitoxin precipitate was made up of mostly antitoxin and this compound consisted of serum globulin. In 1934, Professor Marrack succeeded in attaching a dye to antibodies and through quantitative tests showed that for optimal precipitation, concentrations of antigen and antibody needed to be ideal. Researchers still adhere to this practice today when diluting out concentrates for IHC assays. In 1938, he wrote a book about antigens and antibodies, explaining the relationship between specificity and chemical structure and highlighting his thoughts on the nature of the antigen–antibody complex. In 1971, for pioneering work in the chemical interpretation of antigen–antibody interactions, Professor Marrack received the Distinguished Service Award of the First International Congress of Immunology (Complete Dictionary of Scientific Biography).

The works concerning antibodies and antigens from these early pioneers at the dawn of the twentieth century laid the groundwork for the continued evolution of IHC. The next leap was to bring the technology *in vivo* and observe the antigen–antibody reaction from a morphological viewpoint.

Histology Notions

When a tissue sample is analysed for disease, the first step is gross (macroscopic) examination noting structures and changes to the tissue that are large enough to be visible to the naked eye. Areas of particular interest are sampled and placed into histology cassettes for processing. Routinely, the submitted tissue pieces must be no larger than 25 mm long x 20 mm wide x 4 mm thick. Samples at this size will fix and

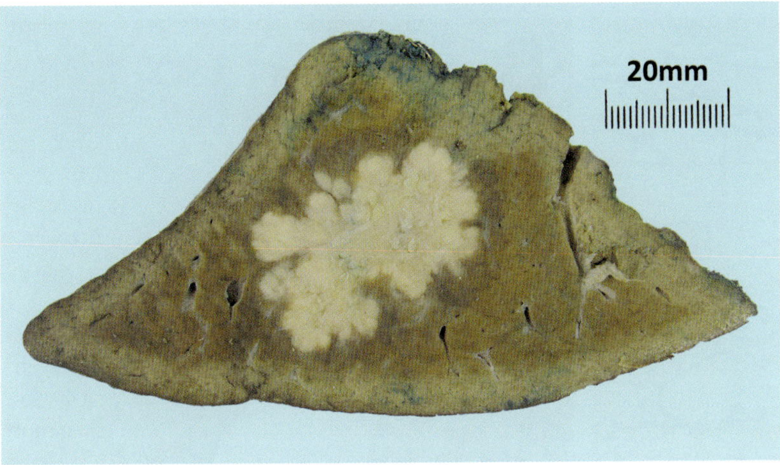

Figure 1.5 Gross macroscopic 'cut-up' is the foundation of anatomical pathology

process optimally on a routine overnight schedule. For formalin fixed paraffin embedded (FFPE) blocks, tissue fixation and processing are fundamentally the most important factors for IHC success. Figure 1.5 shows a section of liver sampled at the macroscopic 'cut-up' to visualize the lesion within the organ. A complete description and measurements are recorded before further dissection into cassettes. The main objectives in this clinical situation are finding answers to questions such as:

- What is the nature of this lesion?
- The description of the morphological features observed under the microscope
- Is this tumour a primary liver cancer or a metastatic deposit from somewhere else in the body?
- Are margins involved? Is there evidence of local spread or metastasis to distant sites?
- What are the prognostic implications for the patient?
- Are specific therapies suitable for this type of cancer?

A series of histological procedures ensues: tissue dehydration and clearing before paraffin wax infiltration, block embedding before microtomy and mounting onto glass slides. Sections are stained for haematoxylin and eosin (H&E), providing the first glimpse of morphology under microscopy. The H&E, using the basic haematoxylin dye to stain nuclear components blue, and eosin, an acidic dye, to stain cytoplasmic components pink, is the gold standard morphology stain in histopathology. A rather simple stain to perform, it highlights significant features of the tissue that if left unstained would be invisible. The subtle hues of the H&E stain allow the trained pathologist to microscopically assess tissue structure and morphology.

Not all structures, however, are demonstrated by the H&E stain. Some structures require the use of special stains to identify and reveal them. As shown in Figure 1.6A, reticulin fibres require silver impregnation to highlight the black type III collagen within organs of the reticuloendothelial system such as the liver. A trichrome stain developed by Dr Pierre Masson is seen in Figure 1.6B. This technique uses a selection of dyes to differentiate muscle from collagen fibres in connective tissue (blue). Other tissue entities such as fibrin and erythrocytes are also identifiable in trichrome stains. Note also the magnification given for Figure 1.6 is 'x40'. This indicates the objective lens on the microscope used to capture the image is rated at x40. The magnification in real terms is achieved by multiplying the objective lens magnification by the eyepiece magnification. For all images used in this chapter and throughout the book, the eyepiece objective is always x10. Therefore the 'real' magnification of images shown in Figure 1.6 is 400x (40 x 10).

The main objective of performing H&E and special stains on tissue sections mounted onto glass slides is to enable the pathologist to observe the morphological picture via microscopy and relate the findings back to the clinical history. A comprehensive illustration of the pathological processes occurring within the tissue specimen is the ultimate aim. Often, details are seen which are not easily recognized or understood. This is because many diseases mimic each other with similar cellular structures but actually differ in their behaviour and how they are treated. Where accurate diagnoses

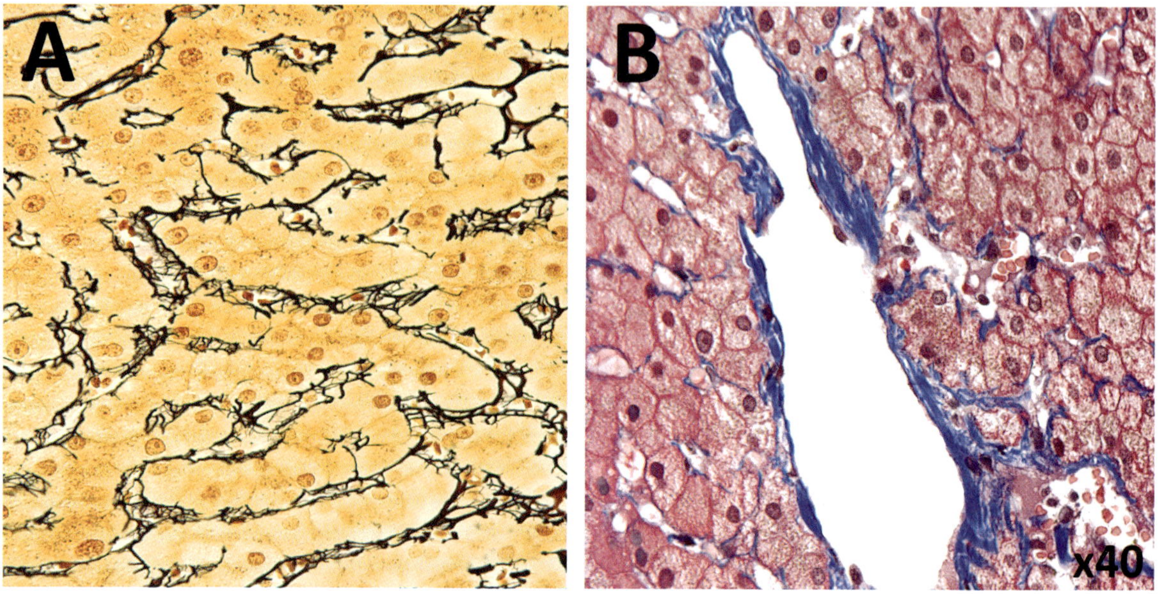

Figure 1.6 Reticulin techniques (A) and trichrome methods (B) are common histology special stains

are concerned, knowing the differences and interpreting them precisely is vital. Immunohistochemistry adds value to this endeavour. It is applied in both diagnostic anatomical pathology and research applications to assist with:

- diagnosis of disease and determining whether a tumour is benign or malignant
- identification of cell type and lineage to histologic origin and primary site of tumours
- identification of prognostic factors and therapeutic indications of some diseases
- identification of structures, organisms and materials secreted by cells
- diagnosis of morphologically non-differentiated neoplasms
- subtyping of neoplasia (such as lymphomas)

Combining immunology concepts to a morphological context is only possible if the investigator can see the reaction. To fulfil this criteria, IHC practice is grounded in the science of chemistry. Without it, microscopic examinations would not be possible.

Chemistry Influences

Performed on tissue sections that are either freshly frozen or FFPE, IHC detects various entities within tissue via a label attached directly or indirectly to an antibody, hence the often-used nomenclature of 'immunolabelling'. The nature of this label dictates the chemistry required to develop and observe the antigen–antibody reaction. The advantage is the spatial information offered, the specific locale within the tissue specimen that is tagged for evaluation via light, electron or fluorescence microscopy. The label can be a fluorophore, chromogenic dye, metal element or radioisotope with each requiring specific protocol development. The science behind two of the most commonly used labels in IHC standard practice is now explored further.

Visualization via Fluorescence

Fluorescence is a phenomenon whereby light at a certain energy (wavelength) has the ability to excite certain compounds to such a degree that when absorbed, it will emit light at a longer wavelength. Naturally occurring substances displaying this marvel are called fluorophores. Dyes and chemicals added to materials to confer fluorescence are known as fluorochromes (Bancroft and Floyd 2008). Immunofluorescence (IF) employs fluorochromes as the label conjugated directly or indirectly to the antibody. However, a specialized microscope different to a conventional optical light set-up is required. Before discussing why this is so, it is pertinent to explore how IF originated.

In 1939, Dr Albert Hewett Coons at Harvard University was investigating the components of Aschoff nodules in rheumatic fever. He studied the nature of antigens and antibodies involved with their formation and wondered if it would be easier to localize the antigen by labelling the antibody molecule with something visible.

Working together with organic chemists Dr Louis Fieser, Dr Hugh Creech and Dr Norman Jones, he coupled anthracene isocyanate to anti-pneumococcal serum and succeeded in agglutinating the pneumococci. The bacteria fluoresced brightly under ultraviolet (UV) light, but this feat was hindered by unwanted background fluorescence seen in many other structures at the blue or red wavelengths. Dr Coons then switched the label to fluorescein isothiocyanate (FITC) to observe the characteristic apple green fluorescence. Visualization of the label was possible via a fluorescence microscope apparatus newly developed by an assistant professor, Allan Graffin, at Harvard's Department of Anatomy. Dr Coon's success with the basic fluorescein-labelling procedure paved the way for diagnostic fluorescence microscopy techniques in bacteriology, immunology and anatomical pathology. For his pivotal work with IF and the discovery that plasma cells make antibodies, Dr Coons received the Albert Lasker Basic Medical Research Award in 1959. He was also the recipient of numerous international honorary academic degrees and awards. These include the Paul Ehrlich Award in 1961, the Passano Award in 1962, the Gairdner Foundation International Award in 1962 and the Emil von Behring Prize in 1966 (American Association of Immunologists).

Fluorescence microscopy is different to conventional light microscopy. The 'light source' must have enough energy to excite the fluorochromes. Commonly, wavelengths in the UV spectrum produced by mercury vapour or xenon gas lamps are utilized. Nowadays, metal halide and light-emitting diode (LED) technology may also be employed to create the required wavelengths. This light is called the excitation wavelength because it is used to excite the fluorochrome. After absorbing the light at the excitation wavelength, the fluorochrome undergoes a change at the atomic level, resulting in a variation to the electron distribution pattern. Energy in the form of emitted radiation is released from the fluorochrome at a longer wavelength and therefore the fluorochrome possesses less energy. This change in energy state is referred to as 'Stoke's shift'. To observe these changes, special filters fitted to the microscope are required. Often termed 'dichroic mirrors', they are designed to transmit light at a certain wavelength to the fluorochrome whilst reflecting away other unwanted wavelengths. These mirrors are often called filter sets and they must be matched to the fluorochrome characteristics. For example, FITC has maximum excitation at 494 nm and emission spectra at 519 nm (Horobin 2002). The dichroic mirror must allow light at wavelength 494 nm through to excite the fluorochrome and then permit light at 519 nm to reach the eyepieces. Notice the reason we see FITC as a green colour is because 519 nm is in the green zone of the visible light spectrum. The path of light after passing through the dichroic mirror to reach the fluorochrome is via the objective lens to excite the specimen and then back up the objective lens again to reach the eyepiece.

To summarize, let's follow the light path. From the lamp source, light in the UV band passes through a dichroic mirror (filter), down through the objective lens and then on to the specimen containing the fluorochrome. It then travels back up the objective lens, through the dichroic mirror again on its way to the eyepiece for visualization. Hence the term 'reflected light microscopy' is often used to mean fluorescence microscopy. To get the most out of fluorescence microscopy, a darkroom is required and since fluorescence fades over time, it is common practice to take digital images for record-keeping. Although it is quite a sensitive marker, fluorescence does have advantages and disadvantages. Fortunately, investigators have other options and technologies with which to 'label' their antibodies.

Visualization via Enzymes

For more than 40 years, IF was considered a powerful diagnostic aid. However, the method clearly had faults. The most frustrating were the need for an expensive fluorescence microscope, the instability of fluorescein over time, autofluorescence in some tissues – especially with formaldehyde fixation – and the failures at the electron microscope (EM) level. Many attempts were made to counteract these issues; some workers used radioactive antibodies while others relied on heavy metals to tag antibodies. In 1966, it was Dr Richard Graham and Dr Morris Karnovsky's studies of enzyme activity that paved the way for others to successfully attach enzymes and confer them as labels conjugated to antibodies.

The enzyme label is visualized by the enzyme's involvement in the chemical reaction with a suitable chromogen inducing a visible coloured or election-dense precipitate with its substrate. The enzyme commonly used for IHC is horseradish peroxidase (HRP). As shown in Figure 1.7, in the presence of the substrate hydrogen peroxide (H_2O_2), HRP drives the oxidation of 3,3'-diaminobenzidine (DAB), resulting in an insoluble, photostable, brown-coloured precipitate at the antigen–antibody site. Addition of nickel, cobalt or copper salt renders the DAB precipitate different shades of brown through to black. Use of enzymes as the label to observe reactions with a conventional optical microscope proved popular. In addition to HRP, different enzymes can be used for different situations, depending on the desired colour for the end product. Other enzymes deployed include alkaline phosphatase, β-galactosidase and glucose oxidase.

Horseradish Peroxidase

This enzyme has a molecular weight 40kDa glycoprotein that consists of 18% carbohydrate isolated from the root of the horseradish plant. Horseradish peroxidase has an iron haem group (haematin) as its active site which forms a complex with the substrate H_2O_2 and decomposing it to H_2O and O_2 when a H^+ donor is available. Chromogens such as DAB are employed as H^+ donors, resulting in an oxidization to form an insoluble brown product. Note the substrate for HRP is hydrogen peroxide (H_2O_2) and not to be confused with the chromogen DAB. Table 1.1 lists alternative chromogens suitable for HRP-based IHC.

Alkaline Phosphatase

This enzyme, derived from calf intestinal alkaline phosphatase (AP), has a molecular weight of 100kDa. The histochemical reaction can be described as a simultaneous coupling or azo coupling whereby the enzyme removes and transfers phosphate groups from organic esters (substrate) by breaking the P-O bond. The esters are hydrolysed to phenolic compounds. The phenols then couple to diazo salts to produce the coloured end product as highlighted in Figure 1.8 using naphthol AS-MX phosphate as the substrate and Fast red as the diazo salt. The reaction product is a red insoluble precipitate but labile to alcohols. Mounting is possible in solvents such as DPX, but the dehydrating steps with alcohol should be avoided and replaced with oven drying.

Other possible substrates include Naphthol AS-BI phosphate, Naphthol AS-TR phosphate and 5-bromo-4-chloro-3-indoxyl phosphate (BCIP). Table 1.2 lists alternative chromogens for AP.

Glucose Oxidase

This enzyme, derived from *Aspergillus niger*, has a molecular weight of 185kDA. Not commonly utilized when compared to HRP and AP, the enzyme facilitates a simultaneous redox reaction in which the substrate glucose is oxidized at the same time as a colourless tetrazolium salt is reduced to a coloured formazan. The colour of the formazan depends on the tetrazolium salt used. Three common salts include:

i. Nitro blue tetrazolium (NBT) = blue reaction product

Table 1.1 A selection of chromogens capable of development with horseradish peroxidase

Hydrogen donors (chromogens)	Colour	Solvent
3,3'-diaminobenzidine tetrahydrochloride (DAB)	brown	resistant
3 amino-9-ethylcarbazole (AEC)	red	labile
2-methyl-2 H-isothiazol-3-one	green	resistant
4-chloro-1-Napthol	blue	labile
p-phenylene diamine dihydrochloride & pyrocatechol in 1:2 ratio (Hanker-Yates)	blue	resistant

Hydrogen donor (DAB) + H_2O_2 $\xrightarrow{\text{Horseradish peroxidase}}$ H_2O+O_2 and oxidized DAB (insoluble brown product)

Figure 1.7 The chemical reaction for diaminobenzidine (DAB) using horseradish peroxidase (HRP)

Naphthol AS-MX phosphate (substrate) + Fast red TR (diazo salt) $\xrightarrow{\text{Alkaline phosphatase}}$ Azo dye (insoluble)

Figure 1.8 The chemical reaction for Fast red using alkaline phosphatase

ii. Tetra nitro blue tetrazolium (TNBT) = brown reaction product
iii. Iodonitro tetrazolium (INT) = red/purple reaction product

β-galactosidase

This enzyme has molecular weight 500kDa and is isolated from *Escherichia coli*. Not commonly used for IHC, it employs the indigogenic histochemical method as highlighted in Figure 1.9.

For standard practice in diagnostic IHC, the two enzyme labels most commonly used are HRP and AP. Although other colours are available, the conventional pairing is DAB with HRP and Fast red with AP. Both pairings are counterstained with haematoxylin for routine optical light microscopy.

Conjugating Antibodies

When the early researchers first bound antibodies to antigens, the specific class of antibodies most often used were immunoglobulin G (IgG) molecules as depicted in Figure 1.3. These molecules have two variable regions specific for antigen binding as well as a constant region where labels can be attached. A quick and short single-step 'direct approach' as highlighted in Figure 1.10 was applied by Dr Coons when he conjugated the label FITC directly to antibodies for attachment to the antigens in his experiments. Using a fluorochrome in this instance, the label can vary with the most popular being an enzyme or metal particle such as colloidal gold. Radioisotopes have also been used.

Even though the direct approach is still in use today due to its simplicity, there are inherent practical shortcomings. The method is insensitive, producing low-signal yields, which necessitates the need for copious amounts of primary antibody to increase the signal-to-noise ratio. This workaround is not always possible, especially with epitopes that are naturally 'low expressors'.

Later research revealed that antibodies could effectively act as 'antigens'. This led to the discovery of secondary antibodies produced against the IgG of the species that made the primary antibody. Secondary antibodies are often produced in larger species offering plentiful sera. Using a two-step 'indirect approach' as highlighted in Figure 1.11, an unlabelled primary antibody reacting with the tissue antigen is applied first, followed by a labelled secondary antibody. The label conjugated to the secondary antibody indirectly locates the epitopes. A big advantage over the direct method is that multiple labelled secondary antibodies can bind with different antigenic sites on a single unlabelled primary antibody, which, in turn, increases the sensitivity of the assay. Another advantage is the ability to use the one labelled secondary antibody with many primary antibodies (clones) raised from the same animal species. Likewise, the secondary antibody can also be conjugated with fluorescent dyes (indirect fluorescence method) or enzymes (indirect immunoenzyme method).

When researching the enzyme–antibody conjugation at the EM level, Dr Stratis Avrameas of the Pasteur Institute in Paris used glutaraldehyde to conjugate peroxidase to IgG. Using these conjugates, in 1971, he developed the enzyme immunoassay (EIA) and enzyme-linked immunosorbent assay (ELISA), both of which are 'close relatives' of IHC and widely used for clinical and research purposes.

While Professor Avrameas worked on enzyme immunoassays, Dr Paul Nakane, an assistant professor at the University of Michigan, also researched immunoenzyme techniques and successfully conjugated peroxidase to IgG with the bifunctional reagent p,p'-difluoro-m,m'-dinitrodiphenyl sulphone. Another

Table 1.2 Chromogens capable of development with alkaline phosphatase

Ester compounds (chromogens)	Colour	Solvent
Fast blue BB	blue	labile
Fast red LB	red	labile
New Fuchsin	red	resistant
Fast Garnet GBC	green	labile
Nitro blue tetrazolium (NBT)	blue	resistant
Iodonitro tetrazolium violet (INT)	purple	resistant

5-bromo-4-chloro-3-indoxyl - β-D-galactoside $\xrightarrow{\text{Enzyme}}$ indoxyl group $\xrightarrow{\text{Azo salt}}$ Azo indoxyl dye (blue)

Figure 1.9 The chemical reaction for β-galactosidase

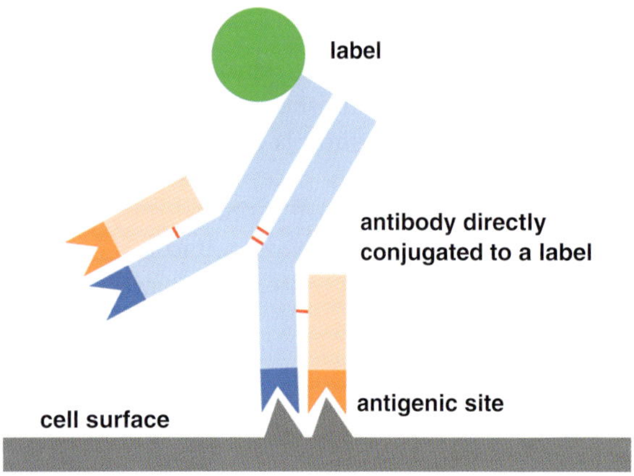

Figure 1.10 Single-step 'direct' immunolabelling

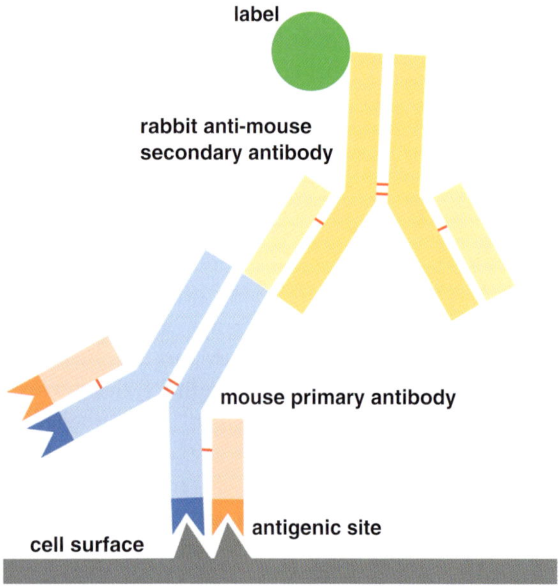

Figure 1.11 Two-step 'indirect' immunolabelling

challenge Dr Nakane undertook was exploring whether immunoenzyme techniques could be applied to the detection of multiple antigens in the same cells or tissues. We now call this endeavour 'double IHC staining' or 'multiplex IHC'. He experimented with a sequential-type multiplex technique using indirect peroxidase labelling on rat pituitary tissue localizing luteinizing hormone, growth hormone and thyroid-stimulating hormone on the one tissue section (Nakane 1968). The method can be summarized as employing the indirect peroxidase technique several times with different primary antibodies each time to locate discrete epitopes and developing them with separate colours. Although primitive compared to today's standards, using multiple sequences with various peroxidase substrates, he and his co-workers established that this could be done.

As a result of further developments in the late 1960s and 1970s to eliminate endogenous enzyme activity whilst maintaining tissue structure, the enzyme-based immunolabelling techniques proved superior to IF methodologies. Less (more diluted) primary antibodies could be used in detecting antigens. The labels did not fade and could be adopted for both the electron microscope and the standard optical brightfield microscopes.

Variations on the Theme

Even though enzyme-immunolabelling techniques were now preferred, there were practical problems still to be solved during the late 1960s to early 1970s. Most prominent was finding solutions to increase the efficiency of labelling and the ability to conjugate enzymes to all antibodies. Three prominent research groups emerged. They were headed by Dr Samuel Spicer from the Medical University of South Carolina, Dr Ludwig Sternberger, a professor at Johns Hopkins University, and Dr Stratis Avrameas of the Pasteur Institute in Paris.

Each team focused on finding suitable alternatives to the use of chemical conjugates for attaching enzymes. They found that anti-peroxidase antibodies can be used as a bridge to introduce the peroxidase enzyme to the assay. This new technology was coined the 'immunoglobulin-enzyme bridge method' by Dr Spicer, the 'unlabelled antibody method' by Dr Sternberger and the 'mixed-antibody method' by Dr Avrameas.

Each research group's technique used indirect immunolabelling in a series of layers, the first layer being the unconjugated primary antibody followed by the second layer of the secondary antibody. The third layer is the anti-peroxidase antibody produced in the same species as the primary antibody. The fourth layer constitutes peroxidase enzyme, which is added to the assay in order to bind to the tertiary antibodies already present in the system. Finally, the fifth layer is added to the system containing the peroxidase substrate H_2O_2. Emphasized schematically in Figure 1.12, this IHC assay was known as the 'sandwich approach' and despite possessing a low-affinity anti-peroxidase-to-peroxidase bridge layer, the method was more sensitive and effective than any before it.

In collaboration with Dr Howard Meyer, Dr Sternberger and co-workers added further refinement to develop the peroxidase anti-peroxidase (PAP) technique. In this assay, as highlighted in Figure 1.13, the third layer antibody to peroxidase is added as a complex with peroxidase enzyme. Compared to the similar immunoglobulin-enzyme bridge technique shown in Figure 1.12, this strategy required fewer steps and also allowed more peroxidase enzyme into the assay, thus increasing sensitivity. With the enzyme being immunologically bound rather than chemically conjugated, the PAP complex was very stable and

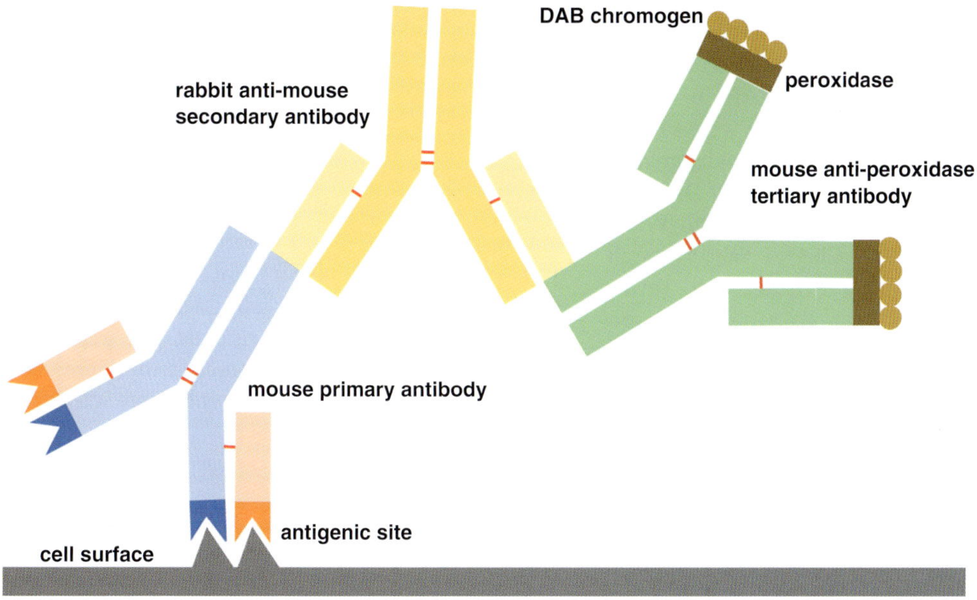

Figure 1.12 Immunoglobulin-enzyme bridge technique

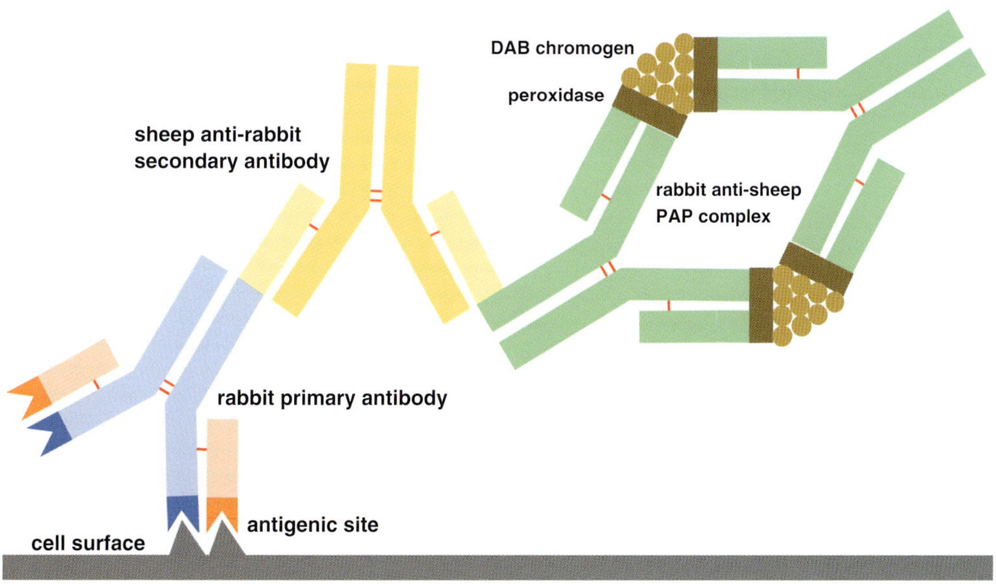

Figure 1.13 Peroxidase anti-peroxidase (PAP) technique

allowed higher dilutions of primary antibody within IHC assays. It was estimated to boost the label's efficiency between 100 and 1,000 times (Sternberger et al. 1970). Other workers successfully adapted this new-found PAP technique to immuno-electron microscopy applications. Moriarty and colleagues (1973) found it more sensitive than radioimmunoassays when working on the hormone adrenocorticotropin.

Colloidal Gold Immunolabelling

The PAP technique seemed a popular choice for immuno-electron microscopy in the early to middle 1970s. Regardless, further improvements were sought, the most promising being the use of colloidal gold as an immunocytochemical label developed by Dr Ward Page Faulk at the University College of North Wales and Malcolm Taylor at the Charles Salt Research Centre in Shropshire in 1971 (Faulk and Taylor 1971). In 1978, Dr Jurgen Roth, Dr Moise Bendayan and Dr Lelio Orci developed protein A-coated colloidal gold which acquired more specific absorption properties (Roth et al. 1978). Figure 1.14 shows an example of Dr Jurgen Roth's protein A-coated colloidal immunogold technique employed to pinpoint the glucosyltransferase enzyme as black electron dense particles (arrows).

Another example of an indirect antibody technique, colloidal gold can be attached to the secondary antibody for binding with the primary antibody as illustrated in Figure 1.15. In this instance, the 'label' is colloidal gold particles instead of a fluorochrome or enzyme.

Another avenue for gold conjugation is employing protein A obtained from *Staphylococcus spp* to react with protein G within the constant region of an antibody. As perfect as it was for ultrathin sections observable as electron dense spots shown in Figure 1.14, the colloidal gold particles used in the 1970s were large and did not penetrate tissue well, labelling only surface antigens on sections. Later years saw the development of smaller gold particles and the use of silver to enhance the label.

Electron microscopy, particularly transmission electron microscopy (TEM), is utilized in highly specialized disciplines of anatomical pathology. More popular in the late twentieth century than it is nowadays, TEM is reserved for specialized investigations of renal, muscle and nerve diseases. Unfortunately, its use is not widespread in routine diagnostic laboratories. The high costs for maintenance and requirement of highly skilled workers to not only operate the machine, but also prepare ultrathin sections has seen TEM units slowly disappear from hospital facilities to find refuge in specific university departments where they also fulfil various research endeavours. As such, the skills attained from immuno-electron microscopy may one day be lost to but a few fortunate scientists.

Correcting Inconsistencies

As the IHC technique improved with each new discovery, there were still practical limitations to overcome. Chiefly among these problems were erroneous results achieved from unreliable protocols. The high probability of unintentional washing away of the antibody–antigen reactants from tissue during the assay rendered the methods inconsistent.

Determined to resolve these issues, in the early 1980s, Dr Su-Ming Hsu of the Department of Pathology at Rhode Island Hospital and Brown

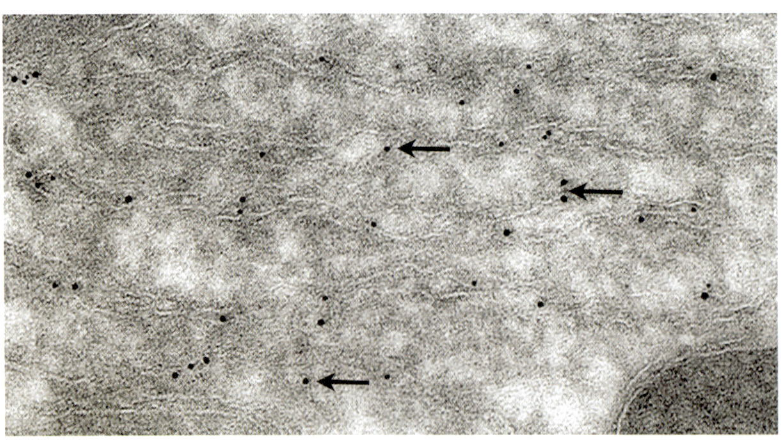

Figure 1.14 Immunogold labelling for glucosyltransferase in the rough endoplasmic reticulum of rat liver hepatocyte. Ultrathin frozen section, protein A-gold technique. Image courtesy of Jürgen Roth, University of Zurich, Switzerland

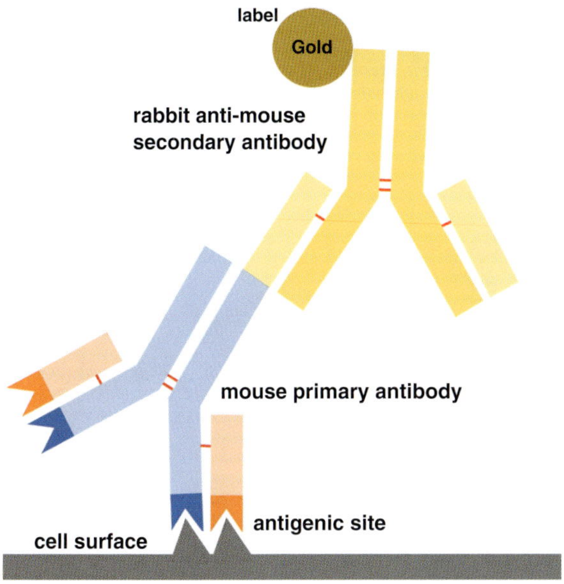

Figure 1.15 Colloidal gold attached to secondary antibody for binding with primary antibody

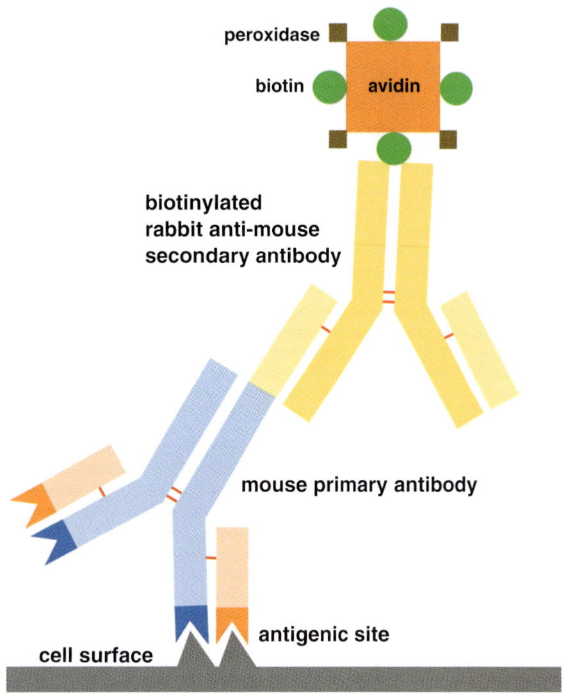

Figure 1.16 Avidin-biotin-peroxidase (ABC) complex

University experimented with avidin. It is a large glycoprotein molecule that has high affinity with biotin, otherwise known as vitamin H. He conjugated biotin to an antibody and linked the peroxidase enzyme to avidin, resulting in an avidin-biotin-antibody-peroxidase complex to the IHC assay. This new avidin-biotin-peroxidase complex (ABC) highlighted in Figure 1.16 develops relatively fast to label the antigen within two hours. Development of the enzyme with DAB then followed in the usual manner to produce the brown-coloured end product. This new technique had several other advantages. The complex was quite robust, able to withstand extremes in temperature, pH fluctuations, exposure to denaturing agents and resistant to enzymatic degradation. Most impressive was the ability to utilize the ABC method to an unlimited number of primary antibodies. The downside is that there are naturally occurring endogenous biotin within tissue that must be blocked. Otherwise, results could be tainted with false positive staining.

Further refinement of the ABC technique centred around the avidin molecule. 'Strepavidin', isolated from the bacterium *Streptomyces avidinii*, allowed the formation of a labelled streptavidin-biotin-enzyme conjugate (LSAB) at the neutral pH of reagents used for IHC assays. The theory is identical to the ABC method, based primarily on biotin having a strong affinity with streptavidin. The same first layer of unlabelled primary antibody is followed by a second layer of biotinylated secondary antibody. The third layer now is an enzyme–streptavidin conjugate in the LSAB technique as shown in Figure 1.17. The technique lends itself to any enzyme label the investigator chooses for chromogenic development and can also be conjugated to a fluorescent dye such as FITC. The main advantage, however, is the higher sensitivity afforded to the IHC assay due to the LSAB complex being much smaller than the ABC compound. Detecting 5 to 10 times more biotinylated antibody on the tissue section when compared to the ABC method results in a 'brighter' signal.

The Modern Era

With such a rich history and many contributors through the years, the question of when exactly the practice of IHC came into the modern era is hard to define and is arguably debatable. The proposal here is that IHC became a 'legitimate' histological technique with the advent of epitope retrieval systems. Even though retrieval methodologies appeared at least 30 years ago, the most profound impact it had on anatomical pathology was that it took IHC practice mainstream and made it available to any histology facility.

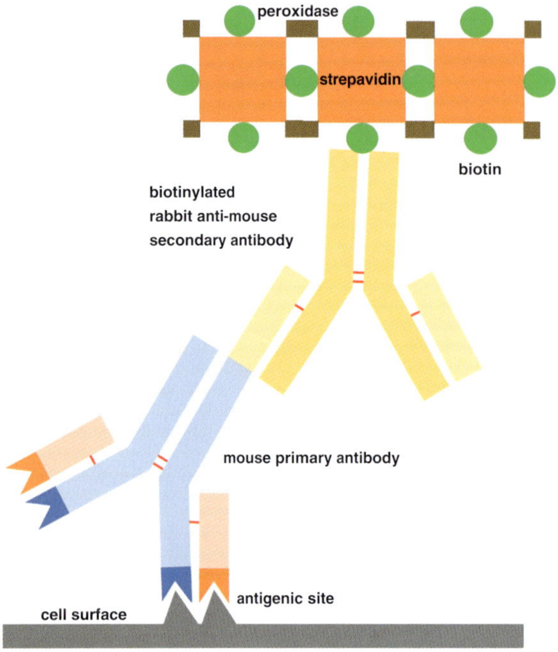

Figure 1.17 Streptavidin-biotin-peroxidase (LSAB) technique

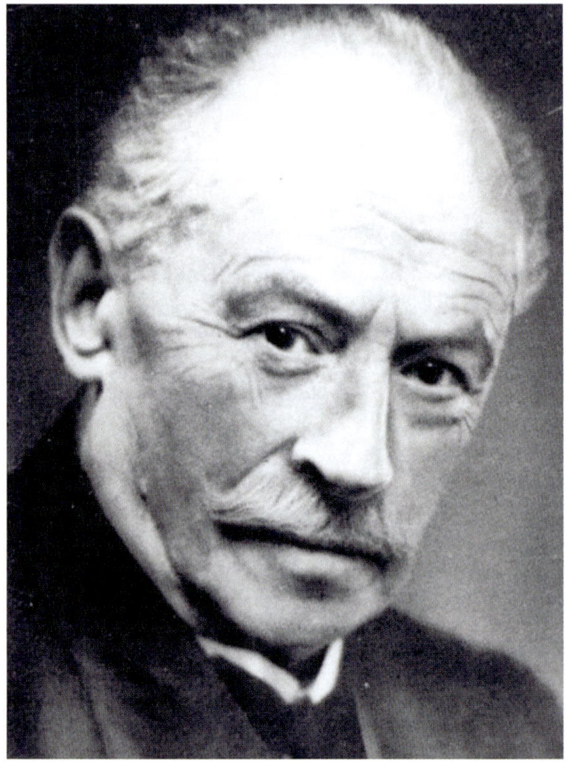

Figure 1.18 Dr Ferdinand Blum (Fox et al. 1985)

The ability to unmask antigens allowed the traditional foundations of histologic technique in the form of FFPE sections to continue, thereby keeping relevant the fundamentals of morphological assessments with H&E staining. In short, this new IHC technology was able to work with existing histology practices, which made it a powerful analytic tool. However, the biggest challenge posed with IHC technology in this modern era was the recognition for IHC practices to follow a standardized stream (Taylor et al. 2010). With so many variables, the consensus was a need for a 'controlled' assay, and the biggest leap was identifying all the parameters into pre-analytic, analytic and post-analytic groups. Chapter 2 continues this standardization theme for IHC within the context of quality assurance.

Unmasking Antigens

In 1893, Dr Ferdinand Blum (Figure 1.18) was approached by the chemical manufacturing company Meister, Lucius and Brunig at Hoechst am Main in Germany to test the antiseptic properties of formaldehyde. In addition to its germ-killing properties, he soon discovered the superiority of the chemical as a tissue fixative when compared to alcohols. In its natural state, formaldehyde is a gas and can be dissolved in water as a 37–40% concentrated solution. For tissue fixation purposes, it is diluted to a 10% working solution containing 3.7–4% formaldehyde, commonly referred to as 10% formalin. This diluted solution has, along with paraffin embedding, become the standard method of tissue preservation in anatomical pathology and is still in use today.

Formalin fixation preserves tissue morphology rather well, highlighted with appropriate staining essential for diagnoses such as the H&E stain. Its mode of action is to form protein cross links in reactive sites via methylene bridges. In doing so, antigenic sites within tissue and their epitopes are altered, effectively masking them from antibodies. These changes lead to a reduction or loss of immunoreactivity of target antigens in formalin-fixed tissue, thereby restricting antigen–antibody binding and limiting their detection. This phenomenon is detrimental for IHC detection, especially with the use of monoclonal antibodies, which recognizes only one epitope.

In 1988, when examining whether the formalin-fixation-induced changes could be reversed and the structure of proteins restored, Dr SR Shi at the

University of Southern California discovered formalin protein cross-linking could be disrupted and the epitopes unmasked by placing the FFPE sections into boiling water (Shi et al. 2001). The use of heat above 100°C for 10–40 min led to further refinements of heat-induced epitope retrieval (HIER) methods using buffers based on citrate, EDTA or Tris saline (Shi et al 1997). Restoration of the antigenic epitopes to their original formation allows antigenic sites to be exposed for antibodies to bind to them. There is a plethora of heating methods utilized for HIER ranging from simple boiling, pressure cooking and microwave irradiation to specialized heating pads. All are suitable, but the main concern is that the distribution of heat energy must be uniform across the entire tissue section and that the heating process is reproducible and consistent day after day.

More experiments focused on breaking up the formalin-protein-methylene bridges revealed a second method for unmasking antigens. Proteolytic-induced epitope retrieval (PIER) uses protease enzymes such as proteinase K, trypsin and pepsin to split the peptides that are believed to mask the epitope (Roth et al. 2000). These enzymes are useful for epitopes which are heat labile and relatively fast acting, but prolonged enzyme digestion incubations may also destroy tissue morphology and epitopes under investigation. The optimal digestion conditions are found by the investigator through trial and error.

The success of the LSAB technique coupled with proven antigen retrieval methods for immunolabelling tissues in both clinical and research situations led to dramatic increases in IHC assays reflected in the vast number of journal publications submitted for peer review. Immunohistochemistry techniques were utilized in many specialties such as molecular biology, surgical pathology, immunology, histology, microbiology and oncology, both in research and in diagnostics. Immunohistochemistry has found a niche in clinical diagnostic endeavours, routinely employed alongside traditional histology stains to answer complex clinical situations.

More refinement to IHC protocols were to be unveiled, coming from the need for greater sensitivities, recognition for assay standardizations and discovery of an ever-expanding list of primary antibodies. Seeking methods to accommodate primary antibodies from different species, alternative labels other than peroxidase enzyme and secondary antibodies to cover IgGs from a wide range of species were the objectives. Ongoing research led to two discoveries that caused great change to the IHC assay in the form of polymer technology and automated staining instruments.

Polymer-Based Detection Systems

The more enzyme label molecules recruited to a localized area, the more sensitivity and improved signal intensity is achieved with the IHC assay. One inspiration uses an inert dextran polymer as a backbone with a large number of antibodies attached and bound to many enzyme molecules. A schematic is highlighted in Figure 1.19 showing the attraction between the rabbit primary antibody and the anti-rabbit antibodies attached to a polymer backbone. Notice the high number of peroxidase enzyme molecules (green circles) attached to the polymer localized in the immediate area, which means a more intense signal development with DAB. Some polymer kits include a 'linker' secondary antibody specific for the primary antibody species of origin. For example, a secondary linker antibody could be of rabbit origin, binding to a mouse primary antibody and then itself being detected by anti-rabbit antibodies on the polymer strand. In this example, there are in fact three layers within the IHC system whereas Figure 1.19 shows a two-layer polymer IHC assay.

Other workers have taken the technology to employ an enhanced polymer one-step (EPOS) IHC protocol (Tsutsumi et al. 1995). Although suitable for rapid IHC assays, it has not found widespread use in diagnostic settings. The main drawback is that each primary antibody must be conjugated to polymer, a practice which is not feasible for a busy IHC facility offering up to 100-plus antibodies.

Regardless, the number of layers in the IHC assay is not important; what matters most is the number of enzymes available to drive the chromogen reaction. Others have found suitable alternatives to this polymer technology. Roche Ventana maximizes enzyme labels within the IHC assay by employing haptens and multimer technology, explained further in Chapter 4. Current-generation IHC detection technology is readily available from many IHC vendors. For ease of use, they are packaged as kits for manual applications or marketed to match proprietary automation platforms. Each detection kit contains the necessary reagents for the IHC assay excluding the primary antibody. A closer inspection of Leica, Roche and Agilent detections kits is provided in subsequent chapters of this book.

The enlistment of polymer technology and its equivalent possesses many advantages over earlier superseded methodologies. The protocols are easier to standardize, the assay is completed in two to three hours, unwanted background staining is minimized, and the one kit works with both mouse and rabbit primary antibodies. In addition, they allow workers to perform high-quality multiplex assays consistently. Figure 1.20 shows both single and double IHC staining typically produced in diagnostic IHC facilities today.

In addition to single and double immunolabelling, IHC can also be combined with special histological stains and *in situ* hybridization (ISH) assays. Polymer technology is flexible, specific and sensitive to be

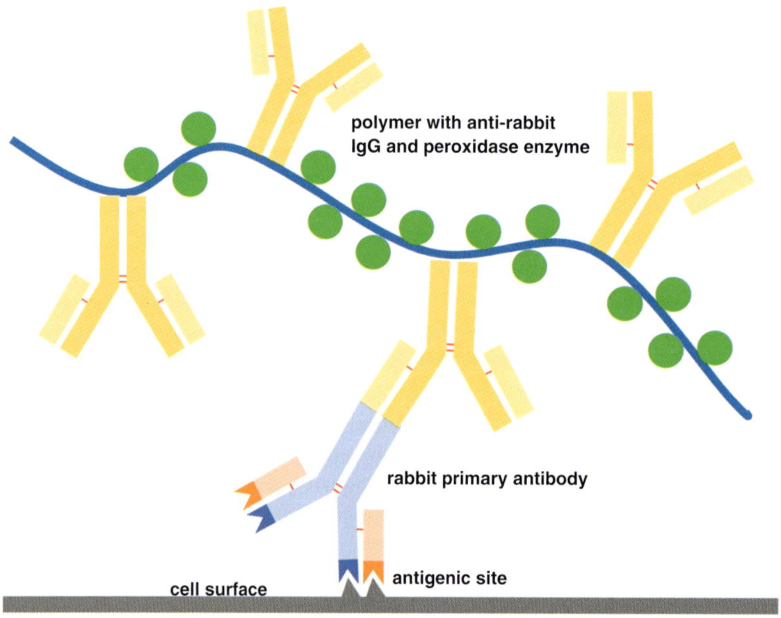

Figure 1.19 Polymer-based detection method

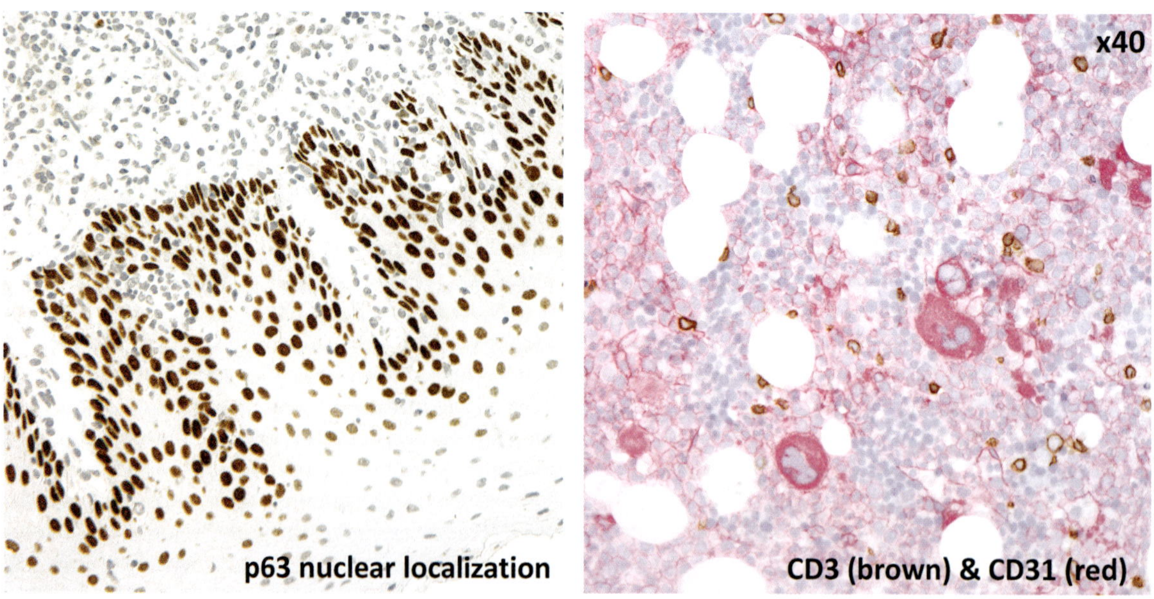

Figure 1.20 Single and dual chromogen immunohistochemistry

deployed in specific clinical situations such as investigating kidney tubulitis, coeliac disease and lymphoma.

Tubulitis is a key histological feature of rejection in kidney transplants and is severely under-detected by conventional H&E microscopy. Although IHC can clearly indicate CD3 positive T-cells in tissue, it is difficult to judge the exact location in reference to the tubular basement membrane. The periodic acid Schiff (PAS) reaction stains tubular basement membranes a magenta colour but cannot reveal T-cell location. Combining the CD3 IHC stain with a PAS on the one tissue section is a useful diagnostic tool to avoid misdiagnosing rejection. Figure 1.21 shows the exact location of a CD3-positive T-cell located within a tubule indicating tubulitis and therefore transplant rejection.

The same assay can also assist the screening of coeliac disease, an autoimmune disorder of the gastrointestinal tract characterized by chronic inflammation of intestinal mucosa. A diagnostic hallmark is observing increased T-cell numbers in the epithelium lining the small bowel. They are the culprits involved in initiating, maintaining and controlling this chronic inflammation. T-cell populations are often difficult to see in conventional microscopy because of the disruption to the intestinal morphology at these sites. As shown in Figure 1.22, IHC staining highlights CD3-positive T-cells and the PAS reaction shows the epithelial basement membrane so that the pathologist can ascertain the exact location of the CD3 positive T-cells. If found in the submucosa, all is normal, but if seen within the luminal epithelium next to glandular structures, this indicates coeliac disease.

An example of combining IHC with ISH is found in a specific lymphoma workup complicit with Epstein–Barr virus (EBV). More than 90% of adults have been infected with EBV, most commonly in B-cells within the tonsils. Epstein–Barr virus is, however, also associated with non-B-cell tumours. When present in T-cell proliferative disorders of childhood, the resulting liver failure and intravascular coagulation may lead to death, so a quick diagnosis is required. Analysis is based on the clonal proliferation of EBV-positive T-cells in liver, lymph nodes and bone marrow. This clonal proliferation can be illustrated via sequential multi-staining to test for EBER ISH and CD3-double-positive cells shown in Figure 1.23 (A). Compare this to a sequential multi-stain of EBER ISH and CD20, a B-cell marker in Figure 1.23 (B).

Automation

Mirroring the evolution of the IHC assay, the story of robotics for IHC applications also began from humble beginnings as simple fluid transfer vehicles to the sophisticated all-in-one systems available today. The arrival of automated staining instruments such as Leica's Bond-III, Roche's BenchMark ULTRA and Agilent's Omnis shown in Figure 1.24 has been met with great enthusiasm by anatomical pathology

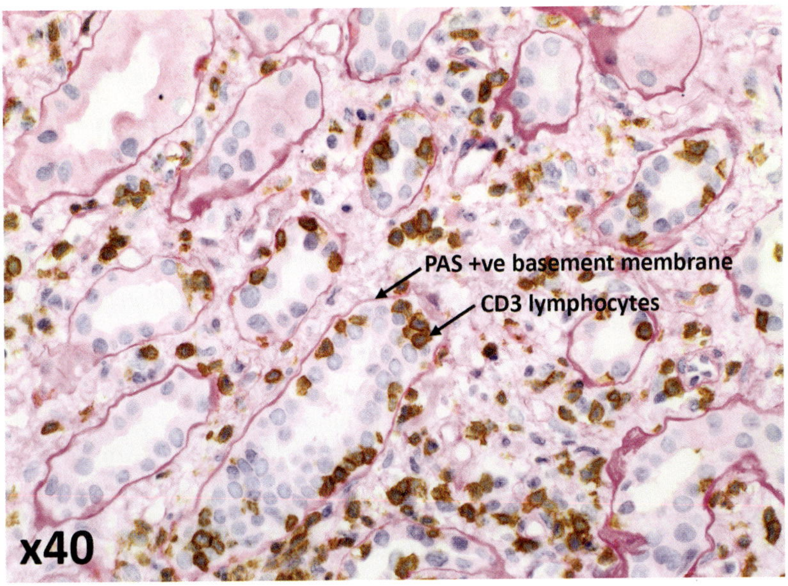

Figure 1.21 CD3-positive lymphocyte (arrow) present inside tubule indicating tubulitis

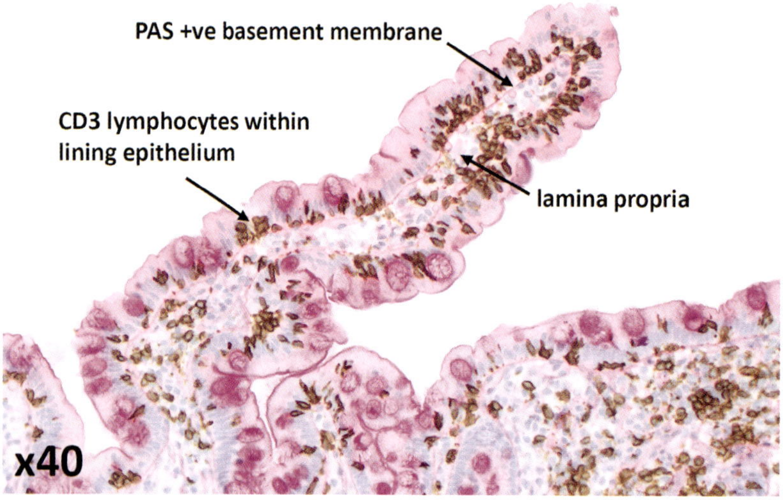

Figure 1.22 Presence of CD3 inside epithelium lining of small bowel

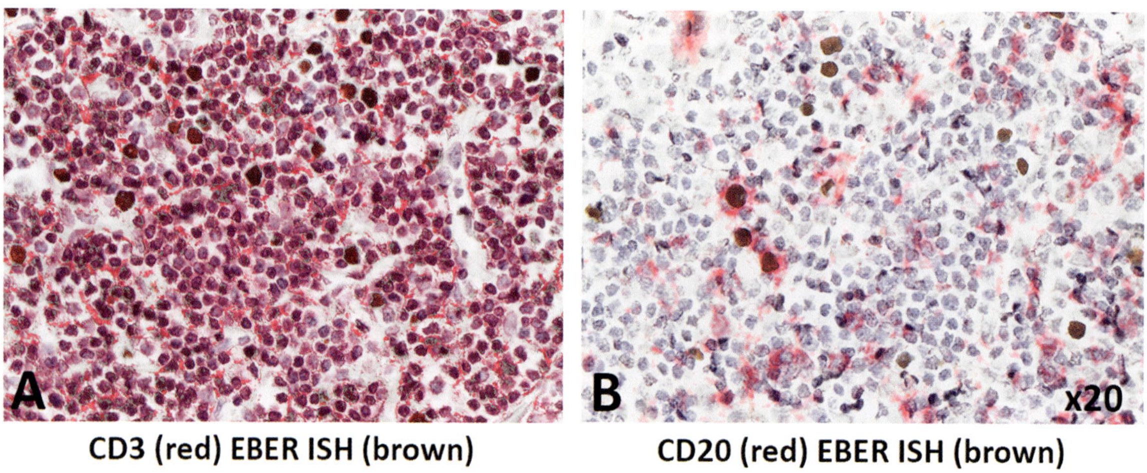

Figure 1.23 (A and B): EBER-ISH (brown) and CD3 and CD20 (red) combinations

laboratories and researchers worldwide. The reasons why and a discussion on each individual vendor's design, attributes and technology are provided in the robotics and automation chapters of this book.

Principally, automation is an improvement over manual staining because it eliminates inter-worker variations and promotes standardized protocols in IHC. Other advantages include:

- Multiple antigen labelling can be performed sequentially using a brown DAB chromogen kit followed by a red alkaline phosphatase kit, or in parallel using a single kit containing both the brown DAB and red alkaline phosphatase chromogens.
- Immunohistochemistry can be combined with *in situ* hybridization (ISH), thus giving information about a particular target both at the protein level and at the DNA/mRNA level.
- Barcode tracking prevents the selection of incorrect reagents and alerts the operator about insufficient reagent volumes.

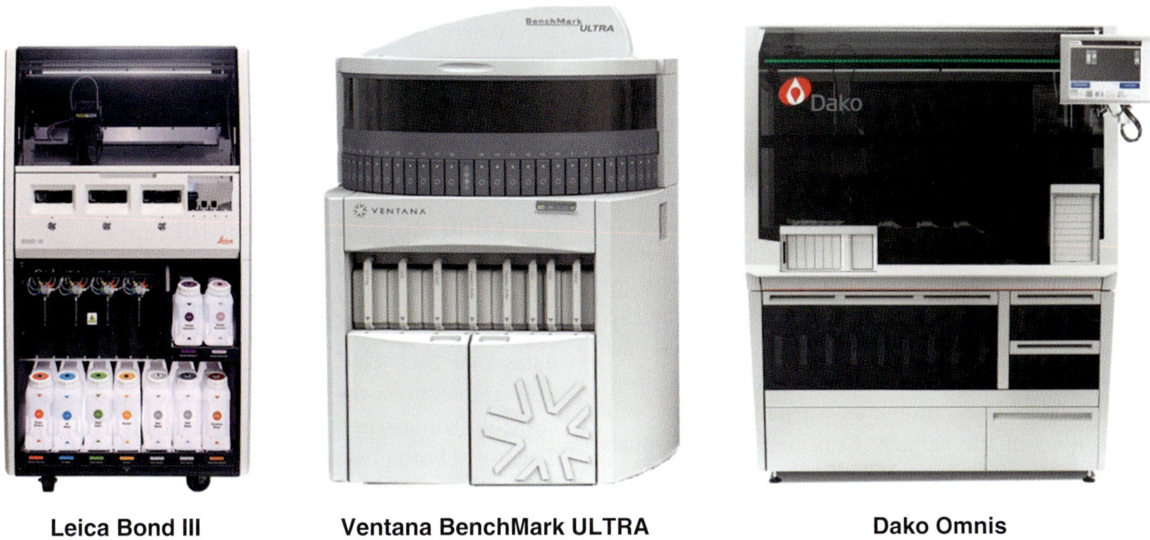

Figure 1.24 Common immunhistochemistry automation platforms (not to scale). Images reproduced with permission Leica Biosystems Melbourne Pty. Ltd, Ventana Medical Systems Inc., Agilent Technologies Inc.

- Computerized software assists with reagent inventory, keeping track of reagent stock and dates of expiry.
- Inbuilt alarms warn about errors such as incorrect temperatures and calibration errors.
- It is less time-consuming for the technologists who are free to complete other duties.

However, as much as automation has advanced IHC, it does have its drawbacks:

- For IHC staining to be optimal, like all machines, these instruments need regular maintenance.
- All breakdowns, whether a blown 50-cent fuse or full module failure, must be attended by qualified service personnel. Any downtime leads to interruption in workflow.
- Vendors 'lock' their systems to insist on the use of their own proprietary reagents.
- The ability to tweak an IHC assay is limited to one or two parameters.
- Due to the 'plug and play' nature of automation, technologists run the risk of being less knowledgeable about the IHC assay and therefore less able to troubleshoot problems.
- Companies may decide to stop supporting a particular model, forcing laboratories to upgrade systems.

Therefore, to get the most out of any IHC platform, the user must be well informed about the science of IHC so that the instrument is used to its full potential. Vendor support applications specialists can only assist in this regard to a certain extent. Optimizing protocols, choosing the appropriate antibody clone and selecting control materials still rests with laboratory staff tasked with providing a reliable IHC service.

The Immunohistochemistry Technique

Thus far, important IHC concepts discussed include references to immunology, histology and chemistry. The various labels acquired and the processes involved to detect them have also been mentioned. Likewise, technologies invented to increase sensitivity and standardization efforts have also been raised. To complete this discussion on the fundamentals of the IHC assay, a closer review is now applied to the primary antibody, control material and the actual IHC protocol.

Choosing the Primary Antibody

Much of the success in IHC staining depends on primary antibodies specifically binding to the target antigen. Therefore, the decision as to the clone, type and class of antibody deployed for staining is an important one. Not all antibodies are created equal, so the IHC technologist will have to spend time researching the literature to choose the most appropriate one for a particular application. Decisions must be made as to whether the protocol will involve direct or indirect methods, the type of label used and the development of the chromogen.

One important factor to consider is the characteristics of the antibody and the species it was derived from. Polyclonal antibodies are attained from immunized animals, giving rise to antibodies produced from different B-cells that have the ability to recognize numerous epitopes of the same antigen. They are renowned for high sensitivity but can be subject to poor specificity. Monoclonal antibodies obtained from hybridomas offer antibodies produced from identical B-cells taken from a parent clone. These antibodies are made to detect only one epitope of the antigen. Conversely, monoclonals have high specificity but may suffer from low sensitivity. Whatever the decision, each antibody needs to be optimized against the staining system used in the IHC laboratory to ensure it is best suited for use.

Primary antibodies have been traditionally available in the concentrated form requiring optimization before use in IHC laboratories. These days, many primary antibodies are also offered as ready-to-use (RTU) predilutes. Each has its advantages and disadvantages. The choice is made by individual laboratory preferences taking into account cost, vendor reputation, consistency of performance, shelf life and ease of use. Some manufacturers also include antibodies conjugated with labels for specific requirements.

Concentrates are adaptable, able to be used in a range of optimal working dilutions in most staining systems, manual or automated. However, time is needed for preparation, optimization and validation. Dilutions made manually could vary from person to person, giving inconsistencies in staining. There is a greater margin for human error. Also, if the expiry date of the concentrate is approaching, the staining quality may deteriorate.

The RTUs are prepared, optimized and validated for use by manufacturers. There is often a stipulation of the parameters required and they are most often tuned for the vendors proprietary IHC platforms. Having one less variable to worry about frees up time for the technologist to better manage reagent and quality control and thus improve laboratory workflow. Elimination of errors via manual dilutions may mean consistent optimal results if all other staining variables are optimal. Unfortunately, these advantages do come at an overall increased cost of the RTU antibodies. However, the most important aspect of RTU antibodies is the prerequisite that pre-analytical parameters such as tissue fixation and processing must have been performed to an acceptable 'standard' and that this standardization of conditions has to be consistently achieved. Otherwise, the IHC assay will produce variable results.

Selecting Appropriate Controls

Because variables such as incubation time, incubation temperature, buffer pH and antibody dilutions can adversely affect IHC staining, standard practice mandates that each IHC run includes positive controls known to express the antigen of interest and negative controls from tissue known not to express the antigen. The use of both positive and negative controls corroborates the results of the test tissue. Chapter 2 dives further into this topic in the overall discussion about quality assurance in IHC.

General Staining Protocol

Taking all the topics that have been discussed and bringing them all together, they can now be summarized into an IHC staining protocol. Generally, the IHC procedure can be grouped into various stages. For FFPE, after baking and dewax, antigens are retrieved first, before application of a primary antibody. If labelling with peroxidase, a blocking step is required to quench endogenous peroxidase activity. The next stage is detection and chromogen development before counterstain and mounting with a coverslip. A summary is provided in Appendix 1 showing the steps of a typical IHC assay using polymer detection with peroxidase as the label and DAB as the chromogen.

In reality, there are many possible variations to this template protocol because IHC is utilized in many scenarios and under numerous situations. Underlying questions include:

- Are the test tissue and animal sera compatible?
- Is the nature of the test tissue fresh, frozen or FFPE?
- Is the label enzymatic or fluorescent?
- Is the detection system avidin-biotin or polymer based?
- Are additional blocking steps required depending on the type of reagents used?

Even though there are many scenarios with their own intricacies, the essentials remain the same.

Thus the core requirements for any IHC protocol include:

- Knowing the nature of the test tissue section
- Ascertaining the animal species that produced the primary antibody
- Requirements for a blocking step or a number of different blocking strategies
- A suitable detection system for the chosen label
- Development and visualization of the label
- Suitable counterstain to contrast with the label
- Mounting and coverslip for permanent storage

Breaking down the IHC assay systematically and addressing each parameter will make the process more manageable. Chapter 6 discusses this in more detail when tailoring IHC to research applications. Obtaining a suitable antibody clone is just the first step in a series of considerations necessary for IHC success.

Conclusion

When IHC is stripped down to basic fundamentals, three categories emerge. Immunohistochemistry borrows concepts from *immunology*, *histology* and *chemistry*. At its core are antibodies employed to tag antigens within a morphological index and to visualize these reactions with chemistry principles. The development of IHC started in the late 1800s and continues to evolve. There are numerous contributors to IHC technology, each one building on the success of their peers. Important discoveries include the realization that antibodies are immunoglobulin proteins and the ability to conjugate them with labels. Then came improved consistencies with the invention of epitope retrieval methods and polymer detection systems. Biomedical engineering marvels brought automation to IHC and the important notion of standardization in IHC assays was realized. Finally, as more protocols were used to determine patient prognosis and therapies, important quality assurance matters needed to be addressed. All of these themes are explored further in this book.

It is hoped that this chapter has served as an introduction to IHC principles and the people credited for its discovery and development. It is such an important tool in research applications and diagnostic endeavours that clinicians, scientists, laboratory staff and managers all need to understand its fundamentals before exploiting its wonders.

Appendix 1 Typical IHC protocol for FFPE using polymer detection for DAB

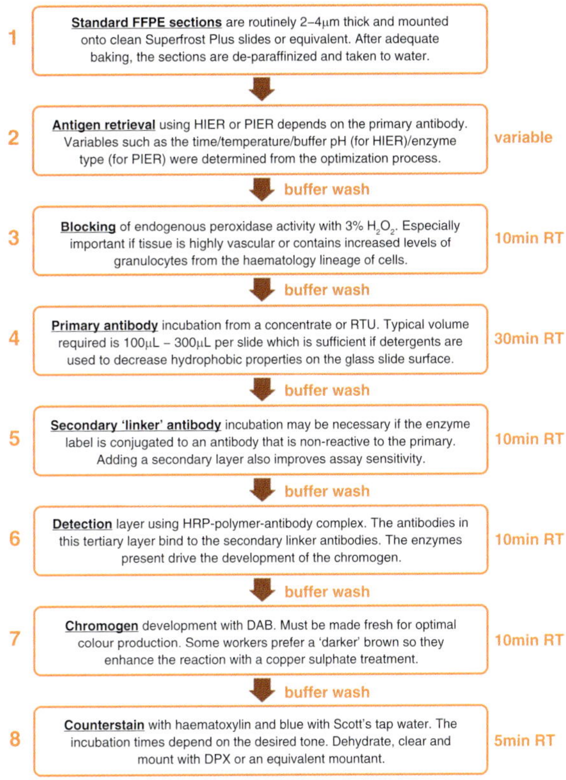

Glossary

Antibody Serum proteins, also known as immunoglobulins, that play a role in the body's defence system. They search for and bind with specific antigens the body recognizes as foreign.

Antigen A molecule or molecular structure targeted by antibodies produced by the body's immune system.

Avidin A tetrameric biotin-binding protein found in streptavidin bacteria and also in the egg whites of

	birds, reptiles and amphibians.
Biotin	A water-soluble vitamin also known as vitamin H produced by the body and involved in the utilization of fats, carbohydrates and amino acids.
Chromogen	A chemical compound used to confer colour to a chemical reaction or assay.
Direct immunohistochemistry	A one-step procedure where the primary antibody is directly conjugated to the label.
Epitope	The specific part of an antigen to which an antibody fastens itself.
Fluorochrome	A dye or chemical added to materials to confer fluorescence. Mostly synthetic compounds, these fluorochromes are employed in immunofluo rescence assays as the 'label' conjugated directly or indirectly to the antibody.
Fluorophore	A naturally occurring chemical compound that absorbs light at a certain wavelength and emits the absorbed energy at a longer wavelength to confer a state of fluorescence.
Immunofluorescence	A technique that uses fluorochromes to visualize antigen–antibody binding via fluorescence microscopy. The antibody can either be directly conjugated to the fluorochrome for direct labelling or unconjugated to be visualized by a multistep assay.
Immunohistochemistry	A procedure that identifies antigens in tissue sections via the conjugating of antibodies to enzymes that produce a coloured reaction visible by light microscopy.
***In situ* hybridization**	The forging of a labelled nucleic acid probe to corresponding sequences of a target nucleic acid (DNA or mRNA) in a fixed specimen. Visualization depends on the nature of the label. Fluorescence assays are known as FISH and chromogenic detection is commonly referred to as CISH. Silver labels are called SISH assays.
Indirect immunohistochemistry	A multistep procedure where the primary antibody is bound by a labelled secondary antibody to give the assay greater sensitivity.
Morphology	The observation and interpretation of cellular processes within tissue. This is made possible with stains and microscopy.
Primary antibody	The antibody enlisted to bind directly to the antigen.
Secondary antibody	The antibody recruited to bind to an unconjugated primary antibody.

References

American Association of Immunologists. Albert H Coons MD brief bio (online). Available at: www.aai.org/About/History/Past-Presidents-and-Officers/AlbertHCoons (Accessed 1 June 2021).

Bancroft JD, Floyd AD 2008. Light microscopy. In Bancroft JD, Gamble M, eds. *Theory and practice of histological techniques*. Churchill Livingstone Elsevier; 33–52.

Childs GV 2014. History of immunohistochemistry. In McManus LM, Mitchell RN, eds. *Pathobiology of human disease*. Elsevier; 3775–96.

Complete Dictionary of Scientific Biography. Marrack, John Richardson (online). Available at: www.encyclopedia.com/science/dictionaries-thesauruses-pictures-and-press-releases/marrack-john-richardson (Accessed 15 April 2021).

De Matos LL, Trufelli DC, de Matos MG, da Silva Pinhal MA 2010. Immunohistochemistry as an important tool in biomarkers detection and clinical practice. *Biomark Insights* **9**(5):9–20.

Faulk WP, Taylor GM 1971. Communication to the editors: An immunocolloid method for the electron microscope. *Immunochemistry* **8**(11):1081–3.

Fox CH, Johnson FB, Whiting J, Roller PP 1985. Formaldehyde fixation. *J Histochem Cytochem* **33** (8):845–53.

Horobin RW 2002. Xanthenes. In Horobin RW, Kiernan JA, eds. *Conn's biological stains: A handbook of dyes, stains and fluorochromes for use in biology and medicine*. Taylor and Francis; 219–52.

Male D, Roitt I 1998. Introduction to the immune system. In Roitt I, Brostoff J, Male M, eds. *Immunology*. Mosby; 1–12.

Moriarty GC, Moriarty CM, Sternberger LA 1973. Ultrastructural immunocytochemistry with unlabeled antibodies and the peroxidase-antiperoxidase complex. A technique more sensitive than radioimmunoassay. *J Histochem Cytochem* **21**(9):825–33.

Nakane PK 1968. Simultaneous localization of multiple tissue antigens using the peroxidase-labeled antibody method: A study on pituitary glands of the rat. *J Histochem Cytochem* **16**(9):557–60.

NobelPrize.org. Emil von Behring: The founder of serum therapy. Nobel Prize Outreach AB 2021 (online). Available at: www.nobelprize.org/prizes/medicine/1901/behring/article/ (Accessed 11 July 2021).

Roth J, Bendayan M, Orci L 1978. Ultrastructural localization of intracellular antigens by the use of protein A-gold complex. *J Histochem Cytochem* **26**(12):1074–81.

Roth J, Ziak M, Guhl B 2000. Non heating antigen retrieval techniques for light and electron microscopic immunolabeling. In Shi SR, Gu J, Taylor CR, eds. *Antigen retrieval techniques: Immunohistochemistry and molecular morphology*. Eaton; 275–85.

Shi SR, Cote RJ, Taylor CR 1997. Antigen retrieval immunohistochemistry: Past, present, and future. *J Histochem Cytochem* **45**(3):327–43.

Shi SR, Cote RJ, Taylor CR 2001. Antigen retrieval techniques: Current perspectives. *J Histochem Cytochem* **49** (8):931–7.

Stacey M 1994. Michael Heidelberger, 29 April 1888–25 June 1991. *Biographical Memoirs of Fellows of the Royal Society* **39**:177–97 (online). Available at: https://royalsocietypublishing.org/doi/10.1098/rsbm.1994.0011 (Accessed 1 June 2021).

Sternberger LA, Hardy PH Jr, Cuculis JJ, Meyer HG 1970. The unlabeled antibody enzyme method of immunohistochemistry: Preparation and properties of soluble antigen-antibody complex (horseradish peroxidase-antihorseradish peroxidase) and its use in identification of spirochetes. *J Histochem Cytochem* **18** (5):315–33.

Taylor CR, Shi S-R, Barr NJ 2010. Techniques of immunohistochemistry: Principles, pitfalls and standardisation. In Dabbs DJ, ed. *Diagnostic immunohistochemistry: Theranostic and genomic applications*. Saunders Elsevier; 1–41.

Tsutsumi Y, Serizawa A, Kawai K 1995. Enhanced polymer one-step staining (EPOS) for proliferating cell nuclear antigen (PCNA) and Ki-67 antigen: Application to intra-operative frozen diagnosis. *Pathol Int* **45**(2):108–15.

Van Epps HL 2006. Michael Heidelberger and the demystification of antibodies. *J Exp Med* **203**(1):5.

Chapter 2

Immunohistochemistry Quality Assurance and Quality Control

Bronwyn Christiansen and Hazel Chambers

Overview

Ask a dozen different people about their thoughts on the meaning of 'quality' and a dozen different replies may be offered. The reason is that this subject is too broad to tackle in one answer and perhaps a better way to address this topic is to raise specific questions:

'How do we achieve high confidence in our immunohistochemistry (IHC) results?'

'Can we remove the doubt of false positives and false negatives from the IHC stain?'

'How does a facility offer many different localization antibodies, each with its unique characteristics, to be used on demand day after day?'

Address questions such as these and eventually the central theme of 'quality' emerges. Accurate and reliable IHC requires a robust quality management system and the ultimate goal of such a system is to eliminate or restrict errors. Quality control, quality assurance and quality improvement are not just buzzwords laboratory managers throw around. Rather they exist as a reference to all the endeavours required when striving for a reproducible, crisp and clean IHC stain. This chapter begins with a focus on the exact nature and make-up of the quality system specifically designed for IHC.

Achieving consistent high-quality IHC staining is possible. The discipline has shifted from something empirical based on observations and personal experience to something now grounded in proven scientific values. With each advancement, theoretical principles were developed to explain what was observed. As the science and knowledge of IHC were disseminated widely, key principles emerged which are now broadly accepted. One such consensus is that the IHC assay has many moving parts. Collectively known as 'variables', they are arranged systematically into pre-analytic, analytic and post-analytic classifications. These parameters and their close relationship to standardization efforts in IHC are explored further in this chapter in order to explain their association within the overall quality framework.

Good laboratory practice involves control tissue and test tissue stained concurrently on the same slide. An explanation as to the reasons why and the underlying circumstances which led to employing this practice is offered. The importance of internal and external controls as well as negative and positive controls is also examined. In much the same way as consumers buy a tin of beetroot at the supermarket, quality assurance dictates that the container not only contains beetroot, but is also of great quality and has the quantity specified.

In addition, organizations in Australia overseeing IHC testing such as the National Association of Testing Authority (NATA), National Pathology Accreditation Advisory Council (NPAAC), Royal College of Pathologists of Australasia (RCPA) and Therapeutic Goods Administration (TGA) are discussed with reference to their function. Equivalent bodies in Europe and the Americas are tasked with the same brief. In addition, non-governmental societies such as NordiQC provide a good resource for best practice. Allusions are offered as to their relevance in today's modern IHC service as they strive to keep pace with new and evolving technologies. *In vitro* diagnostic tests, the advent of companion diagnostics/personalized medicine and the special partnership with molecular techniques are cited as case examples. The chapter concludes with a glimpse into the near future and highlights the challenges quality assurance programs may encounter. After all, the main aim of quality control in IHC is to ensure reproducible and clean staining of the intended target which ultimately confers patient safety.

Quality Management System

The set of tools available to survey, assess and record the performance metrics of an IHC facility is often referred

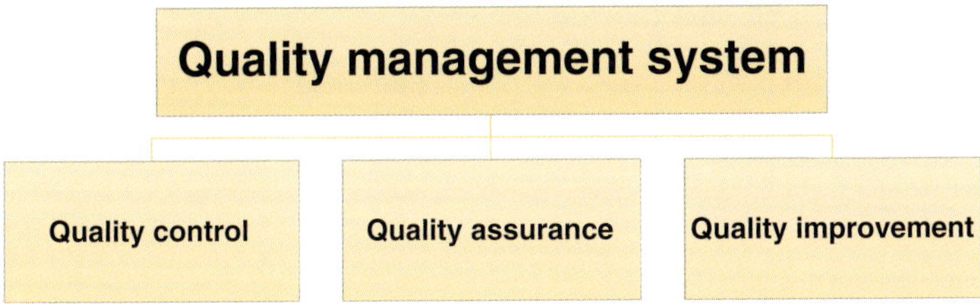

Figure 2.1 The key elements of a quality management system

to as the quality management system. It is made up of three main aspects (Figure 2.1) and designed to monitor the IHC laboratory's overall performance.

Quality Control

The College of American Pathologists (2017) defines quality control (QC) as 'the aggregate of processes and techniques so derived to detect, reduce and correct deficiencies in analytic process'. This broad, sweeping statement means that in practical terms, QC is mainly concerned with the actual IHC test, otherwise known as the 'assay' or the staining procedure. This is the 'analytic phase', and in order to ensure that the IHC stain is valid, a combination of events and procedures must be satisfied. These include:

- Daily assessment of tissue controls to ensure appropriate staining.
- Documentation to indicate the person responsible for accepting the IHC stain and signing off. Recorded either manually within record logbooks or electronically within the instrument software or laboratory information system (LIS).
- A record of the nature and origin of control tissue.
- Equipment maintenance and annual review as defined by the manufacturer.
- Records of validation and/or verification of new antibodies and assays.
- Stringent antibody and reagent storage inventory measures.

Both positive and negative forms of control from the perspective of the tissue as well as the reagent within the IHC assay are summarized in Table 2.1. A positive 'tissue' control contains the epitope which the antibody should recognize. These controls have an expected positive staining result, ideally with low and moderate intensities to aid in the identification of inconsistent staining which therefore warrants further investigation. A dark and intensely positive stain, although 'pretty' to observe, will be more difficult to detect any subtle changes that would indicate suboptimal assay conditions. Negative controls will have expected non-staining of tissue. There are two strategies to achieve this. First, specific negative tissue controls do not have the epitope present and second, the antibody reagent is substituted for diluent only. Most diagnostic IHC laboratories routinely employ positive and negative tissue controls by way of a multi-block. Using diluent-only reagent as a negative control measure to detect unwanted background staining is not routine practice in diagnostic laboratories but should be routinely employed in pure research settings. It is deemed unnecessary in diagnostic work because of the added costs involved with very little overall benefit. Besides, assessment of non-specific background staining does not conclude with substitution of antibody with diluent only. To conduct a full investigation of the cause of unwanted staining, there ought to be replacement and substitution of the secondary antibody and tertiary detection reagents as well. To employ all of these negative controls for a single IHC assay is not feasible.

Quality Assurance

Slightly different to QC, quality assurance (QA) is the practice of assessing IHC performance in all aspects of the laboratory testing cycle. Not only is the analytic stage scrutinized, but the pre-analytic and post-analytic phases are also inspected in order to promote excellent outcomes in medical care. Figure 2.2 is an example of a QA tool used at the Royal Children's Hospital (RCH) Melbourne. This log can be used to track possible causes of suboptimal IHC results. For instance, the QA number 0910 (failed IPX stain) may be due to QA numbers 0210 (insufficient formalin) and 0303 (badly fixed specimen) which was logged previous to the IHC stain being done.

Other examples of QA activities include staff training and enrolment into competency programmes, regular calibration processes, updated standard operating procedures (SOPs) and precise record-keeping (College of American Pathologists 2009). Where QC examines the IHC test, QA surveys the overall bigger picture in order to ensure the IHC

Table 2.1 Types and purpose of daily quality control within the immunohistochemistry laboratory

Control	Tissue	Reagent	Rationale
Negative	No staining expected because the epitope is absent. With nothing to bind to, the primary antibody should be washed away.	Substitute primary antibody reagent with diluent only. Any staining present is due to unwanted background reactions.	To determine the specificity of the assay and to measure non-specific staining which can lead to false positive results
Positive	Staining is expected because antigen is present. Ideally, both low and high levels of expression are available in a multi-block.	Ensure retrieval solutions, secondary antibody 'linkers', detection kit and chromogen are all optimized for the assay	To establish the sensitivity of the assay and its ability to detect antigenic sites so false negative results are not attained

QUALITY ASSURANCE ISSUE LOG

Lab number   Logged by: Date:

QA number	QUALITY ISSUE LOG	QA number	Errors which * require escalation	QA number		QA number	
01	**REQUEST**		**CUT-UP cont**	**05**	**EMBEDDING**	**09**	**IMMUNOPEROXIDASE**
0101	Incomplete request form	0308	Decal inadequate – more	0501	Incorrect orientation	0901	Incorrect antibody applied*
0102	Mislabelled request form*	0309	Incorrect colour cassette	0502	Re-embedding required	0902	Transcription error IPX label*
0103	Mislabelled specimen*	0310	Mislabelled cassette*	0503	Re-waxing required	0903	IP control missing
0104	Incorrect sticker*	0311	Tissue put in wrong cassette*	0504	Carryover of tissue b/w cases*	0904	IP control failure
0105	Labelling discrepancy*	0312	Inadequate block selection	**06**	**MICROTOMY**	0905	Incorrect IP control used
0106	Specimen count unequal	0313	Sutures left in specimen	0601	Poor cutting	0906	IP control cut through
0107	Empty specimen container*	0314	No tissue in cassette*	0602	Block not full face	0907	IPX background excessive
0108	Specimen lost*	0315	No sponges in cassette	0603	Block over trimmed	0908	IP slide dirty
0109	Registration errors (skels etc)	0316	One sponge only in cassette	0604	Block cut through	0909	IP slide moved from platform
		0317	Tissue lost from cassette*	0605	Block damaged	0910	Failed IPX stain
02	**SPECIMEN TRANSPORT**	0318	No lid on cassette*	0606	Recut wrong block		
0201	Specimen delayed in transit	0319	Tissue section too thick	0607	Section cut onto wrong slide	**10**	**EM/IF**
0202	Delay between collection/FS	0320	Tissue very fatty	0608	Fold and/or knife marks	1001	EM processing failure
0203	Specimen to wrong dept*	0321	Tissue block too large for cassette	0609	Thick section	1002	No glomeruli in EM
0204	Specimen arrived fresh	0322	Sponge used when should wrap	0610	Instructions not followed as per request	1003	No epidermis in skin IF
0205	Specimen autolyzed*	0323	Block over-inked	0611	Waterbath contaminants		
0206	Specimen not opened	0324	Block not described	0612	Dirty slide		
0207	Specimen leaking formalin	0325	Embedding orientation not clear				
0208	EM spec in formalin not glut	0326	Block lost *	**07**	**FROZEN SECTIONS**		
0209	Muscle/IF spec in saline	0327	Carryover of tissue b/w cases*	0701	Freezing artefact		
0210	Insufficient formalin			0702	Poorly quality F/S		
0211	Too long in transport medium			0703	F/S code not added		
0212	IF specimen not halved			0704	Discrepancy F/S and P/S	**11**	**TRANSCRIPTION**
0213	IF/muscle block dried out			**08**	**ROUTINE STAINING**	1101	Major transcription error
		04	**PROCESSING**	0801	Overstained	1102	Minor typo/spelling error
		0401	Poorly processed tissue	0802	Understained	1103	Delayed sign-out
03	**CUT UP**	0402	Tissue reprocessed	0803	Floaters	1104	Case mislaid report > SO
0301	Specimen delayed at cut up	0403	Processor failure	0804	Restain required		
0302	Wrong specimen code used	0404	Processor left on clean cycle*	0805	Incorrect stain	**12**	**DIAGNOSIS**
0303	Badly fixed specimen	0405	Wrong processor program*	0806	Unsatisfactory control	1201	Minor diagnostic error
0304	F/S alert not entered	0406	Tissue found outside cassette*	0807	Mislabelled slide	1202	Diagnostic error > correction
0305	Request wrongly dictated	0407	Tissue lost in processing*	0808	Air bubbles under coverslip	1203	Significant error with Rx imp*
0306	Specs dictated wrong order	0408	Tissue did not survive processing	0809	Crooked coverslip	1204	Discrepancy Frozen/paraffin
0307	Wrong decalcification protocol			0810	Squames contaminating	1205	Incorrect SNOMED code

QA number marked with an * must be escalated to scientist in charge/relevant medical head for immediate action. OFI/VHIMS numbers are to be recorded here:

Figure 2.2 A quality assurance log as used at the Royal Children's Hospital Melbourne

test is correct. Listed next are standards of QA measures which laboratories need to perform:

- Assess, investigate and report analytic (staining) problems.
- Identify reasons for repeat stains and record trends (if any).
- Maintain and assess turn-around time logs.
- Prospective monitoring and review of IHC stains for recently validated (new) antibodies.
- Instigate a surveillance programme for infrequently ordered IHC assays.
- Participation in external proficiency testing programmes such as RCPA QAP or UK NEQAS.
- Review and update IHC SOP manuals for the methods being performed.
- Implement and record corrective actions.
- Assure continuing education and competency of staff performing IHC (Figures 2.3 and 2.4).
- Provide adequate specialized training for new staff.
- Use updated SOPs to provide a mechanism for training and competency assessment of staff.
- Perform regular audits of pathology reports (Figure 2.5).
- Ensure there is appropriate coverage of trained personnel to perform IHC. The roster should have contingencies to cover sick and annual leave.

Anatomical Pathology Competency Indicators – Knowledge, Skills and Conduct				
Procedure	**Initial training and competency performed**	**On-going competency level obtained**	**Tasks observed or verbal description**	**Reviewed By**
AP-P-800 – IMMUNOHISTOCHEMISTRY	❑ Yes ❑ No ❑ Not Applicable	❑ Competent ❑ RETRAIN ❑ Not Applicable	❑ Knowledge: Principals of antigen retrieval ❑ Skill: Completion of ISH staining ❑ Conduct: Troubleshooting failed staining	

Competency Statement – The competency of the above-mentioned staff member has been assessed and:

❑ **The staff member is deemed competent in Anatomical Pathology Tasks as indicated on pages 2–5 (no further action)**

❑ The staff member is required to complete competency standards for Anatomical Pathology tasks as indicated on page 1 by..........................(date).

Comments:

Signature of Staff Member: Date:

Signature of Assessor: Date:

Figure 2.3 Training and annual competencies of staff at the Royal Children's Hospital Melbourne

At the RCH Melbourne, IHC staff competencies are reviewed annually as per NATA accreditation for ISO 15189. Documents such as those in Figure 2.3 show certification of staff members deemed competent by way of observation or verbal discussion of their knowledge. Another method to employ is to challenge staff to successful completion of assessments in the form of a quiz as shown in Figure 2.4.

Regular audits are necessary to examine the integrity of the systems and procedures within the laboratory. Internal audits are conducted within the organization whereas external audits usually involve a visit from a third party. Often termed 'vertical' audits, a simple strategy is to follow a specimen that has been processed by the laboratory starting from receipt and accessioning and moving through the various stages towards diagnosis. Figure 2.5 highlights such an audit via a worksheet used at the RCH Melbourne. Conducting these audits may uncover weaknesses within the quality system such as staff not following SOPs, suboptimal staining or other events which preclude inaccurate diagnoses. As faults are detected, the laboratory can proceed to find remedies.

Quality Improvement

As QC and QA systems may have inherent limitations and failings, quality improvement (QI) seeks to find workable solutions. Quality improvement is the practice of continuously assessing and adjusting performance using statistically and scientifically accepted procedures (College of American Pathologists 2009) and may include:

- QA/QC reports to laboratory quality management committee.
- Report proficiency testing results to quality manager or laboratory director.
- Report audit results to quality management committee.
- Evidence of continuing education participation.
- Review volume of specific IHC assays.
- Compare IHC results with reported data within literature.
- Protocol standardization.
- Evaluation of new platforms and reagents (antibody clones, detection systems etc.). (Cates and Troutman 2015)

The RCH Melbourne laboratory collates quality issues for incorporation into regular education sessions. Items such as failed stains due to user error, instrument failure or wrong controls are shown and discussed so that all staff can gain knowledge to both recognize the issue and to prevent it from occurring again. Figure 2.6 is an example of quality issues collated at the RCH Melbourne for discussion in laboratory meetings using information sourced from the previously mentioned quality log shown in Figure 2.2.

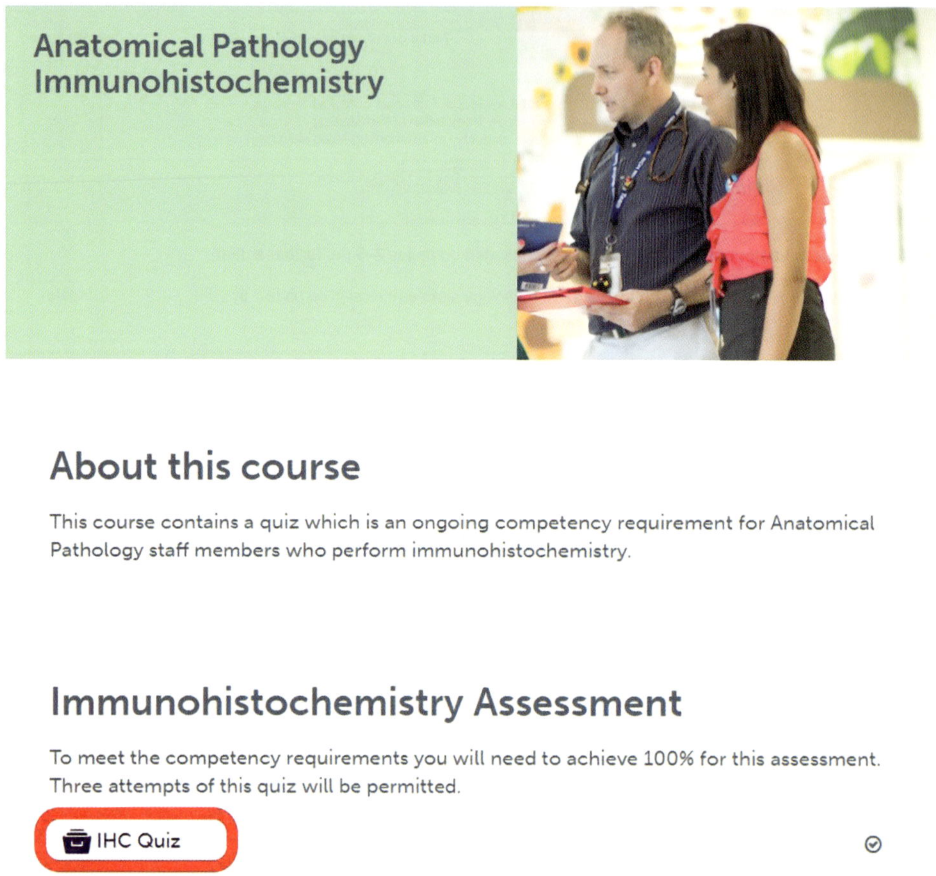

Figure 2.4 Online quiz for staff competency at the Royal Children's Hospital Melbourne

Another critical part of QI is recognizing when a protocol requires change. For instance, if a laboratory receives a borderline or an unsatisfactory result from a quality assurance programme (QAP) proficiency testing for a particular antibody, the staining method for that antibody needs to be investigated. The laboratory may also seek to improve the staining even if a satisfactory result is obtained. Regardless, if there is a change to a previously validated protocol, it must be documented, and the new method requires authorization and sign-off by a pathologist before being utilized on patient samples.

Factors Influencing Immunohistochemical Staining

To explore the factors that influence IHC outcomes, it is pertinent to first investigate factors which influence the science of histology in a general sense. Many parameters can impact IHC staining. By convention, such factors are neatly categorized into three distinct groups: pre-analytic, analytic and post-analytic.

However, a discussion involving these terms of the pre-analytic, analytic and post-analytic phases can be confusing. The reason is there may be a lack of context when explaining this concept. Consider the flow chart in Figure 2.7 highlighting the steps involved to achieve a histological diagnosis. In this concept, events within the pre-analytic phase are considered out of the control of the histology laboratory. There is no input from the laboratory in what happens to the tissue before it is received. Once the tissue is formally accessioned, the facility determines how it proceeds with the tissue analysis. This includes sharing tissue for flow cytometry, microbiology culture and sensitivity studies or molecular studies etc. Once tissue is selected for histological processing and testing requirements, the analytical phase commences. After

ANATOMICAL PATHOLOGY AUDIT WORKSHEET

CASE DETAILS					
Accession number*					
Specimen type					
Number of specimens		Number of blocks			
Set up	Embedded	Cut by		Sent by	
Number of slides					
Registrar		Pathologist			
Received (date)		Validation (date)			
T.A.T : Received to validated					
PRE-ANALYTICAL/DATA ENTRY ISSUES					
Labelling of specimen matches request?	Yes	No	Requesting Dr details correctly entered?	Yes	No
Clinical history provided?	Yes	No	Copy to Dr/s correctly entered?	Yes	No
LABORATORY ISSUES					
Re-cuts or re-stains required?	Yes	No			
Quality of staining	Good	Problems Details:			
Other laboratory issues?	Yes	No Details:			
REPORT					
Typographical errors	Yes	No Details:			
Diagnosis	Concur	Disagree Details:			
Classification of errors	- N/A				
	- Minor non-clinical minor typographic error etc which do not present any risk of patient harm, yet nonetheless can detract from laboratory efficiency or client perceptions of the report.				
	- Minor clinical Report contained errors which could alter patient management but did not place the patient at risk of immediate harm.				
	- Major clinical Report contained errors which could potentially have resulted in immediate harm to the patient.				
SNOMED coding	Present: Yes No Correct Incorrect				
OUTCOMES					
Audit outcome	- No action required				
	- Review by reporting pathologist				
	- Corrected report recommended				
AUDIT					
Auditing pathologist					
Date of audit					
Time taken to perform audit					

Figure 2.5 Internal audit as used at the Royal Children's Hospital Melbourne

completion of the 'test', the interpretation of the result, formal reporting and every task thereafter (from block filing to tissue disposal) is considered post-analytical. Note that the events described thus far pertain to general histology analysis, in which IHC is one of many techniques available.

Compare this flow chart to Figure 2.8, where there is a slight shift in the activities making up the pre-analytic, analytic and post-analytic stages discussed from the viewpoint of the IHC assay alone. Processes before the actual IHC method are now considered pre-analytical and include section thickness, decalcification and type of fixation, for example. These processes were considered 'analytic' from a general histology point of view. This contextual shift from a general histology viewpoint to that of the IHC assay has changed the thinking around the factors making up the three phases.

Consider a histology reference laboratory tasked to perform IHC from another facility. Commonly unstained sections are sent to the reference laboratory requesting a specific antibody that the original laboratory does not offer. For the reference laboratory, the type and length of fixation and the nature of microtomy in terms of section thickness and drying time, as well as the brand of 'sticky' slides, are all considered pre-analytic factors because it has no control over these variables. The reference laboratory can only apply its own tissue controls on the slide and proceed with the IHC stain. The tissue

01	REQUEST	
0101	Incomplete request form	
0102	Mislabelled request form*	
0103	Mislabelled specimen*	
0104	Incorrect sticker*	
0105	Labelling discrepancy*	
0106	Specimen count unequal	
0107	Empty specimen container*	
0108	Specimen lost*	
0109	Registration errors (skel etc)	1
Total 01 errors		1
02	SPECIMEN TRANSPORT	
0201	Specimen delayed in transit	
0202	Delay between collection/FS	
0203	Specimen to wrong dept*	
0204	Specimen arrived fresh	
0205	Specimen autolyzed*	
0206	Specimen not opened	
0207	Specimen leaking formalin	
0208	EM spec in formalin not glut	
0209	Muscle/IF spec in saline	
0210	Insufficient formalin	
0211	Too long in transport medium	
0212	IF specimen not halved	
0213	IF/muscle block dried out	
Total 02 errors		0
03	CUT UP	
0301	Specimen delayed at cut up	
0302	Wrong specimen code used	
0303	Badly fixed specimen	
0304	F/S alert not entered	
0305	Request wrongly dictated	
0306	Specs dictated wrong order	
0307	Wrong decalcification protocol	

	CUT-UP cont	
0308	Decal inadequate - more	
0309	Incorrect colour cassette	
0310	Mislabelled cassette*	
0311	Tissue put in wrong cassette*	
0312	Inadequate block selection	
0313	Sutures left in specimen	
0314	No tissue in cassette*	
0315	No sponges in cassette	
0316	One sponge only in cassette	
0317	Tissue lost from cassette*	
0318	No lid on cassette*	
0319	Tissue section too thick	
0320	Tissue very fatty	
0321	Tissue block too large for cassette	
0322	Sponge used when should wrap	
0323	Block over-inked	
0324	Block not described	
0325	Embedding orientation not clear	
0326	Block lost*	
0327	Carryover of tissue between cases	
Total 03 errors		0
04	PROCESSING	
0401	Poorly processed tissue	
0402	Tissue reprocessed	
0403	Processor failure	
0404	Processor left on clean cycle*	
0405	Wrong processor program*	
0406	Tissue found outside cassette*	
0407	Tissue lost in processing*	
0408	Tissue did not survive processing	
Total 04 errors		0

05	EMBEDDING	
0501	Incorrect orientation	
0502	Re-embedding required	
0503	Re-waxing required	
0504	Carryover of tissue between cas	1
Total 05 errors		1
06	MICROTOMY	
0601	Poor cutting	1
0602	Block not full face	1
0603	Block over trimmed	
0604	Block cut through	
0605	Block damaged	
0606	Recut wrong block	2
0607	Section cut onto wrong slide	
0608	Fold and/or knife marks	
0609	Thick section	
0610	Not followed as per request	1
0611	Floaters from waterbath	1
0612	Dirty slide	
Total 06 errors		6
07	FROZEN SECTIONS	
0701	Freezing artefact	
0702	Poorly quality F/S	
0703	F/S code not added	1
0704	Discrepancy F/S and P/S	
Total 07 errors		1
08	ROUTINE STAINING	
0801	Overstained	
0802	Understained	
0803	Floaters	
0804	Restain required	1
0805	Incorrect stain	
0806	Unsatisfactory control	
0807	Mislabelled slide	2
0808	Air bubbles under coverslip	3
0809	Crooked coverslip	
0810	Squames contaminating	
Total 08 errors		6

09	IMMUNOPEROXIDASE	
0901	Incorrect antibody applied*	
0902	Transcription error IPX label*	1
0903	IP control missing	1
0904	IP control failure	4
0905	Incorrect IP control used	2
0906	IP control cut through	1
0907	IPX background excessive	
0908	IP slide dirty	
0909	IP slide moved from platform	
0910	Failed IPX stain	6
Total 09 errors		15
10	EM/IF	
1001	EM processing failure	
1002	No glomeruli in EM	
1003	No epidermis in skin IF	
Total 10 errors		0
11	TRANSCRIPTION	
1101	Major transcription error	
1102	Minor typo/spelling error	2
1103	Delayed sign-out	
1104	Case mislaid report > SO	
Total 11 errors		2
12	DIAGNOSIS	
1201	Minor diagnostic error	
1202	Diagnostic error > correction	
1203	Significant error with Rx imp*	
1204	Discrepancy frozen/paraffin	
1205	Incorrect SNOMED code	
Total 12 errors		0

Total 01 errors	REQUEST	1
Total 02 errors	SPECIMEN TRANSPORT	0
Total 03 errors	CUT UP	0
Total 04 errors	PROCESSING	0
Total 05 errors	EMBEDDING	1
Total 06 errors	MICROTOMY	6
Total 07 errors	FROZEN SECTIONS	1
Total 08 errors	ROUTINE STAINING	6
Total 09 errors	IMMUNOPEROXIDASE	15
Total 10 errors	EM/IF	0
Total 11 errors	TRANSCRIPTION	2
Total 12 errors	DIAGNOSIS	0

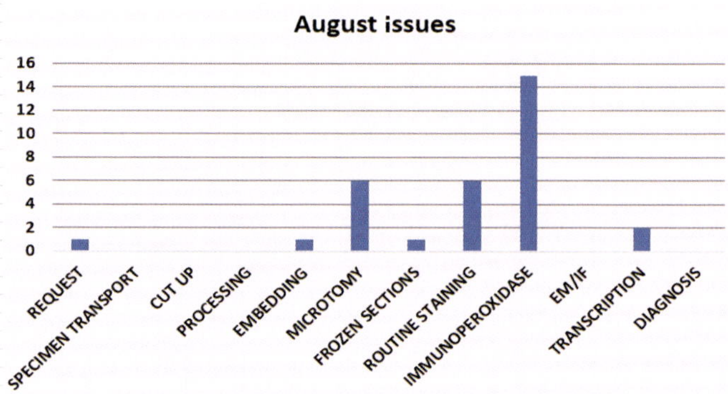

Figure 2.6 A record of quality issues for the month of August 2020

controls only determine staining success according to the reference laboratory's set parameters and there must be an understanding that interpretation of the test tissue should proceed with caution because of the possible variances in pre-analytic factors between the requesting laboratory and the reference laboratory. The important notion of 'standardization' of histological techniques has now become evident as laboratories grasp the need to employ standard techniques being fundamental for success. The take-home point is that context must be set out clearly when discussing pre-analytic, analytic and post-analytic factors influencing IHC or general histology.

Ultimately, it is the lack of 'standardization' which leads to failed or inconsistent IHC staining. So many parameters are involved in IHC that if a certain 'standard' for each was not adopted, then the likelihood of success would be remote. Adopting a 'standard setting' incorporates both intra- and inter-laboratory processes. Within the IHC facility, a consistent effort in attaining optimal fixation, epitope retrieval and incubation conditions, for example, will provide every opportunity for success. Similar sentiment must also be shared between separate laboratories if IHC is distributed across multiple facilities. A few important variables from the pre-analytic, analytic and post-analytic stages are discussed with reference to adopted standard practices.

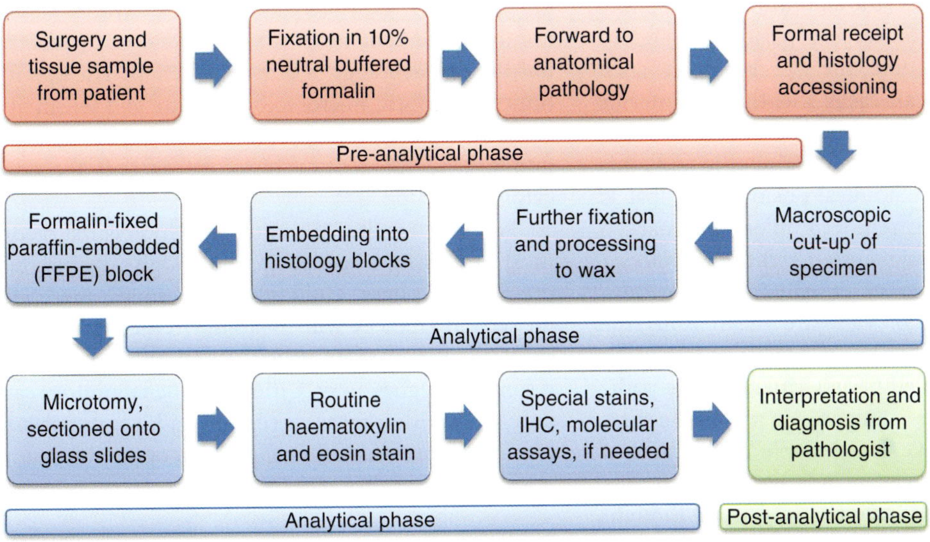

Figure 2.7 A stepwise approach to general histological analysis of tissue specimens

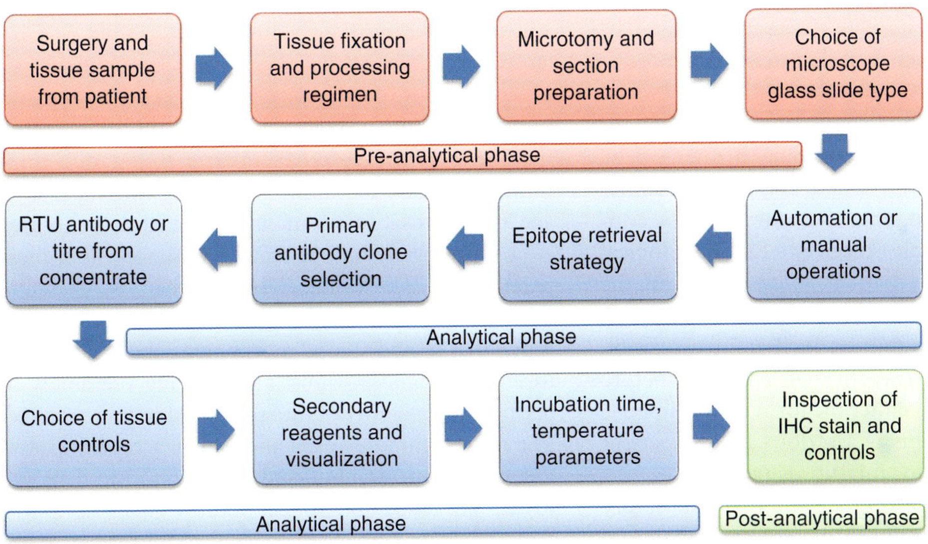

Figure 2.8 Pre-analytic, analytic and post-analytic variables from the immunohistochemical perspective

Pre-analytical: General Histology

As alluded to previously, this group encompasses all the processes from the time a laboratory request is made until the specimen is analysed in the laboratory. In diagnostic histopathology, there is usually no input from the laboratory as to how the tissue is sampled, the specific conditions under which the specimen is acquired or the quantity supplied.

Tissue Procurement

The clinician and/or surgeon plays a major role in supplying the laboratory with optimal tissue for analysis. For instance, the tissue removed must contain the lesion under investigation. If the specimen is a skin lesion, for example, the surgical margins should be clear macroscopically. The laboratory understands that sometimes it is difficult to achieve good representation, especially in awkward and hard-to-reach parts of the anatomy. However, the laboratory must be able to interpret the type of surgery performed and to reconstruct and orientate the specimen in such a way that clinicians can easily identify the inferior or superior aspect of the specimen or which way is left and right, anterior and posterior. Being able to do this is important because anatomical positions are lost as soon as the body part is removed unless it is marked by a suture or clip to designate left/right side, superior or inferior aspect and so on. Equally important from the laboratory's point of view are the reasons the surgery was performed.

Accurate clinical history as written on the pathology request form goes a long way in aiding the steps taken for analysis. Take for example a resection of bone. Possible pathologies include bone density disorders, osteoarthritis or malignancy. Careful thought is needed if anticipating malignancy because of the necessary decalcification process. Acid-based reagents are known to affect certain localization antibodies for IHC whereas a more gentle approach using calcium chelators such as EDTA will preserve epitopes better, but their action is slower than that of acid.

An important point that is sometimes overlooked is the adequate labelling of specimens. Patient details on the specimen container must match that of the pathology request form, a simple concept but sometimes not fully followed. The laboratory must be confident that the sample received for histological analysis belongs to the patient as described on the label. If there is a mismatch between the request form and specimen container, further investigation is required so as to ascertain the correct details before proceeding. Sometimes either the form or specimen is received unlabelled. This is a serious risk to patient safety as the potential for mix-ups is magnified.

If there is an anticipation of multiple laboratory investigations, the quantity of tissue supplied should match the demand. Take lymphoid tissue as an example. For lymphoma queries, flow cytometry is a valuable ancillary test, but the tissue cannot be subjected to formalin fixation. The tissue should be fresh or held in a transport medium such as RPMI solution. What if the tissue sampled is not lymph node because the surgeon missed the lesion? The conundrum here is whether histological analysis is performed first to confirm and warrant flow cytology or whether the laboratory proceeds with flow cytometry concurrently with histology. Not first ascertaining whether the sampled tissue is suitable for flow cytometry may lead to a waste of resources. Consider an enlarged lymph node removed and sent for histology and flow cytometry but the real aetiology is due to infection. The opportunity to perform microbiology culture and sensitivity studies has passed since the fresh tissue has been placed into fixative for routine histology or sent for flow cytometry.

For best results, the clinician/physician/surgeon must be willing to assist the pathologist during this pre-analysis phase. Unlike blood samples, there are no second chances with histology. Once a lesion is surgically removed, there isn't another one to supply if something goes awry. Ultimately the laboratory can only work with what was received and it is important to start the pre-analytical stage in an optimal fashion.

Fixation

Optimal fixation of tissue is **essential**. This statement cannot be stressed enough as the fixation process preserves cellular components, prevents autolysis and displacement of cell constituents, stabilizes cellular materials against deleterious effects of subsequent procedures and facilitates conventional staining and immunostaining (Hayat 2002). In addition, other fixative properties are that it is fast acting, non-toxic to humans, easy to handle with straightforward storage and disposal requirements and affordable to use.

Unfortunately no one fixative possesses all of these parameters. The choice of fixative is therefore a compromise and the fixative most laboratories utilize is one that provides good morphological detail in order to enable diagnosis whilst also offering the ability to perform the majority of the specialized testing required. The most commonly used and widely accepted fixative today is 10% neutral buffered formalin (NBF) deployed to act on tissue for 10–24 hours (Shi et al. 1991). Formaldehyde is the active chemical ingredient and is actually a gas in its natural state. It is dissolved in water as a concentrate at around 40% w/v and then diluted out to a 10% (4% formaldehyde) working solution. This is how it is known as 10% formalin. Some laboratories do not apply buffer solutions to keep the reagent at neutral pH whilst others add sodium chloride so as to replicate physiologic conditions at the cellular level. The RCH Melbourne's standard tissue fixative is 10% formalin buffered to neutral pH. Although there is widespread acceptance of 10% NBF as the 'industry standard' fixative, it is not perfect because it doesn't satisfy all of the previously mentioned criteria. However, it is the closest to an 'ideal' fixative. In addition, there are antibody clones which are incompatible with formalin-fixed paraffin-embedded (FFPE) tissue. Frozen sections may be required or an alternative marker to the epitope of interest may be sought. Fixation in acetone can assist in preserving some epitopes but can lead to problems in interpretation due to poor morphology (Shi et al. 2008). Soluble antigens can also be destroyed or denatured during tissue processing. It is also worthwhile noting that formalin fixation can also lead to problems with artefactual sequence alterations when performing polymerize chain reactions (PCR). C-T and G-A base substitutions occur in approximately 1 in 500 base pairs following formalin fixation (Williams et al. 1999).

Traditionally, histology has been concerned with morphology and microanatomy of tissue architecture. There is now an additional emphasis on molecular technologies to supplement traditional histological analysis. During tissue procurement it is important to avoid degraded morphological effects due to ischemia (lack of blood supply) in tissues as it will also lead to damaged RNA and DNA. The detrimental effects of autolysis and enzyme destruction on unfixed tissues exposed at room temperature for a number of hours can be observed microscopically. The time taken between anaesthetizing a patient to submerging their opened specimen into fixative impacts both morphology and gene expression. Implications of suboptimal fixation range from an altered ki-67 index in breast-wide local excision specimens to distorted expression of genes for molecular applications. Slices of tissue that are well fixed around the periphery but poorly fixed in the centre can show differences in IHC staining and heterogeneous gene expression. Figure 2.9 shows the fixation front indicated by black arrows, as 10% NBF works its way from the periphery of the tissue to the centre in this sample observed by the colour difference. Best practice would have this sample 'bread-loaf' sliced for optimal fixation. It increases the surface area in which the fixative can perform. The importance of optimal and even fixation on resection specimens cannot be emphasized enough.

Other fixatives such as glutaraldehyde are not endorsed due to their reactivity and speed, and they can seriously interfere with both antibody and lectin binding, causing considerable non-specific staining. In addition, it is difficult to remove excess glutaraldehyde from tissue components. Bouin's solution should also be used with caution as a fixative as IHC staining and some molecular techniques can be negatively impacted with its use (Ananthanarayanan et al. 2005).

Prompt opening of a specimen and an adequate fixative volume are essential for consistent, even staining. Certain antibodies are highly sensitive to uneven fixation. The mismatch repair proteins MLH1, MSH2, MSH6 and PMS2 are particularly susceptible whereas other antibodies such as Vimentin and CK20 within the same panel may show even, crisp staining. Figure 2.10 shows highly variable IHC staining of oestrogen receptor (ER). Observing the whole slide scan at x1 magnification (A), the image resembles a bubble artefact. Closer inspection of the tissue periphery, however, shows the staining boundary contours with the tissue (arrow). A bubble artefact would not

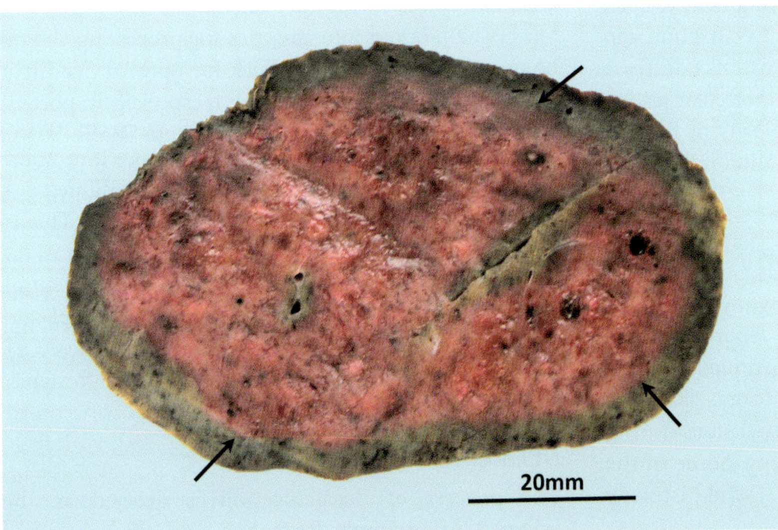

Figure 2.9 Fixation front (arrows) as 10% neutral buffered formalin penetrates the tissue

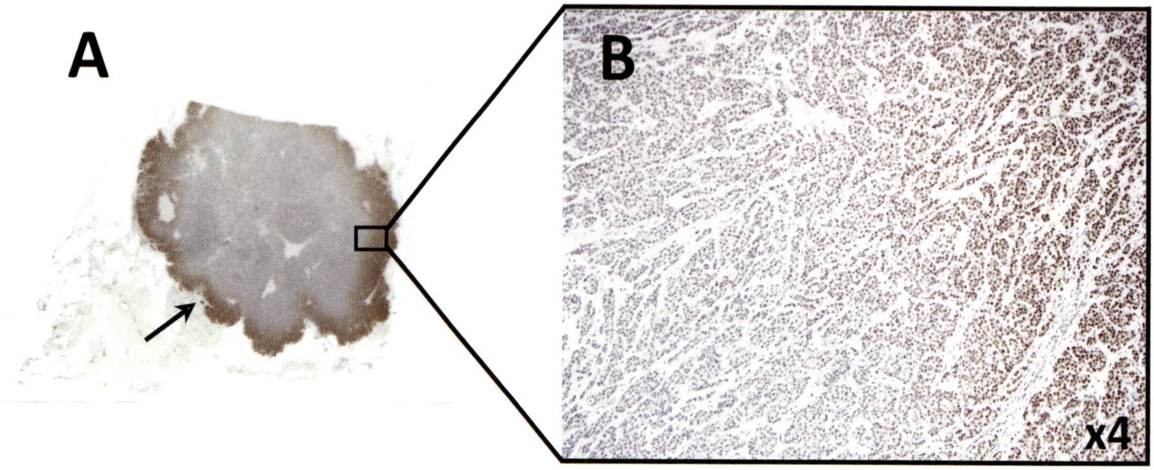

Figure 2.10 Heterogeneous immunohistochemical staining due to suboptimal fixation

behave this way and being a spherical object does not follow the tissue boundary. When the image is zoomed in at x4 magnification (B), note the adequate nuclear labelling towards the periphery contrasting to poor staining at the centre of the tissue. A result like this points to suboptimal tissue penetration of the fixative. The cause may be failure to 'open' up the tissue for fixative penetration or the fixation time is too short.

The specimen type usually dictates the length of fixation before tissue processing to paraffin wax. Clinical demand often places undue pressure on histology laboratories to push through samples for rapid turn-around result times. It is important for pathology departments to educate clinical teams on the importance of fixation in order to avoid compromising specimens and preventing downstream testing failures such as molecular assays (NCCLS 1999). Over-fixation can also be a problem when irreversible crosslinks decrease the amount of usable nucleic acids for molecular testing (Miyatake et al. 2004). By far, the majority of fixation problems are contributed to under-fixation rather than over-fixation.

Analytical: General Histology

This stage involves all of the processes after the tissue specimen is formally received in the laboratory. The 'macro cut-up', tissue sampling, continued fixation and processing to paraffin, microtomy, staining, mounting and coverslip are the essential steps during the analytical stage of general histology. Some of the important parameters critical for successful histology are highlighted.

Thickness of Tissue Sampled at Macro Cut-up

When selecting tissue at cut-up for processing to a FFPE block, it is important to consider physical properties such as penetration rate of the fixative in use. Upon receipt of a large specimen or organ such as liver, uterus or bowel resections, it is imperative to expose a large surface area of the sample to the fixation reagent. The recommended fixation strategy for solid organs is via repetitive slicing much like slicing a loaf of bread whilst taking care not to destroy the integrity of the overall organ or damage orientation markers. For large tubular organs or tissue with a natural cavity, the sample is carefully 'opened' to allow the inner aspects adequate contact with the fixative.

Tissue blocked into cassettes for processing should be no more than 3–4 mm thick for optimal overnight automated tissue processing. This is especially important for dense tissue like fibroids or uteri (Rolls 2016). Likewise, the width of the tissue within the processing cassette should not touch the sides. A perimeter of 3–5 mm from the edge of the tissue to the edge of the cassette ensures optimal fluid transfer (Carson and Hladik 2009; Hewitt et al. 2008). In other words, do not squash tissue into cassettes like a can of sardines because they will not process successfully. Figure 2.11 shows examples of poor selection of tissue for processing.

Decalcification

The process of decalcification is defined as the removal of minerals from bone or other calcified

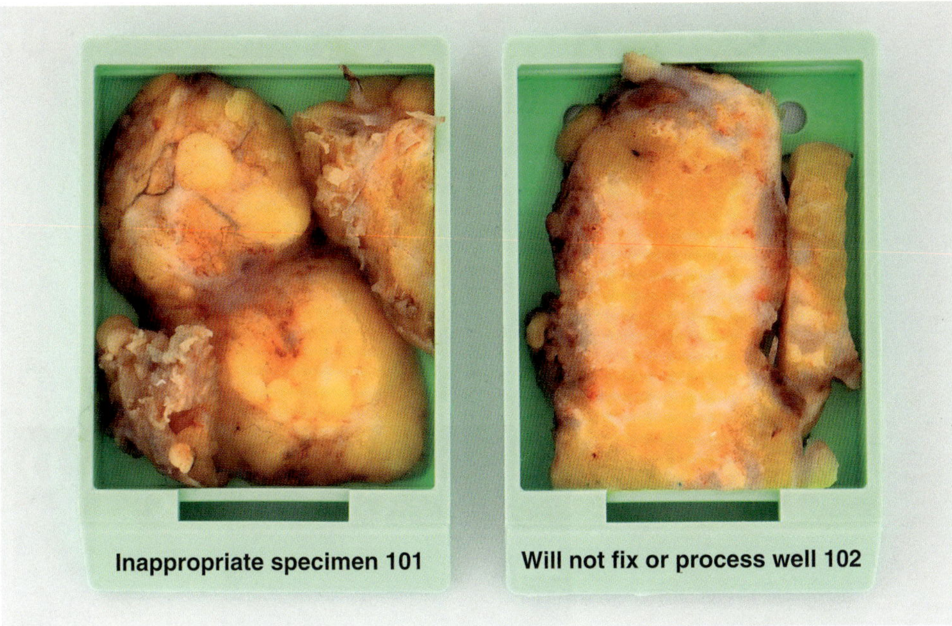

Figure 2.11 Overfilling of cassettes with tissue at cut-up

tissues so that high-quality paraffin sections can be prepared whilst preserving all of the essential microscopic elements. It is crucial that this process is undertaken following complete fixation of the tissue specimen. Poorly fixed tissue subjected to decalcification may end up macerated with inferior morphology and will confer feeble staining properties. A few decalcification strategies are available using different types of decalcifying fluids.

(1) Strong mineral acids such as nitric acid and hydrochloric acids. These reagents are most rapid in action but can lead to detrimental effects in tissue if decalcification is prolonged.
(2) Weak organic acids such as formic acid. A slower-acting reagent but less likely to interfere with routine stains due to their gentle action.
(3) Chelating agents such as ethylenediaminetetraacetic acid (EDTA). Decalcifying with a calcium chelator is very slow with the process taking weeks for some specimens. However, they excel at maintaining molecular information for ISH/PCR and for achieving high-quality morphology (Rolls 2013).

Some reports have shown that decalcifying can lead to false negative IHC results in surgical specimens (McMahon 2018). Consider a scenario where the control tissue used for IHC did not undergo decalcification but the test tissue did. After obtaining a negative IHC result, it is important to ascertain whether the IHC stain is a 'true' negative because in this instance, the control tissue and test tissue have not been treated in a standardized manner. It is important to acknowledge and communicate to the reporting pathologist that decalcification has been used in the tissue processing schedule and subsequent downstream assays have not been validated or verified. Results should be interpreted with caution given the likelihood of false negativity on decalcified specimens.

Tissue Processing

As discussed earlier, the size of tissue sections processed in cassettes will dictate the overall morphology and quality of IHC. Room must be available for the processing reagents to circulate within cassettes during the processing cycle. Similarly, the tissue section should fit comfortably onto a glass slide without overhanging edges in order to ensure the entire section is protected by the glass coverslip.

Adequate processing is achieved by using reagents and cycles of suitable length to fully process tissues, ensuring full penetration of solutions especially towards the centre of the tissue. The reagents used should be fresh, clean and pure for maximum effectiveness. Prevention of water contamination during

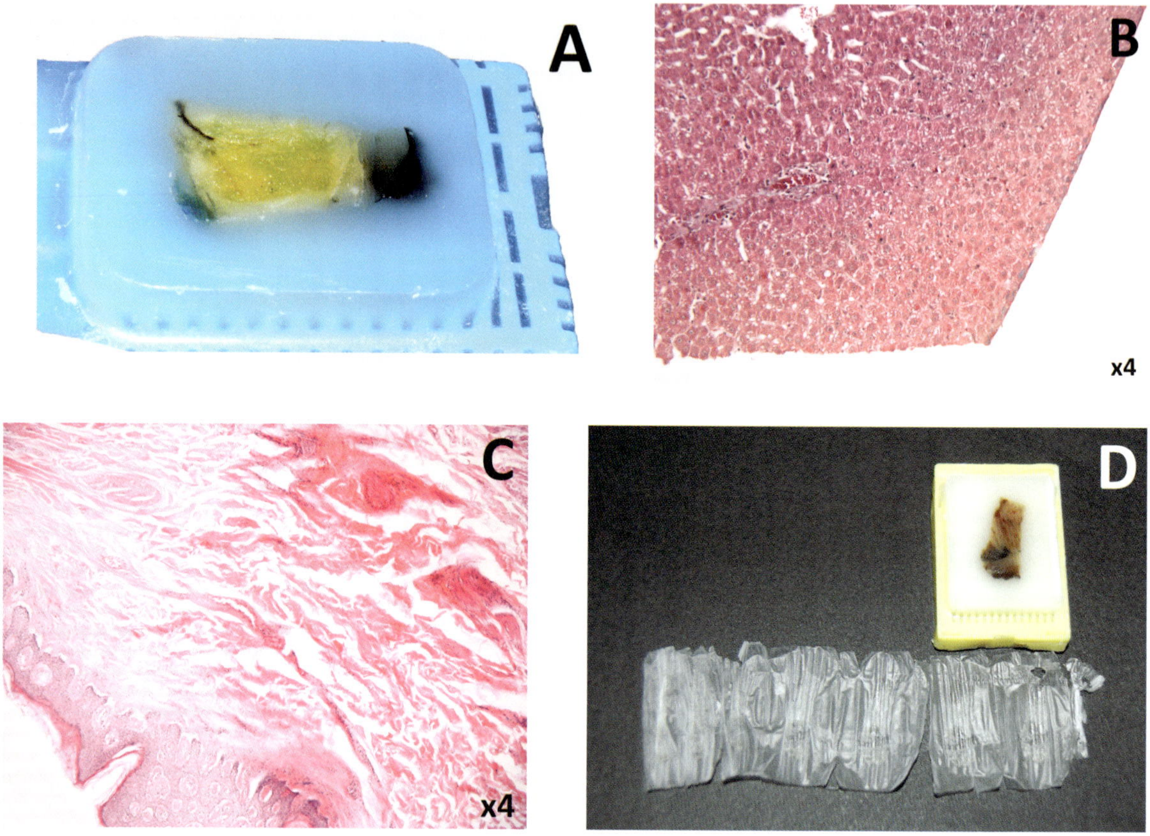

Figure 2.12 Factors determining high-quality tissue processing (Rolls 2019). Images reproduced with permission Leica Biosystems Melbourne, Pty. Ltd.

processing is of utmost concern because of the detrimental effects on tissue component morphology as well as IHC and ISH. Some groups have had increased success with enhanced immunostaining by increasing the temperature of the processing steps from room temperature up to 45°C whilst also lengthening the dehydration and wax infiltration steps (Williams et al. 1997). Figure 2.12 shows examples of the results of poor tissue processing.

A: Under-processed adipose tissue: A fatty specimen will not section appropriately if under processed. Because fat possesses a high lipid/triglyceride content and low protein index, its adequate fixation and processing require a three-pronged approach of cross-linking proteins, alcohol coagulation and suitable 'clearing' of lipid content with xylene. Deficiencies in any one area will not allow adequate infiltration of wax for FFPE.

B: Zonal fixation: When fixation is not uniform across the tissue section different 'zones' emerge. In this example, the outer edge is fixed with formalin whereas the inner and deeper aspects of tissue show the effect of alcohol fixation. The formalin penetrates from the periphery of the tissue. Whilst morphology may still be diagnostic with the hematoxylin and eosin (H&E) stain, it can be disastrous for many IHC stains and molecular assays due to decreased antigen and DNA preservation.

C: Using old and exhausted reagents: The old saying 'garbage in, garbage out' is true for tissue processing. If the quality of the reagents is poor, the resulting morphology will also be poor. To achieve optimal tissue processing, ensure reagents are high quality and they are replenished regularly so as to prevent contamination and chemical exhaustion. The fixative, dehydrating reagent, clearing solvent and paraffin wax must all be surveyed

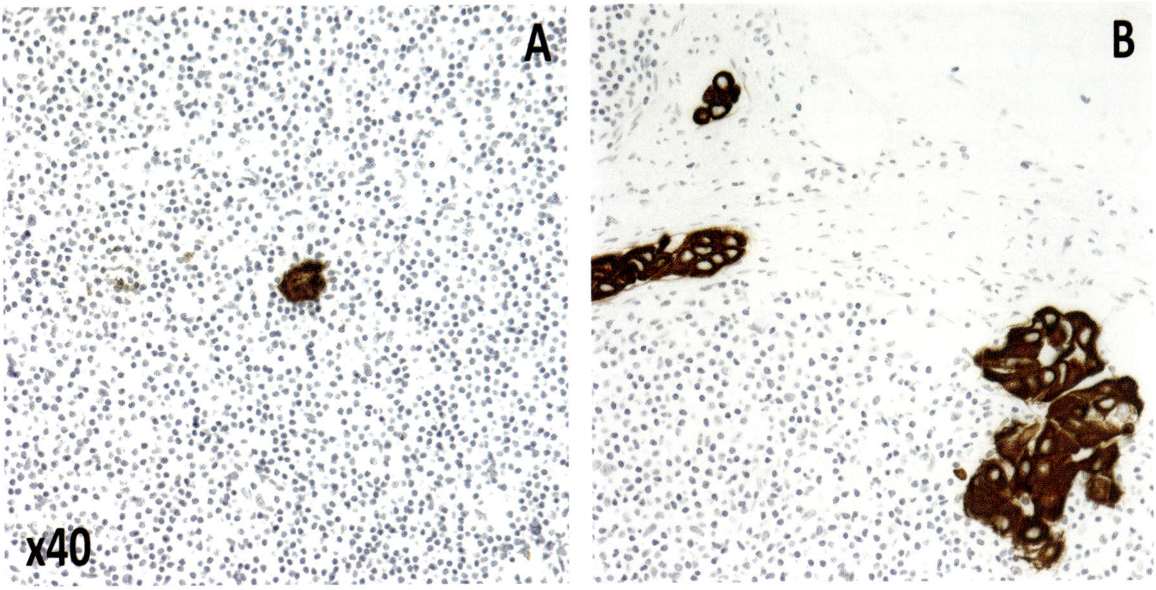

Figure 2.13 Lymph node CK AE1/3 immunohistochemical assay with an interfering 'squame' (A) and metastatic carcinoma (B)

because they are interconnected. If one solution is suboptimal, the whole process is adversely affected.

D: Poor wax properties: Always use high-quality wax because inadequate wax quality will provide difficulties during infiltration and using wax which has an inappropriate melting temperature can render blocks impossible to section. Ease of ribboning, the degree of compression and the wax 'hardness' are all attributed to the quality of paraffin used and whether the tissue has been optimally 'cleared' before infiltration.

Sectioning Formalin-Fixed Paraffin-Embedded Tissue

Although seemingly obvious, good sectioning practice is essential for a quality IHC slide. If sections are of low quality before being stained – possessing rips, compression and folds, for example – the IHC process will not improve on what was provided. The IHC stain is an expensive assay relative to the humble H&E stain when factoring in the types of antibodies used, platforms acquired, number of errors and repeat staining if needed. It is therefore prudent to ensure unstained slides for IHC are of the highest quality. Sections for IHC should be cut using quality consumables and include clean adhesive slides so sections are not prone to lifting off the slide during the IHC process. Certain processes such as breast SISH are prone to artefactual silver deposition and it can be warranted to use specific slides in order to avoid this problem.

Microtome blades should be sharp so as to ensure tissue sections are not heavily scored. The water bath should be at a suitable temperature for the wax used and must be clean and free of contaminants and floaters. Figure 2.13 shows CK AE1/3 IHC stain demonstrating squamous contamination shed from a staff member's fingers (A) closely mimicking metastatic carcinoma (B). This artefact may harbour a false positive result and can also obscure the section if present at high levels. This case was a sentinel lymph node biopsy sectioned at certain levels so the assay cannot be easily repeated.

Section thickness on average is around 3 μm with the exception of renal and lymphoid tissues being sectioned thinner at 1 μm. Thick sections can be prone to improper dewaxing, leaving patches of absent staining or entrapment of reagents under sections seen as large patches of brown diaminobenzidine (DAB) deposit. Figure 2.14 highlights a spectrin IHC assay on a fresh frozen section. The pattern localization is membranous, but notice the brown patches indicating DAB chromogen trapped underneath the cryostat section. In addition, thick tissue sections have been demonstrated to influence the Her2 IHC scoring algorithm changing from 1+ to 2+. This 'overcalling' of HER2 IHC results leads to inappropriate requests for molecular testing (McCampbell et al. 2017).

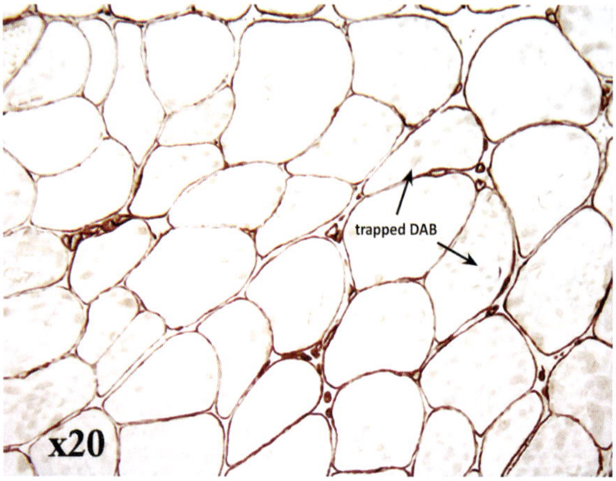

Figure 2.14 Spectrin immunohistochemical (IHC) staining showing trapped diaminobenzidine (DAB)

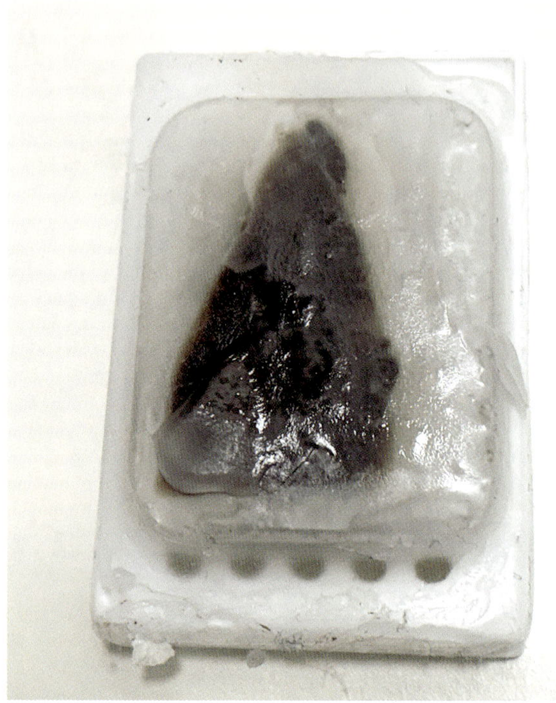

Figure 2.15 Paraffin block coated in wax in order to preserve tissue antigenicity

The sections must be dried prior to staining. A variety of methods are available to achieve section drying; the most common include using an oven at a preset temperature, placing slides onto a hot plate or leaving them to air dry in ambient temperature. Care must be taken when utilizing ovens and hot plates for prolonged periods of time. Antigenicity is lost with extended heating at 60°C. Slides left in the oven overnight at 60°C should be recut even if staining is observed because this staining may be unreliable (Jacobs et al. 1996).

Block and Slide Storage

It is important that processed paraffin blocks are stored under optimum conditions. They should be kept in a cool, dry place and be protected from heat, moisture and physical damage. Some laboratories may elect to 'reseal' paraffin blocks prior to archiving in order to safeguard against potential tissue damage. The block face is dipped into a shallow depth of molten wax and allowed to set as can be seen in Figure 2.15 showing a thin film of wax covering the surface. This wax seal prevents tissue shrinkage and other deteriorating effects during prolonged storage. Some laboratories pre-cut controls as an efficiency tool, both to reduce the time taken to prepare slides for staining and to get the most out of the control block without having to realign the block to the microtome each time a section is needed. It is worth noting that some studies have found antigenicity in pre-cut control slides to decrease on storage, leading to unreliable results (Bromley et al. 1994; Prioleau and Schnitt 1995). It is thought that sections stored for lengthy periods of time and exposed to air can oxidize and lose antigenicity. It is common practice for research projects to cut all of the sections within a cohort at once and store the slides prior to staining. A recommended protocol in this situation is to hold the slides at 4°C or in frozen storage in order to mitigate lost antigenicity (Engel and Moore 2011).

Pre-analytical: Immunohistochemical Assay

Turning our attention to the actual IHC assay methodology, all of the pre-analytic and analytic factors discussed earlier in this chapter in relation to general histology can now all be considered pre-analytic for IHC. The laboratory may or may not have input to how the tissue is sampled, the fixation and processing regime, exposure to decalcification reagents and tissue sectioning.

Glass Slides

In addition, the quality of the microscope slide for IHC purposes is as important as the antibody clones. They must be clean, stored per manufacturer's recommendations and purchased from a reputable vendor. Slides for IHC needs to be 'sticky' in order to help the tissue section adhere to the glass slide during high-temperature epitope retrieval. The main method to infer the necessary adhesive property to microscope slides is to coat them with a suitable reagent producing electrostatically charged surfaces.

Historically laboratories would make 'silanized' slides using 3-aminopropyltriethoxysilane in house but this practice has largely been abandoned due to health and safety concerns. It is more feasible to purchase commercially available 'SuperFrost Plus' or 'Matsunami' slides for IHC. The type preferred would also be treated for hydrophilic properties in order to aid the spread of reagents over the entire glass surface.

Pre-cut Controls

For efficiency gains, standard practice for most laboratories is to prepare slides complete with control section prior to sectioning the test section. The custom of using pre-cut controls can be contentious as some practitioners believe cutting fresh controls matches the fresh test section prepared for IHC, making the assay results more robust since this pre-analytic condition is identical for both control and test tissue. Others question the merit of this logic as they point to the possibility of a mismatch in fixation and processing of control tissue and test tissue anyway. Take, for example, the fixation parameters of control tissue obtained from post-mortem procedures and how vastly different it would be when compared to a simple excision.

Real-world experience suggests most pre-cut controls used on a daily basis seem adequate for diagnostic IHC. The more appropriate question, however, is the age of these pre-cut controls and the limit to their viability. Similar to how some antibodies are not affected by decalcification while others are, the same rationale can be applied to pre-cut controls. The IHC laboratory quickly works out the threshold of each antibody and puts in place a suitable strategy. Laboratories keen to bring in a form of 'standardization' may impose a set timeline in which pre-cuts are used. A recommendation of two weeks is quite acceptable whilst stipulating minimal exposure to light is common practice.

Analytical: Immunohistochemical Assay

The analytical variables from the viewpoint of an IHC assay involve the protocol and directly include the baking and dewaxing steps, instrument platform, pretreatments for epitope retrieval, antibody preparation, incubation times and temperatures, type of detection method and chromogen development as well as counterstain. Notable consideration must also be paid to the competency of the testing personnel (Lin and Chen 2014). Common errors attributed to assays developed 'in house', otherwise known as laboratory-developed tests, are variations associated with the staining protocol and cannot be traced back to a 'standard' that causes irregularities (Bogen 2019).

Unlike pre-analytic factors which the IHC facility may or may not control, analytical factors pertaining to the IHC assay can be modified and controlled within the IHC laboratory. Much of the downfall with IHC is that many proponents believe that the ability to control analytic variables and to change parameters as the need arises is all that is required for high-quality IHC staining. This is a fallacy because it is also equally important to have controlled and standardized pre-analytic parameters for consistent results. Regardless, the important analytical parameters critical for successful IHC are now highlighted.

Pretreatment

Often referred to as epitope or antigen retrieval, various pretreatment strategies are available. The two main methods are via heat energy or enzyme digestion. Heat-induced epitope retrieval (HIER) can be achieved with water baths, microwave irradiation, pressure cookers, heating pads or on board a fully automated IHC stainer. Common proteolytic enzymes include Proteinase K, Pronase, Pepsin and Trypsin. It is also possible to combine HIER and enzymes if required. Under- and over-retrieval significantly affect IHC quality. The challenge is therefore finding the optimal epitope retrieval settings for each individual antibody.

Heat-Induced Epitope Retrieval

A number of methods can assist in unmasking epitopes within tissue sections. Back in the early 1990s, Shi and colleagues (1991) discovered enhanced IHC staining by using HIER. Before the advent of HIER, a large number of tissue epitopes could not be demonstrated with FFPE. The group showed that by using microwave irradiation to heat solutions (containing metal) up to 100°C, there was a significant change in the ability to demonstrate IHC staining in FFPE tissue. In addition, enzyme digestion of tissue could be omitted and antibody titres could be increased in some instances. Overall, antibodies previously unreactive with FFPE tissues now showed excellent staining with HIER.

Yamashita and Okada (2005) demonstrated antigen retrieval performed at pH9 afforded a much stronger IHC staining than those sections treated with solutions at pH6. They postulated that the main mechanism of HIER is the disruption of the cross links and that optimal pH level is an essential factor for appropriate refolding of epitopes – and therefore makes them detectable with antibodies. Figure 2.16 shows formaldehyde action altering the protein structure and the hypothesized return to structure following HIER, allowing IHC antibodies to bind.

Kakimoto and colleagues (2008) also proposed that the need for HIER depends on the location of the epitope. Figure 2.17 shows two clones of oestrogen receptor. The MC-20 clone recognizes the antigen located on the surface and is relatively unhindered by the protein cross links. The 6F11 clone, however, recognizes the epitope which is located deep inside the molecule. As heat is applied, the unravelling exposes binding sites to 6F11 clone for IHC detection. The MC-20 clone is able to bind to epitopes with or without HIER because of its surface position.

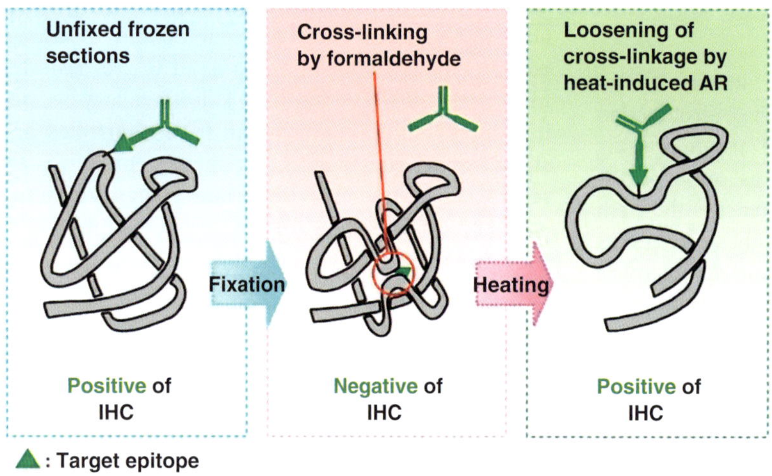

Figure 2.16 Formalin fixation masks epitopes within tissue (Kakimoto et al. 2008).

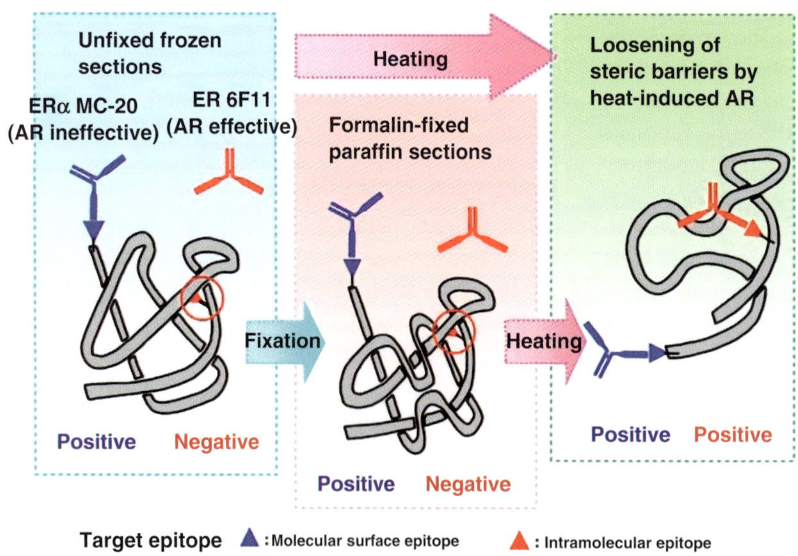

Figure 2.17 Epitopes are affected by formaldehyde fixation due to location (Kakimoto et al. 2008).

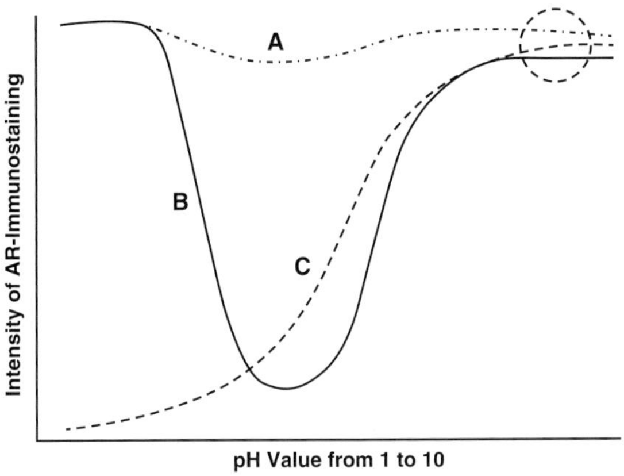

Figure 2.18 Intensity of staining versus pH (Shi et al. 1995)

If pretreatment is determined necessary to 'retrieve antigens', its effectiveness is dependent on several key elements:

- The pH of the retrieval solution.
- Maximum temperature achieved during incubation.
- Time period of the sustained heat temperature.
- Nature of retrieval buffers (EDTA, Citrate, Tris etc.).

Shi and colleagues (1995) studied the effects of various pH solutions on the intensity of IHC staining achieved. The group published a chart showing the intensity of staining on three different antibodies with varied pH levels (reproduced in Figure 2.18). Note all three antibodies have relatively high staining intensity when the retrieval buffer is at around the pH9–pH10 level. There were vastly different staining results at pH levels below this.

Leong and colleagues (2002) also described the use of high temperatures to assist with antigen unmasking. The group used different temperatures to retrieve tissue antigenicity and the most consistent success was obtained at 98°C via pressure cooker. It is also worth noting that some antibodies, whilst preferring HIER, do so at a lower temperature (Shi et al. 2002). In reality, no set pretreatment parameters will work for all the antibodies available. The astute immunohistochemist can find the best set of retrieval conditions for each antibody so high-quality staining can be achieved consistently. In terms of selecting the correct pretreatment parameters in which to perform HIER, the recommended strategy is trial and error via a 'test battery' approach. Different antigens require different conditions for retrieval (Shi et al. 1997).

Common examples of retrieval solutions include:

- 0.01 M citrate buffer pH6
- 0.01 M PBS buffer pH7
- 0.05 M EDTA pH8
- 0.05 M Tris-EDTA pH9
- 0.05 M Tris-HCl (pH1 – pH12)

Proteolytic Enzymes

The goal of using enzymatic digestion as a pretreatment method in IHC is to break the covalent cross links within tissue as a result of formalin fixation. Proteolytic enzymes act by cutting and cleaving amino acid sequences within peptide chains. This has the intended consequence of improving reagent penetration into tissue and also restoring the epitopes of interest for antibody binding. Proteolytic-induced epitope retrieval (PIER) can be achieved with protease, proteinase K, trypsin or pepsin, as highlighted in Table 2.2. Other enzymes such as chymotrypsin and pronase have also been employed to restore immunoreactivity to tissue antigens with varying degrees of success. These enzymes may also inadvertently destroy epitopes and tissue morphology. The laboratory must optimize enzyme concentration and duration of digestion so adverse effects do not occur in the tissues. Ramos-Vara and Beissenherz (2000) noticed cytokeratins tend to prefer enzyme digestion pretreatment in most instances. The PIER can be a suitable alternative to difficult epitopes sensitive to heat energy. An analogy often cited is that epitope retrieval is similar to a tangled ball of thread. To untangle and expose the epitopes trapped within, 'physical' heat energy (HIER) can be used or precise 'scissor cuts' (PIER) can be applied.

Combination of Heat-Induced Epitope Retrieval and Proteolytic-Induced Epitope Retrieval

In some instances a suitable approach to unmask antigens is to use a combination of enzyme and HIER. Some antibodies, whilst staining adequately with one method, can show enhanced intensity when both methods are combined (Singh and Sood 2017). This combined method is especially useful when performing double or triple labelling of two or more antigens simultaneously. However, care should be taken when using two retrieval methods as it may cause an erroneous result manifesting in a false negative or false positive staining in one of the two antibodies or cause a tissue section to detach from the slide after a long retrieval process.

Table 2.2 Common digestion enzymes for PIER (Jackson and Blythe 2008; Agilent 2021)

Enzyme	Working concentration	Buffer	Digestion condition
Trypsin	0.05% to 0.1%	0.1% Calcium chloride adjust to pH 7.8 with 0.1 M NaOH	37°C (10 min–40 min)
Protease	0.1% (Sigma type XXIV)	Distilled water adjust to pH 7.8 with 1 M NaOH	37°C (5 min–10 min)
Proteinase K (Dako)	Ready to use reagent	0.05 M Tris/HCl at pH 7.5	ambient room temp (5 min–20 min)
Pepsin	0.4%	0.01 M Hydrochloric acid. Optimal activity at pH 2	37°C (30 min–180 min)

Note: Parameters such as concentration, temperature and incubation period are indicative only and these settings must be determined via an optimization process.

Automation

Common types of available IHC automation platforms are investigated in Chapters 3, 4 and 5 of this book. It is important when deciding to employ automation for IHC that the needs of the department are taken into consideration. The technologies used for retrieval, reagent delivery and ability to edit protocols should all be accounted for. The decision to purchase an IHC instrument needs to be driven by questions relating to capacity, quality and consistency of the stains, performance in external QAP proficiency testing, turnaround time, reagent use, waste disposal, ability to run multiplex or *in situ* hybridization techniques and integration into laboratory information systems (LIS) as applicable. High-quality applications specialists and troubleshooting services from the vendor are invaluable to the IHC laboratory. The manufacturer's knowledge of the machine, expertise and support are all requirements for a successful IHC service. The instrument should also exhibit a high degree of 'user friendliness' so laboratory staff are comfortable working with it. The cost for this implementation is also very important with business plans showing how the instrumentation will provide high-quality outcomes to patients compared to the current methods often required.

Antibody

Antibody choice or, more precisely, the selection of a specific clone requires careful thought before implementing it into a laboratory's repertoire. A request for a new antibody is usually at the discretion of the pathologists within the department. It is wise to determine if the new antibody will be used enough to warrant it being included in the service or if it would be more cost-effective to request a referral to another department for staining. Once a decision is made to incorporate new antibodies into the laboratory's repertoire, decisions are made whether to select concentrates or ready-to-use (pre-diluted) antibodies, monoclonal or polyclonal varieties and the animal the antibody is derived from. These are some of the factors lab clinicians should consider before implementing a new antibody into the service.

Validation and Verification

These two terms are very similar and are often used interchangeably. Strictly speaking, there is a point of difference. The discussion and explanation given here lies within the context of anatomical pathology and may differ slightly for other disciplines such as biochemistry and haematology. Pertinent to histopathology and especially to IHC testing is the concept of validation and verification of 'subjective methods'. These are procedures where the results are based on interpretive decisions or a degree of subjectivity. For example, microscopic identifications of tissue morphology come under the auspice of being a subjective method. 'A subjective test method is one where the experience and expertise of the analyst(s) or examiner(s) is a significant determinant on whether or not samples or test items are said to meet certain criteria' (NATA 2018).

With this in mind, the term 'validation' in the context of IHC occurs with all new antibodies and must be performed before its use in patient testing (NATA 2019). Antibodies used for patient treatment management are validated in accordance with published guidelines. The testing facility offering the IHC assay must always place the antibody through a validation process. A pertinent question here is 'what constitutes a validation process?'

Initial validation of a new antibody should be performed in accordance with the laboratory's local quality management protocols. Some laboratories specify a minimum number of cases to be used. NATA recommends a minimum of seven samples to compare and familiarize the antibody performance. A representative cohort should include negative and positive cases of differing intensities (low expressors and high expressors), all of which can be externally verified by a reference laboratory. Quality of staining is assessed via review of internal and external tissue controls. Tissues (both control and test) selected for validation with the new antibody should be processed in the same manner regarding fixation and tissue-processing schedules. The importance of standardization procedures of these pre-analytic variables has been discussed previously. Likewise, if the antibody is to be used to demonstrate staining in cytology specimens, the method for validation should include samples prepared in the same way as potential patient samples. For example, if cytology samples are routinely fixed in methanol, 95% ethanol or processed as cell blocks, these are the same conditions the antibody should be tested in. A similar approach is required if decalcified tissues are used. Regular external proficiency testing should be performed in order to ensure accurate testing and interpretation.

Validation parameters which should be considered are:

- Precision and accuracy.
- Repeatability/reproducibility. Evidence of repeatability could include:
  - The level of agreement between two different analysts or examiners who have assessed the same evidence of performance for a particular method (i.e. inter-analyst or examiner reliability).
  - The level of agreement of the same analyst or examiner who has assessed the same evidence of performance but at different times (i.e. intra-analyst or examiner reliability).
- Probability of detection and/or potential error rate. This is the likelihood that a test methodology will correctly identify the measurand. It is often determined through proficiency testing studies.
- Critical (or risk) analysis. This includes identification of possible sources of errors and process variations. Once the sources are identified, their impact on the process needs to be evaluated.
- Collaborative exercises such as inter- and intra-laboratory comparison testing.
- Quality control: Test methods should include procedures for the inclusion of negative and positive controls whenever possible.
- Competency levels of staff involved. The expertise of the analyst is a vital component. Therefore validation must depend to a large extent on testing the expertise of the worker. Ongoing verification of competency is needed.
- Level of acceptance of test method. Considerations might include whether the technique has been subject to peer review and published in a recognized journal. Has the technique been generally accepted within the relevant scientific community?

Note that not all parameters need to be assessed for all methods. The validation method should ensure the method is sound and will provide the outcome necessary for the need of the test.

If for any reason the reagents involved in the testing regime change – for instance, antigen retrieval solutions, detection systems or tissue processing instrumentation – a revalidation process must be performed so as to ensure the quality of the IHC is not impacted. All of the validation testing must be documented in accordance with NATA accreditation requirements. 'It is the responsibility of the facility to choose the validation or verification procedure and protocol most suitable for the desired outcome. However, it is important to remember that the main objective of validation or verification of any testing method is to demonstrate that the method is suitable for its intended purpose' (NATA 2018).

The technical circular continues:

> Facilities need to keep comprehensive records of method validation, including the procedures used for validation, the results obtained and a statement as to whether the method is fit for purpose. Facilities must also continually check that a method of analysis meets the values for the performance characteristics documented in connection with validation. This can be achieved by for example tracking the behaviour of internal quality control samples over time. Should the method no longer produce results consistent with the original validation data, the method may be rendered unfit for its intended purpose.

'Verification', on the other hand, is a term often related to manufacturers of antibodies and the way they market a particular clone for an intended use under specific conditions. Take, for example, Roche Ventana's PDL1 SP263 clone. The intended use of this clone is for the workup of PDL1 status in patients with non-small cell lung carcinoma (NSCLC) on the BenchMark ULTRA IHC platform. The manufacturer (Roche) still must do all of the necessary validation processes for the PDL1 clone SP263 before approving it to be specifically used for NSCLC. By offering the antibody as an RTU, Ventana has also 'locked' the protocol to make it an *in vitro* diagnostic (IVD) product. In doing so, Roche has 'validated' this product for only a specific set of conditions. The laboratory (end user) then proceeds the verification process on its own control tissue. Testing the antibody through this verification process is likened to a somewhat limited validation process, (remember the protocol is locked by the manufacturer) and the primary purpose is to ascertain if the antibody is fit for purpose because pre-analytic variables may affect the performance of the antibody.

On the other hand, if the laboratory purchases a PDL1 concentrate to be diluted and used, the testing laboratory becomes the 'manufacturer' of this in-house IVD assay and the antibody must undergo full validation. In this context, the difference between validation and verification is that manufacturers validate whereas end users verify.

Antibody suppliers such as Roche have zero input in how the in-house control or test tissue is fixed and processed. In fact, the expectation from commercial vendors is that each laboratory conforms to a 'standard' in that the tissue is not under-fixed or subjected to a lengthy cold ischaemic time. In the context of IHC testing, it is understood that any deviation from the suggested parameters outlined by the manufacturer as supplied in the package insert renders the IHC assay an 'in-house IVD' test.

Choosing an Antibody

In an ideal world, possessing several different IHC platforms from different vendors would give the IHC facility freedom to select the proven best-performing antibodies and implementing them into their service. Unfortunately, not all laboratories have this luxury (apart from large reference IHC facilities) and realistically most laboratories would have just the one IHC platform.

A good starting point for selecting a new antibody clone is to research previous external QA results from organizations such as NordiQC, UKNEQAS, RCPA QAP and IQPATH. Although it is not an exhaustive list, the best-performing clones, protocols and controls are highlighted for each vendor's IHC platforms. The free information is authored by reputable and highly regarded IHC professionals and is also a great resource for teaching and training.

Another consideration is whether to use an antibody in concentrate form or ready to use (RTU). This is largely dependent on the budget of the laboratory and how much flexibility the department requires. Concentrates can be cost-effective for high-use antibodies. However, if used at very low dilutions such as 1:5 or 1:10 ratios, concentrates can become a very expensive exercise. As laboratories become busier, efficiencies must be made and diluting out antibodies can be time-consuming for scientists (with increasing documentation requirements) and an opportunity for human error (diluting incorrect antibodies). These risks can be mitigated by using RTU products, but they can be expensive per test and lack flexibility. However, their 'plug and play' nature offers maximum efficiency and convenience. An added bonus is the tedious record-keeping which is no longer required as all information is controlled on board the instrument for accreditation purposes. Beware that some RTU antibodies can perform poorly despite being run to the exact conditions found in the package inserts, evidence perhaps of a difference in pre-analytic conditions tuned for by the vendor due to a lack of required pre-analytic standardizations.

Storage Considerations

The accepted convention is to store antibodies at 4°C when not in use. Some workers advocate the practice of aliquoting out concentrates and storing them frozen. Others elect to mix aliquots of the antibody with glycerine, which prevents the formation of ice crystals during storage, to greatly extend the shelf life of the antibody. However, it is important to record expiry date and lot numbers related to the aliquots. Compliance with the manufacturer expiry date is compulsory on automation platforms. These machines will not allow the use of expired reagents in IHC assays. Manually, the reagents are carefully monitored for fluctuations in their performance from the staining results and appropriate action is taken when staining falls out of the expected QC. Storage of aliquots in frost-free freezers should be avoided as the regular freeze-thaw cycles can damage the antibodies and affect their performance in patient testing (Sanderson and Zardin 2013).

Monitoring Performance

Managing stock levels and avoiding the use of expired antibodies can be difficult. The importance of same-slide controls for immunohistochemical critical assay performance controls (ICAPCs) enables the laboratory to validate each IHC slide and verifies that the staining criteria are met. As each slide undergoes QC after staining, it is relatively simple to observe shifts in IHC assay behaviour. A trend of decreasing stain intensity or a pattern of erratic results requires investigation. Appendix 1 highlights common IHC staining scenarios and their possible remedies.

Detection

The visual end product of routine IHC is determined by the use of a detection system. The vast majority of routine IHC antigen expression is visualized chromogenically by converting a substrate into an insoluble end product at the site of the antigen–antibody binding. An antibody can be directly labelled and visualized; however, using an indirect method increases the sensitivity and amplifies the signal so that minute levels of antigen expression can easily be demonstrated.

The most common substrate used is 3,3'diaminobenzidine (DAB), which is converted to a brown insoluble product with the enzyme horseradish peroxidase (HRP) in the presence of substrate hydrogen peroxide (H_2O_2). Diaminobenzidene is the most common chromogen used because it is insoluble in alcohol and xylene and does not fade with sunlight. Double staining is made possible by using a secondary detection system with a contrasting colour such as red.

A limitation of chromogenic IHC is multiplexing. Dual and triple staining are commonly used in routine IHC applications using two chromogens with two or three antibodies respectively. Target co-localization is not possible due to dual signals blending together, making interpretation difficult. Targeting the nucleus and cell membrane with one chromogen and the cytoplasm with another chromogen is extremely useful for multiplexing on tiny core biopsies with limited tumour or on prostate core biopsies using the PIN4 cocktail.

For routine applications, the benefits of chromogenic detection far outweigh the pitfalls. They offer the ability to visualize by routine light microscopy and the slides can be permanently stored and reliably work with routine FFPE tissue.

Detection systems are available from numerous vendors; however, choice is mainly dictated by the IHC platform used and budget constraints. Note some diagnostic IHC platforms have limited utility in research applications because the detection systems are designed for human samples with mouse or rabbit antibodies. Vendors do cater to research applications with specific automation models that aren't as 'closed' as the diagnostic versions and the availability of specifically designed kits for these purposes. There is no flexibility with research detection systems for handling xenograft tissues, though.

Early-generation detection systems used avidin biotin complexes (ABC) before polymer- and biotin-free detection systems were introduced. Figures 2.19 and 2.20 replicate the schematics of the IHC assays based on avidin biotin complex and polymer technology as seen in Figures 1.16 and 1.19. The current-generation detection systems have replaced the avidin biotin molecules and replaced them with polymer technology. These systems are highly sensitive and specific, not prone to non-specific background staining, and have crisp, strong, intense staining with the addition of proprietary enhancers as part of the kit. A variation on the polymer theme is the use of haptens to intensify the signal demonstrated in Figure 2.21.

Counterstaining after detection gives contrast to the IHC signal. Haematoxylin is most commonly used

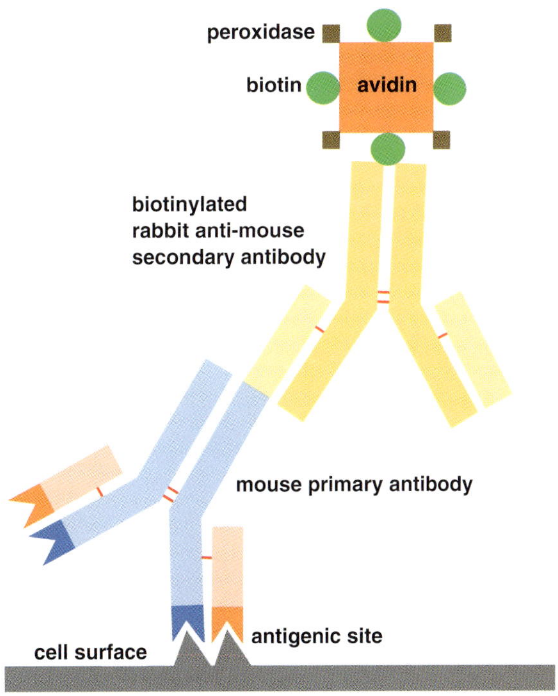

Figure 2.19 Avidin biotin complex immunohistochemical method

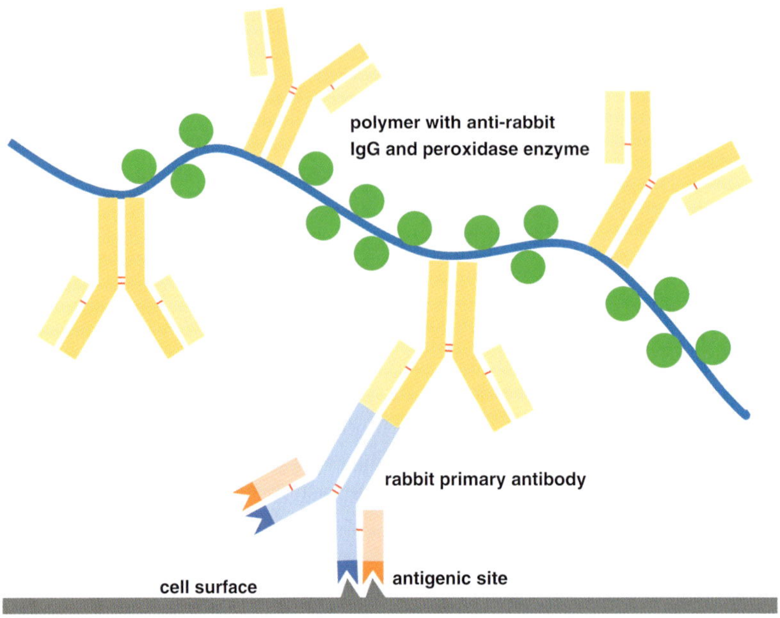

Figure 2.20 Polymer with enzyme molecules attached along with multiple secondary antibodies

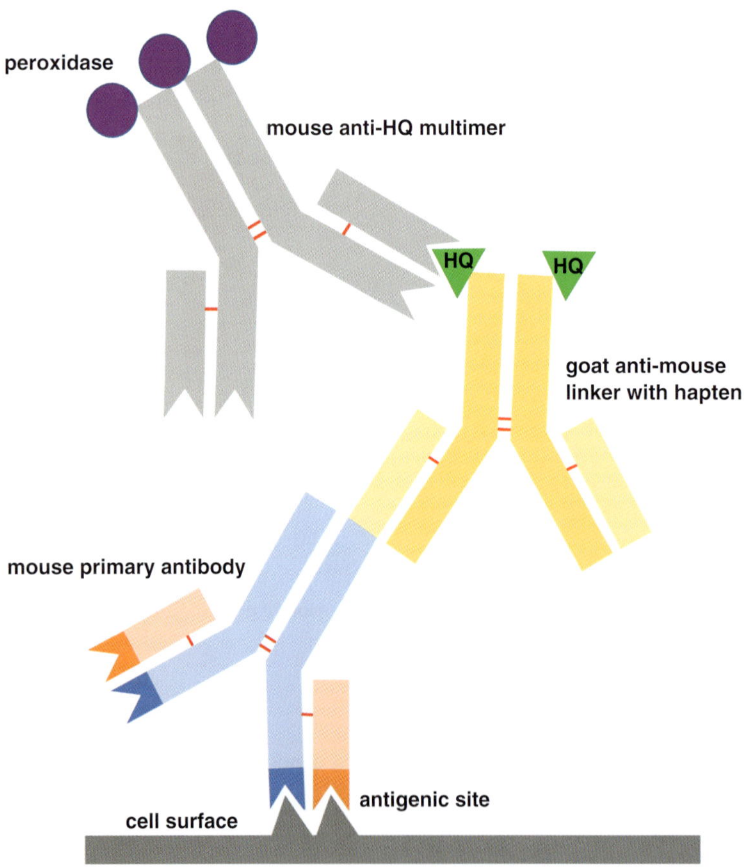

Figure 2.21 Diaminobenzidene detection using high-quality haptens linked to a secondary antibody

for DAB chromogenic IHC. The intensity of the counterstain must be controlled so as to ensure it is balanced without being so intense that it masks the signal or is so weak that the blue colour can barely be discerned. Counterstaining can be performed on board the staining platform or off board. The choice is dependent on budget and laboratory preference.

If an alcohol-soluble chromogen has been used, slides must not be dehydrated in alcohol as the IHC stain will be lost. The DAB reaction is alcohol and xylene resistant and can therefore be routinely dehydrated, cleared and mounted with a coverslip. Double-stained chromogenically developed IHC slides must be air dried before being cleared in xylene and coverslipped if one or both chromogens are alcohol fast. Lastly, it is important to check if the mounting media is compatible with the detection system as some may cause fading.

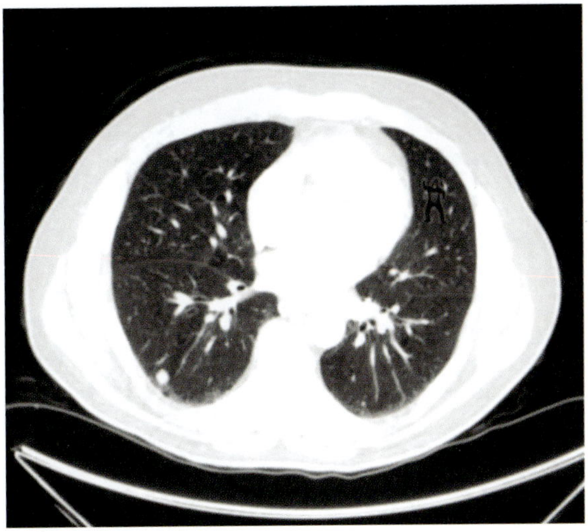

Figure 2.22 The invisible gorilla (Drew et al. 2013)

Post-analytical: Immunohistochemical Assay

Referring back to Figure 2.8 of the flow chart, the post-analytic phase predominantly consists of the interpretation of the IHC results and formulation of a report and findings. Laboratory technical staff should not consider these tasks solely for the pathologist. In fact, it is necessary for the laboratory worker to scrutinize every IHC stain produced by the facility before the slides are given to the pathologist for reporting.

Immunohistochemical Interpretation

In order to interpret staining results, the technical staff providing assurance for the IHC assay having passed QC and the pathologist offering a diagnosis must be trained to understand the staining characteristics for the IHC marker of interest. For instance, inspecting a TTF-1 IHC stain and observing cytoplasmic staining instead of the expected nuclear labelling from this antibody should trigger warnings that require further investigating. Likewise, observing lymphocyte staining for a CK20 IHC marker may mean that the CD20 antibody may have been mistakenly used.

Another advantage of inspecting every IHC slide produced is it affords the facility to closely monitor antibody performance. A 'drift' in staining characteristics can be identified and dealt with swiftly by close examination of the tissue controls. As the same tissue controls are used repeatedly for each antibody, they become a surrogate standard to which subsequent staining can be compared. For example, take an antibody such as E-Cadherin. If there is any doubt of its performance today, than a slide stained last week can be retrieved and compared if the same control tissue was used from the same FFPE block for both slides.

Mandating both technical staff and pathologist to analyse every IHC stained slide is good laboratory practice. In much the same way as radiologists can miss dancing gorillas 'hidden' in MRIs as illustrated in Figure 2.22 (look towards the top right corner of image), pathologists may also miss key criteria in stained slides even though they have undergone many years of training to diagnose cancer and disease.

The training in their registrar years and into their consultant years requires attendance at conferences and applying their knowledge at various continuing education programmes throughout the year. Interestingly, a study has shown that pigeons can diagnose breast cancer too (see Figure 2.23 (Levenson et al. 2015)). In other studies, it is also worth noting that diagnoses were overlooked by pathologists working in laboratories which did not routinely see certain conditions (Evans et al. 2013).

Internal QA programmes, peer reviews and multi-header sessions with difficult and complex cases are all important aspects of routine learning. Participation in external QA programmes also assists with learning opportunities and helps to cement diagnostic criteria. External opinions from experts can also help to support a diagnosis in instances where a consensus

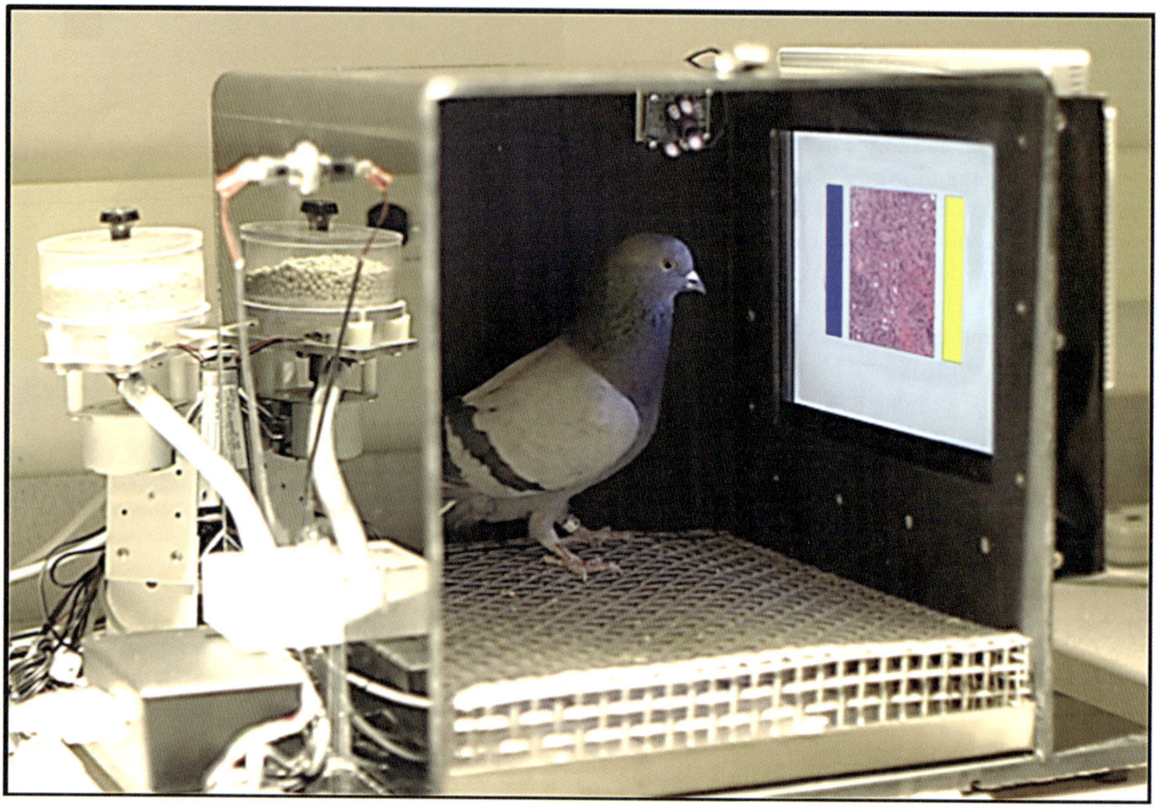

Figure 2.23 Pigeon selecting images showing breast cancer (Levenson et al. 2015)

cannot be reached. However, pathologists also understand the value of a good IHC stain and the effects pre-analytical, analytical and post-analytical variables can all have on interpreting a stained slide (Gown 2016). Another tool at the pathologist's disposal is image analysis. Technologies such as artificial intelligence and whole-slide scanning can assist in a variety of ways such as provision of cell counts for Ki67 staining. They may also be employed to assist in the assessment of intensity and percentage of staining as in ER and PR cell counts.

Report Generation

Reporting of IHC assays can take many forms. The result may include a mention of positive versus negative stain such as S-100 positive or HMB45 negative. Another aspect of reporting may be descriptive of the intensity and amount of staining within a certain cellular population, as per the RCPA breast synoptic reports highlighted in Figure 2.24. It is at the pathologist's discretion whether the IHC results are mentioned in the final pathology report. Certainly the companion diagnostic markers and antibodies which offer certain treatment regimens such as ER, PR, Her2 and Ki67 should be incorporated. Likewise semi-quantitative scores should be included.

Controls

In a similar vein to scientific experimentation in general, IHC controls are employed in order to validate results obtained from such experiments. These controls and in particular, their quality and consistency have become an important facet of IHC specifically with the emergence of theranostic IHC markers whereby patient treatment is based on the IHC results because other confirmatory tests are not available or not used. A case in point is the PDL1 IHC assay for non-small cell lung carcinoma. A positive PDL1 IHC result directs the patient to monoclonal antibody therapy. Controls used in IHC ensure we are comparing 'apples with apples'. A significant contributor to QA measures, controls can be classified

Ancillary test findings

S4.01 Oestrogen receptors

- [ ] Not performed
- [ ] Pending
- [x] Performed

Percentage of nuclei staining

90 % to 95 %

Predominant staining intensity

- [ ] 1+ Low
- [ ] 2+ Intermediate
- [x] 3+ High

ER result

- [ ] Negative
- [x] Positive

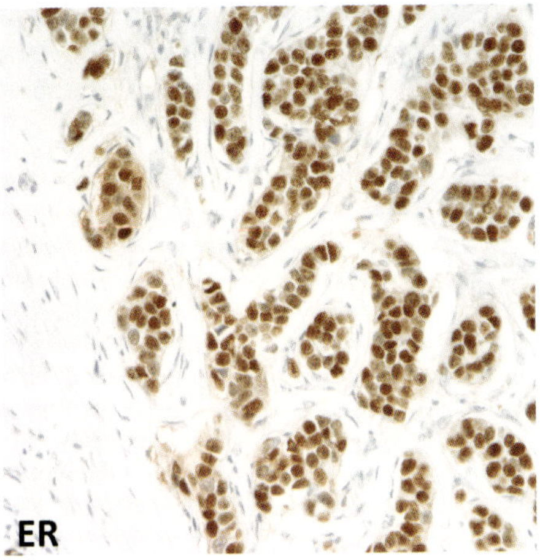

Progesterone receptors

- [ ] Not performed
- [ ] Pending
- [x] Performed

Percentage of nuclei staining

90 % to 95 %

If >0 record:

Predominant staining intensity

- [ ] 1+ Low
- [ ] 2+ Intermediate
- [x] 3+ High

PR result

- [ ] Negative
- [x] Positive

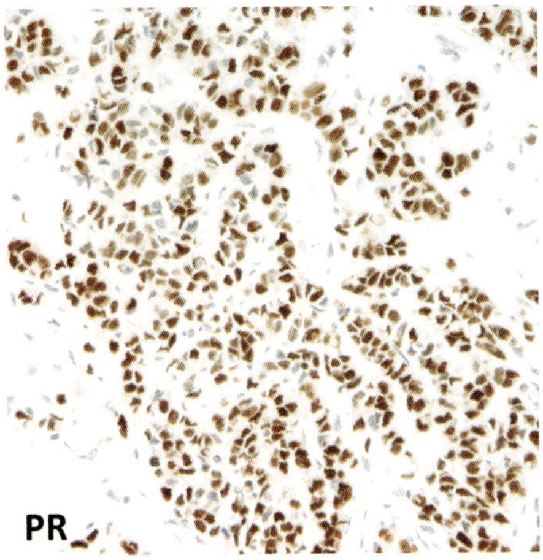

S4.03 Her2 (ISH)

- [ ] Not performed
- [x] Pending
- [ ] Performed

Number of copies of Her2

Number of copies of CEP17

- [ ] Not assessed OR

Her2 Result

- [ ] Amplified
- [ ] Non-amplified diploid
- [ ] Non-amplified polysomic
- [ ] Indeterminate

Her2 IHC (if performed)

- [ ] 0
- [ ] 1+
- [ ] 2+
- [x] 3+
- [ ] Not performed

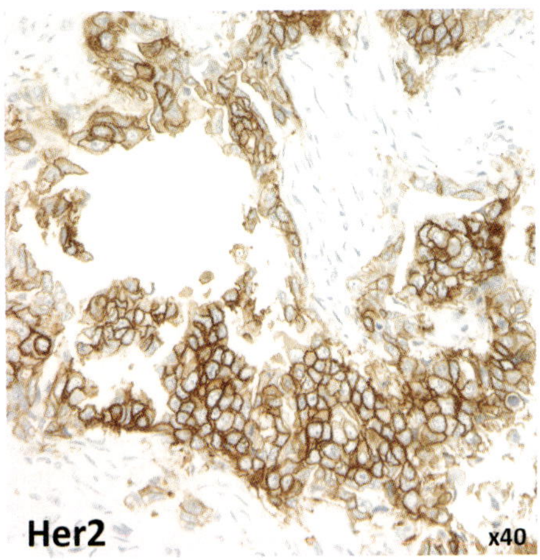

Figure 2.24 An example of a breast synoptic report (RCPA 2019)

into internal and external categories. Nominated as internal are all QC activities the laboratory conducts within the IHC facility without outside influences. External QC are events originating from outside the organization which contribute to the IHC facility's QA programme.

Internal Quality Control

There are many facets to a facility's internal QC endeavours. Some directly involve the IHC assay itself while others incorporate a laboratory-wide approach. Listed next is a summary of the challenges a diagnostic IHC facility must meet and overcome.

Tissue Controls

Employing tissue controls for IHC means selecting specific tissue to stain in parallel with patient test tissue. These controls may or may not contain the epitope to which the antibody is matched. For example, a suitable tissue control for TTF-1 is one that harbours a lung adenocarcinoma. Interestingly, not many laboratories would use thyroid tissue (it is a thyroid transcription factor after all) because most clinical applications of TTF-1 would be ascertaining if a tumour originated in the lung. Tissue controls determine whether the IHC stain is valid. Utilizing these controls and effectively managing their logistics is crucial for a reliable IHC service and a feat that may prove quite challenging. Every control block with its individual components should be traceable back to the original specimen. In other words, the IHC facility knows exactly the nature and origin of the control tissues being used to validate each IHC stain. Another important concept with using tissue controls is that they should be fixed and processed with the same conditions as the 'test' or patient surgical specimens. This will ensure the results are directly comparable.

Excess or surplus tissue sourced after report authorization is a useful means to bank tissue for control use. This practice is commonplace and accepted as standard practice. Unfortunately, there are various reasons not every specimen can be harvested for controls. The tissue or lesion may have been processed in its entirety, the sample may have been stored for an extended period of time in formalin or the tissue sample is too small to harvest as a control block.

Another valuable source of control tissue is the actual test FFPE block. With permission obtained from the reporting pathologist, samples can be taken from archived blocks. The benefit of standard fixation and processing attributed to these FFPE blocks cannot be overstated, but the material may be thin due to the block being subjected to trimming for routine H&E sections and perhaps multiple IHC markers. The RCH Melbourne IHC facility employs both methods for control tissue harvest. For example, when collecting HER2 breast samples from surplus tissue, 3+ and 1+ tumours are easier to find than the 2+ variety. In this instance, 2+ cases are located from the archives and permission sought from the reporting pathologist to effectively 'sacrifice' the original FFPE block.

Identifying potential control tissue is best achieved during the quality check of each IHC slide. When a large lesion with good morphology and appropriate staining is seen, the reporting pathologist can be notified for permission to harvest the excess lesion within the original tissue sample when they are satisfied that additional sampling is not required.

Multi-block controls are versatile and can cover a large proportion of the laboratory's antibody repertoire. Ideally, all of the components of multi-block controls should be sourced in house in order to ensure fixation and processing is kept consistent. If possible, use normal tissue to ensure consistent staining because tumour material may have inherent heterogeneous and inconsistent staining intensities. Some facilities employ tissue cores as a 'mini tissue micro array' for their multi-block controls. Observed as small circles on the slide, these can be arranged very close to each other so that a dozen cores can be easily created in one tissue control block. The construction of such blocks can be onerous if they are made manually. The tissue core selected may only contain necrotic debris which is useless for control material. There is potential for wastage especially if the tumour selected as a control is heterogeneous or if the selected cores are at different depths within the block as shallow cores will be exhausted first. Regardless, all tissue blocks made for IHC control purposes need to be tested and validated as fit for purpose before use in diagnostic testing capacities.

'Same-slide controls' should be standard practice so as to ensure every slide is validated before being issued to the pathologist. This is important even when the test tissue contains internal positive elements. For consistency in QA, observing the same tissue control every time an antibody is used is the best way to judge if the IHC assay is performing optimally. There is no other way to guarantee the process has worked as each slide run on an automated IHC platform is its own reaction. Modern IHC instruments run slides individually, so essentially every slide is its own reaction and must have its own control (Torlakovic et al. 2015).

Dynamic Range Controls

Dynamic range controls should be used where a range or intensity level is being assessed such as Her2 status in breast or gastric cancer. ER, PR and PDL-1 are other notable examples of antibodies which benefit from the use of dynamic range controls. It is important to include wherever possible low-level positive tissue elements – often termed 'low expressors' – to help in detecting calibration errors because these are the first to be affected in suboptimally calibrated IHC assays. Ultimately, they prevent laboratories from reporting false negative staining and assist the pathologists in comparing patient tissue staining to verified control tissue.

Table 2.3 shows an example with CD4 and recommends the type of tissue to gauge low expression (LE), high expression (HE) and no expression (NE). Although CD4 antibody is often used for T-cell subset classification, it is also important to observe the weak to moderate expected staining of CD4 for liver sinusoids and germinal centre lymph node macrophages. Using LE controls will highlight errors in protocol performance faster than using HE controls alone. Low-expression controls are incorporated into immunohistochemical critical assay performance controls (ICAPCS) and include, for example, using Kupffer cells in the liver as an LE for leucocyte common antigen, otherwise known as CD45 (Torlakovic et al. 2015). Described by NordiQC, ICAPCS is a system of gold standard controls for individual antibodies that demonstrate NE, LE and HE. The aim is to provide guidance to laboratories to set up, calibrate and monitor protocol performance. Other examples include tonsil as a LE marker for oestrogen receptor and p63 in scattered lymphocytes. Approximately 20 ICAPCS are available and most can be incorporated into a routine diagnostic IHC laboratory's multi-block controls using normal tissue.

Negative Controls

The use of negative controls in routine diagnostic IHC facilities can be contentious. The question often asked is, 'What is the point of a negative control and when are they of use?' The purpose of a negative control is to demonstrate that the IHC reaction observed is due to the interaction of the epitope of the target molecule and nothing else (Hewitt et al. 2014). Negative controls can be in the form of negative tissue controls as well as negative reagent controls (Torlakovic et al. 2014).

Negative tissue controls include tissues known to not contain the epitope of interest. Hence the IHC result will show no staining because the antibody employed for that specific epitope will have nothing to bind to. These negative tissue controls can also be engineered from tissue culture, guaranteeing confidence that the cell lines are known not to exhibit the antigen of interest.

There are two types of negative tissue controls – internal and external. The control is regarded as internal if the control element is a portion of the patient's test sample. It is intrinsic or built in, and it is often used because it exists conveniently within the test tissue. A sound knowledge of histology morphology is required to observe naturally occurring muscle tissue not staining for CD31 as an example. External negative tissue controls are usually found as part of the external (usually on-slide) control, which contains both positive and negative cell types or tissues. These are sections deliberately selected by the laboratory known to show no reaction to the antibody and include using tonsil (lymphoid) tissue for TTF-1 marker as a typical example.

Negative reagent controls are used to validate the specificity of the primary and secondary antibodies. The overall purpose is to show that the antibody–antigen reaction is due to expression of the target of interest. A common 'negative control' many laboratories employ is to stain two slides concurrently, one with the primary antibody and the other slide with the primary antibody omitted. A positive IHC result in the negative control shows the non-specific binding of the antibody (Hewitt et al. 2014). Most workers substitute the antibody with antibody diluent for the negative control slide, but a true negative reagent control is substitution with serum or isotype-specific immunoglobulins from the same animal at the same protein concentration as the primary antibody (Hewitt et al. 2014). This is especially important if the antibody is polyclonal and comes from a non-commercial supplier.

Table 2.3 An example of dynamic range controls. Reproduced with permission Soren Nielsen, director of the Institute of Pathology, Aalborg University Hospital

CD4 (M)	Appendix	Liver	Pancreas	Tonsil
High expression [right antibody]	The majority of T-cells in lamina propria must show a moderate to strong, distinct predominantly membranous staining reaction.	Dispersed T-cells and Kupffer cells must show a moderate to strong, distinct predominantly membranous staining reaction.	Dispersed T-cells must show a moderate to strong, distinct predominantly membranous staining reaction.	The majority of T-cells both in the inter-follicular T-zones and in the germinal centres must show a moderate to strong, distinct, predominantly membranous staining reaction.
Low expression [right sensitivity]	Dispersed intra-epithelial T-cells must show an at least weak to moderate, distinct predominantly membranous staining reaction.	The vast majority of the endothelial cells of the liver sinusoids must show an at least weak to moderate, distinct predominantly membranous staining reaction.	The majority of T-cells in lamina propria must show a moderate to strong, distinct predominantly membranous staining reaction.	The germinal centre macrophages must show an at least weak to moderate predominantly membranous staining reaction.
No expression [right specificity]	No staining reaction must be seen in the columnar epithelial cells.	No staining reaction must be seen in the hepatocytes.	No staining reaction must be seen in the epithelial cells of the exocrine pancreas or the endocrine cells of the islets of Langerhans.	No staining reaction must be seen in the B-cells.

Similar to negative tissue controls, there are also two types of negative reagent controls. The first one is against the primary antibody. For monoclonal antibodies, the primary antibody is replaced by a monoclonal antibody of the same species, isotype and concentration but having no known reactivity against the target tissue. For polyclonal antibodies, the primary antibody is replaced by a dilution of whole normal/non-immune serum of the same animal source at the same immunoglobulin concentration. The other type of negative reagent control is against the detection system when the secondary/linker or labelling antibody (or other component) is replaced by antibody diluent or culture medium (McCoy tissue culture medium is commonly used) or buffer. Torlakovic and colleagues (2014) suggest using serial sections for the omission of each reagent within the protocol with a suitable alternative. For example, to detect unwanted endogenous peroxidase labelling, switch the enzyme to alkaline phosphatase and to detect background biotin, use a polymer detection instead. Negative reagent controls are recommended for laboratories which utilize avidin-biotin detection systems.

Routine use of negative controls, either reagent or tissue based, in diagnostic facilities is commonly not performed. This is standard practice and is mainly due to the additional resources needed for staining extra slides per patient. It is especially relevant for automated instruments where the valuable space is taken by negative slides on the machine. Separate negative reagent controls are recommended when optimizing non-commercial antibodies for research projects and should be employed in these scenarios. Scrutiny of internal negative tissue controls is done to observe evidence of antibody deterioration (increased background) and to ensure correct antibody titration application.

Specific Controls for Specific Situations

In some instances a wide choice is available to select the tissue control for a particular antibody. A good example are the epithelial markers such as CK7. Both breast and lung cancers are expected to display positivity. In other situations, there is a need to have specific controls for a particular antibody. These controls can be employed to show a loss of expression in a certain condition. For example, INI-1 staining loss is indicative of central nervous system atypical teratoid/rhabdoid tumours, renal medullary carcinoma and rhabdoid tumours. In other examples, specific controls are used to prove expression of a particular protein – for example, ROS1 IHC positivity in lung cancers. Manufacturers often specify recommended positive controls to be included in the IHC assay. It is up to the laboratory to act on the advice or find a suitable alternative. For example, at the RCH Melbourne, the recommended tissue control for PD-L1 clone SP263 is placenta, but the pathologists would like something more attune to the tissue types being stained. A good compromise is that both options are endorsed and included as a multi-block control.

Cytology Specimens

Diagnostic laboratories worldwide are commonly asked by pathologists to perform IHC on cytospin or FNA-prepared slides. Practically and theoretically, IHC can be done, but it is important to have appropriate QC and QA measures in place. First, there are sampling issues to contend with. For example, FNA sample preparations are difficult to reproduce on multiple slides. The nature of the sampling method is that if there is a good yield of cells on the first pass, the second pass may not be as fruitful. The sampling is inherently heterogeneous when compared to serial sections of FFPE tissue blocks. This comes into consideration when multiple antibodies are requested on FNA samples. Second, are the existing control measures suitable for confidence and validation of the IHC assay in this situation? Applying the IHC principles strictly discussed thus far, a supply of validated cytology prepared slides, not FFPE tissue, should be the control material used in this instance. Otherwise, a comparison of apples with apples is not achieved and therefore the IHC test is not valid. This is a conundrum because it is difficult to procure and maintain control material for cytology preparations. Ideally, specific cell lines are generated for control material from tissue culture for the antibodies that are to be used for IHC investigations. In a practical and financial sense, this is not feasible.

One method many laboratories employ to overcome this issue and to have the same comparison material for cytology IHC testing is to prepare cell blocks from the cytology sample and process it to paraffin. The cells within the cell block will have been fixed, processed, embedded and sectioned in the same fashion as FFPE control blocks and will also be undergoing the same IHC treatments such as antigen retrieval. Common methods to prepare cell blocks include the use of agar or plasma and thrombin.

Renal Immunohistochemical Controls

Renal IHC controls present another example of a real conundrum in diagnostic IHC. In theory controls for renal IHC should be performed because controls are necessary to validate the IHC, so there should be a consistent approach for IHC staining of renal biopsies. The limitations are the size of the biopsies. They are often thin cores sampled to detect glomerular immune deposits in kidney disease, and using archival tissue from patients as controls is not suitable as the cores will often be cut out of the block very quickly if used for control material. Explant tissues are rarely available to be used as they are processed very differently to core biopsy.

Some sites performing IHC have reported using tonsil tissue for the verification of immune complexes such as IgG, IgM and IgA IHC staining. As renal biopsy tissue is not used as a control, tonsil tissue is seen as a 'surrogate control' showing staining in plasma cells rather than glomerular deposits. The practicalities are questioned further when typical working titres for renal biopsies are in the order of thousands. Dilutions of 1:20,000 are common and there is doubt that at these large working titres there will be any staining in the plasma cells. For demonstration of fibrinogen, C3 c and C1q, finding 'like for like' control material is more difficult. Some sites have reported using archival renal biopsies with noted success. However, this option is rarely available at all sites performing renal IHC.

For these reasons some IHC facilities stain their renal panels with a negative control but no positive controls. When this is the case, renal IHC performance should be carefully monitored in house. Any issues identified by staff or raised by pathologists regarding the performance of renal IHC staining should be investigated by referral of unstained sections to an NATA-accredited laboratory for duplication of staining.

Tissue Control Banks

In this context, a control bank does not mean purposefully harvesting tissue to be stored at −20°C. It's the procurement of surplus FFPE tissue for use as tissue controls for IHC staining after histological analysis has been finalized. In this regard, it is beneficial and common practice for laboratories to assist other laboratories with control material and vice versa. Human tissue cannot be 'bought and sold' as federal law prohibits financial transactions of this nature. Alternatively, human tissue used for control material can be given and received amongst laboratories for the purposes of pathology testing. Under these circumstances, tissue used for control material is exempt by law. The RCPA (2018) states: 'Material may be archived as slides or blocks during diagnosis and therapy for use in research, training or evaluation of medical or laboratory procedures, such as to fulfil laboratory accreditation requirements or to meet laboratory standards.' The tissue shared from an external source should be tested in order to ensure staining criteria is met and traceable back to its original source.

Specialist hospitals are relied upon as a good supply of specific tumour banks. For example, a children's hospital would be the best place to ask for paediatric tumour samples for tissue controls. Likewise, a general hospital would have easy access to organs such as appendixes and tonsils. Laboratories are now closely aligned in their histology fixation and processing protocols that receiving FFPE tissue to be used within a different facility does not pose any problems. The high level of inter-laboratory histology practice standardization achieved, and its importance realized, means the pre-analytic problems of the past do not apply to today's modern IHC method.

Staffing Controls

When the term 'controls in IHC' is mentioned, most workers would go straight to the 'nuts and bolts' of the IHC test such as the reagents, the tissue etc. In fact, there are other controls associated with the IHC test such as staffing controls.

Behind every IHC assay is a laboratory-trained user to 'run' the test. Whether the IHC is manually performed or is automated, consideration needs to be given to operational requirements such as rostering and supervision of the IHC facility. Does the organization have multiple people trained in the technique or is the IHC area operated by a solo person? How are annual and sick leaves covered? How is competency maintained across all trained personnel? These are questions every IHC facility needs to address so as to ensure the outcome of the IHC stain is not biased towards the person performing the test. Although automation and robotics are employed to impose a level of impartiality to the results, ensuring adequate staffing arrangements at all times can be challenging.

Most commonly there is a designated IHC supervisor who is usually a senior scientist to oversee the IHC service of the anatomical pathology department. The logistics of staffing, up-to-date training of staff and adequate leave cover falls within their responsibilities to safeguard the integrity of the IHC so that the situation where 'Hazel's CD3 stain is always better than Bron's' does not occur.

Inventory Controls

Often overlooked but equally important is the ability to effectively manage stock levels. The IHC facility may have the slickest instrumentation on the planet, but if it doesn't manage reagents and consumables appropriately, it's just an expensive waste of space! There must be a robust system of checking the inventory stock levels. Ordering too little and risking running out of reagent before the next delivery is a reality. Ordering too much may risk the reagents expiring before getting a chance to use them. The RCH Melbourne performs a weekly stocktake checking a list of minimum quantities for each item against actual stock counts as can be seen in Figure 2.25. Laboratories may have external staff such as hospital stores personnel to perform regular consumable checks and supply stock as required. Standard practice is to assign a member of staff this logistical responsibility whereby the minimum stock level required for each reagent is known and requisitioned by demand. Another possible strategy is knowing the amount of stock the facility uses per month and placing a standing order for those products.

Items required to be stored in a particular way must be kept according to the manufacturer's instructions. As such, temperature monitoring of freezers and fridges is vital to ensure the optimum operation of the IHC reagents. Most laboratories invest in external alarms or paging systems for temperature failure incidents. Once again standardization is the key to guaranteeing successful IHC. A fridge/freezer failing on the eve of a four-day weekend of 30°C plus will likely affect the IHC staining of patient tissue.

Equipment Controls

Similar to contingency planning for worldwide haematoxylin shortages, there must also be a backup plan for laboratories choosing to use automation technologies. Is there redundancy with multiple machines available to continue staining the same antibody panels?

Product	Minimum quantity	Current stock	Ordered
UltraView DAB detection	1 in use + 1 backup		
OptiView DAB detection	2 in use + 2 backup		
ISH iView detection	1 kit		
OptiView amplification	1 kits		
UltraView amplification	1 kit		
EZ prep	2 bottles		
LCS	9 bottles		
SSC	2 bottles		
Reaction buffer	6 bottles		
CC1	3 bottles		
Ab diluent	>100mLs		
EBAR label kit	1 in use + 1 backup		
ISH protease 3	1 in use + 1 backup		
Protease 1	1 in use + 1 backup		
CA 125	1 in use + 1 backup		
CEA	1 in use + 1 backup		
Cerb-2/Her-2	1 in use + 1 backup		
CK (AE1/3)	1 in use + 1 backup		
CK 7	1 in use + 1 backup		
CK 20	1 in use + 1 backup		

IHC/VENTANA ORDERING CHECKLIST

Figure 2.25 An ordering checklist showing minimum quantities

For laboratories with a single machine in the event of a breakdown, what are the possible outcomes to minimize the impact on IHC services? Some laboratories will temporarily send out their slides for IHC staining to other accredited laboratories. Some will revert to validated manual methods while others will wait for the engineers to fix the issue and accept the delayed turnaround time. It is important that whatever the path chosen, it is documented in the laboratory's quality manual and laboratory contingency plans.

The scenarios outlined previously are all unplanned occurrences. Preventative maintenance, servicing and system upgrades are occasions which can be planned and managed according to the facility's operational requirements. The amount of downtime is usually known and with some careful consideration can be accommodated within the laboratory's schedule without severely impacting the IHC service. Good laboratory practice ensures appropriate documentation and record-keeping of each episode of maintenance and breakdown callouts from the service engineer. The IHC automation platforms today are built with extreme accuracy and calibrated accordingly so that even the smallest instrument errors must be investigated in order to guarantee the integrity of the IHC output.

Intrinsic Tissue Controls

Commonly known as internal tissue controls, many normal tissues contain components which also react when incubated with an antibody of interest. For example, Figure 2.26 shows a melanoma positive with melan A antibody (A). The internal control lies in the natural melanocytes found at the basal layer of the epidermis (arrows). Likewise, TTF-1 antibody stains the lung adenocarcinoma (B) as well as the normal pneumocytes (arrows). Internal positive controls such as these provide evidence that the test tissue was fixed and processed in an adequate manner confirming a valid IHC test (Sanderson and Zardin 2013). The key to developing a successful strategy with internal controls is to have a thorough grounding in normal tissue histology. For example, when investigating for rhabdomyosarcoma and the desmin antibody is employed, zero staining of normal muscle within the section means a failed IHC assay and a remedy is required.

There are occasions when the allocated control for a specific antibody is not used. Most commonly, it is from a mistake made when selecting control tissue for an IHC assay. The conundrum here is the most appropriate course of action for this situation. In some instances, this scenario will imply an automatic repeat of the IHC assay especially for markers such as ER and PR. The reasons are twofold. First, it is difficult to ascertain natural intrinsic positivity in normal tissue with these markers as not all ductal cells are guaranteed to be ER or PR positive. Second, if there are internal positive cells within the ducts, there is no reliable method to differentiate them as ER or PR as both markers display nuclear reactivity. In some cases IHC assays using 'incorrect' control material can still

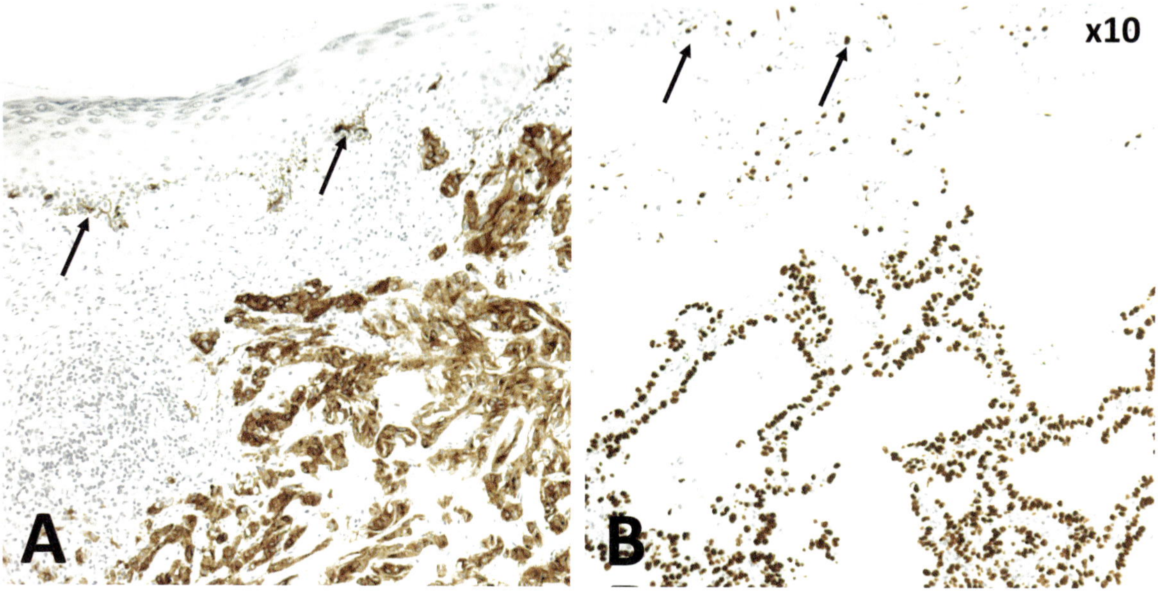

Figure 2.26 Internal controls (arrows) for Melan A in skin (A) and TTF-1 in lung (B)

be valid. Take, for example, a situation where the S100 protein is employed for melanoma studies but lymph node tissue was mistakenly applied as the control tissue. Since the naturally occurring dendritic cells within the lymph node stain positive for S100 and the lymphocytes are negative, the IHC assay can be released for reporting. However, this episode should still be documented as a move away from the SOP and followed up accordingly.

Immunohistochemical System Control

A common strategy some laboratories use to monitor the overall IHC system is to apply Vimentin in a 'canary in the mine' role. Canaries were used as a warning in coal mines of increasing carbon monoxide and other toxic gases. In much the same way that a silent canary is evidence of a problem in a coal mine, a negative Vimentin stain can also be interpreted as a problem with the IHC assay. Being ubiquitous, Vimentin stains almost every tissue element, so for any test section stained with this antibody, there should be some elements within it that are positive. For occasions when there seems to be a string of negative IHC results, it is useful to run a Vimentin to ascertain that the overall assay is working. It is a surrogate validation exercise to check all the reagents in the IHC system including dewaxing, retrieval, detection kit and chromogen development.

External Quality Control

Although many regard external quality control as a 'necessary evil', it is important to remember that laboratories are required to show participation and adherence to external quality assurance (EQA) programmes. Not only are they necessary for accreditation, these activities provide many useful functions. They allow inter-laboratory comparison of performance and results, serve as a warning system for problems, identify systematic kit problems, provide objective evidence of laboratory quality, act as an indicator of where to direct improvement efforts and identify training needs (Vyberg et al. 2005). External quality assurance is also of increasing importance because of the direct therapeutic consequences of detection of stand-alone markers such as ER, HER2 and CD117 (Vyberg and Nielsen 2016).

External Quality Assurance and Proficiency Programmes

Worldwide, there are a number of EQA schemes from numerous countries. They all have the same core goal and that is to standardize and improve the results laboratories achieve with their IHC testing. NordiQC (Europe), UK NEQAS (Europe), RCPA QAP (Australasia) and CAP (Americas) are the most renowned EQA organizations offering modules and services independently of each other.

The main roles of these organizations are to:

- Educate members, the public and participants to identify and use best practice guidelines to achieve consistent high standards.
- Act independently of economic or political interests.
- Provide clinical governance.
- Provide proficiency testing.

Some EQA organizations such as RCPA QAP are multidisciplinary, covering all aspects of laboratory disciplines and their subspecialties whilst groups such as NordiQC focus solely on IHC. To satisfy accreditation in Australia, RCPA QAP would be the chosen EQA to assess the full diagnostic and technical components of accreditation, but it is also common for laboratories to enrol in multiple EQA schemes with the purpose of achieving excellence in their IHC service.

Nordic Immunohistochemical Quality Control Programme

Based in Denmark, the Nordic immunohistochemical quality control (NordiQC) programme is a subscription-based programme for laboratories that want to participate in assessments of their IHC. Similar to proficiency modules in other countries, unstained slides are sent out to laboratories for staining of a particular antibody and then returned for critical assessment. A report is generated for that laboratory discussing the overall quality achieved based on reference NordiQC ranges and also compared to other laboratories. The advantage of NordiQC's programme is that non-members also have access to the published survey results. The best-performing protocols, recommended antibody clones and suggested control tissue are discussed and available for any IHC professional to compare along with high-quality images. It is for this very reason that the website www.nordiqc.org is recommended when researching a new antibody or different clone for use in the laboratory. These programmes highlight the highest-scoring submission method which can be used as a base for optimization in your own laboratory. Although the range of antibodies assessed to date is impressive, it is not exhaustive and may not contain the specific antibody you are interested in. The NordiQC also coordinates regular IHC workshops in diagnostic IHC.

International Quality Network for Pathology

The International Quality Network for Pathology (IQNPath) is an organization based in Luxembourg. Its primary aim is to gather the various QA groups around the world to share expertise and knowledge in all facets of tissue biomarker testing. Member organizations include UK NEQAS (United Kingdom), NordiQC (Denmark), ESPQA (European), AIOM (Italy), Gen&Tiss (France), DGP (Germany), CAP (USA), CIQC (Canada), CCPI (China) and RCPA QAP (Australia). The IQNPath was established in 2015 and focuses on the implementation and quality assessment of new molecular and IHC biomarkers for precision medicine. With such a vast representation from all corners of the globe, the main topics of discussions are centred around standardization of proficiency programmes and quality matters for emerging biomarkers. The recommendations and findings from IQNPath would form the basis of local geographical external QA programs.

Royal College of Pathologists of Australasia

The Royal College of Pathologists of Australasia Quality Assurance Programme (RCPA QAP) is an NATA-accredited service responsible for the organization, preparation, result gathering and review of all the various surveys sent each year. For anatomical pathology, the program covers a range of diagnostic and technical modules. Immunohistochemical proficiency testing is similar to NordiQC in that unstained slides are sent to laboratories to stain a marker of interest and submitted back for assessment. The number of surveys sent out to participants each year depends on the number of modules enrolled.

In 2021, the RCPA QAP offers the following IHC proficiency programmes:

- ALK Translocation for non-small cell lung carcinoma (NSCLC).
- Immunohistochemistry breast markers.
- Immunohistochemistry general.
- Immunohistochemistry lymphoma markers.
- Immunohistochemistry PD-L1 for non-small cell lung carcinoma (UKNEQAS).
- Neuropathology immunohistochemistry and technical.
- ROS1 translocation for non-small cell lung carcinoma (NSCLC).

Whilst a wide variety of programmes are available, not all will be applicable to all laboratories. For example, some laboratories may have a uniquely gynaecological focus and routinely test for p16 IHC which may not be covered in the general module and there is no dedicated programme for gynaecological antibodies. In these instances inter-laboratory slide exchange is recommended. Facilities can compare their IHC staining with another NATA-accredited laboratory and verify that the results are comparable. In instances where the staining is deemed not satisfactory, the laboratory should refer the slides for staining to an external facility until the staining is deemed satisfactory.

Online Resources

It is worthwhile noting that while NordiQC assessments and reports are free to access online, not all organizations allow viewing of material without paid membership subscriptions. For instance, www.immunoquery.com requires subscription whereas www.pathologyoutlines.com and www.e-immunohistochemistry.info are free resources. The www.proteinatlas.org website contains a wealth of knowledge for workers in human peptide research. Many IHC vendors provide educational guides and webinars whilst marketing their products. Thus the amount of information available on the Internet can be overwhelming. There are resources for antibody clones and IHC methodology as well as interpretation guides. Most will not have been peer reviewed and it is incumbent on the reader to be diligent about the accuracy of content and whether they 'trust' the author or organization behind the website.

Regulatory Framework

The use of antibodies as a 'stain' in anatomical pathology has largely been unregulated in the past. Some might say it was like the 'Wild West' where laboratories had free rein to adjust, manipulate and control staining protocols to suit their tastes. It was apparent that there was a need for standardization and regulation, especially when IHC is used to determine patient treatment strategies. In Australia, the Therapeutic Goods Administration (TGA) in association with the NATA provides this regulatory framework for diagnostic IHC.

When purchasing reagents for IHC, reputable vendors offer a plethora of information on the label. Essential details such as volume, lot numbers, protein concentration and expiry dates should be clear. It is also important to note the manufacturer classification of the reagent because this notifies the user as to the purpose and intended use of the product. Figure 2.27 shows a sample label from Cell Marque. Reagents are marked as 'research use only (RUO)', 'investigational use only (IUO)', 'analyte-specific reagent (ASR)' or '*in vitro* diagnostic (IVD)'. This notification dictates the final classification of the IHC assay as either IVD or in-house IVD use.

'While RUO, IUO and ASR products may be commercially supplied, they are not intended by the manufacturer to be used for an in vitro diagnostic purpose and will not be included on the Australian Register of Therapeutic Goods (ARTG). Therefore, the use of these items to develop a test for the purpose of reporting clinical results for a patient means the test would be captured by the in-house IVD regulations' (TGA 2018).

Therapeutic Goods Administration

The IVD medical device regulatory framework came into full effect in Australian laboratories on 1 July 2017.

Figure 2.27 Differences between an IVD (A) and an RUO (B) antibody label

Reproduced with permission from Merck KGaA, Darmstadt, Germany and/or its affiliates

Administered by the TGA, the framework is designed to ensure all IVD medical devices, including in-house IVD medical devices, are to be notified to or registered with the TGA following a level of scrutiny commensurate with the risks associated with their use. The practical outcome of the IVD medical device regulatory framework is that post 30 June 2017, unless otherwise exempt, laboratories will not be able to offer testing using Class 1–3 in-house IVD medical devices unless that test is NATA/RCPA or NATA accredited and the laboratory has complied with the requirements for notification to the TGA. Note the regulations apply to in-house IVD medical devices which have been developed from first principles, developed or modified from a published source and/or commercially supplied which have undergone modifications.

In addition, commercially supplied products sold as 'Research use only' used by laboratories to test and report on patient samples are considered in-house IVDs (as they can affect diagnosis, treatment or management of a patient). In these circumstances the laboratory must validate the assay as an in-house IVD for diagnostic use in line with the NPAAC requirements. The use of disclaimers does not preclude the need for the laboratory to validate the assay (NATA 2016). Essentially, this means the NATA can, in the course of assessing a laboratory's accreditation, notify the laboratory of its obligations to meet the regulations where it has failed to register Class 1, 2 or 3 in-house medical devices with the TGA. If a laboratory has failed to notify the TGA of a class 4 in-house IVD, the NATA will advise the TGA directly of the breach and order cessation of manufacturing and testing of that device. In addition to TGA registration, class 4 in-house IVDs may also warrant registration with the ARTG (NPAAC 2018).

Immunohistochemistry Is a Medical Device

The TGA defines the term 'medical device' as any instrument, apparatus, appliance, material or other article (whether used alone or in combination, and including the software necessary for its proper application) intended, by the person under whose name it is or is to be supplied, to be used for human beings for the purpose of one or more of the following:

(1) Diagnosis, prevention, monitoring, treatment or alleviation of disease.
(2) Diagnosis, monitoring, treatment, alleviation of or compensation for an injury or disability.
(3) Investigation, replacement or modification of the anatomy or of a physiological process.
(4) Control of conception. (Therapeutic Goods Act 1989)

Relating this to IHC testing, the method in which it is used to diagnose disease renders IHC a form of medical device. There are two types of medical devices, IVD or in-house IVD, with four classifications for each type.

In Vitro Diagnostic and In-House *In Vitro* Diagnostic Tests

The difference between these two medical devices, according to the TGA, is that 'in-house' IVDs are pathology tests that have been developed (or modified) within a laboratory (or laboratory network) to carry out testing on human samples, where the results are intended to assist in clinical diagnosis or be used in making decisions concerning clinical management (TGA 2018). An in-house IVD medical device means an IVD medical device that is:

(a) within the confines or scope of an Australian laboratory or Australian laboratory network:
    i. developed from first principles; or
    ii. developed or modified from a published source; or
    iii. developed or modified from any other source; or
    iv. used for a purpose, other than the intended purpose assigned by the manufacturer; and
(b) not supplied for use outside that laboratory or laboratory network. (Health 2020)

The laboratory is the 'manufacturer' of the medical device (IHC stain) and needs to show good laboratory practice (GLP). Conversely, IVDs are purchased to be used under the manufacturer's specified conditions without deviation from the laboratory. If a method has been changed from the manufacturer's recommended protocol, the IHC assay 'loses' its IVD standard and becomes an 'in-house' IVD requiring registration with the TGA. In general terms, the facility will need to state what the assay IVD conditions were, how these have been changed by the laboratory and that the changes made have been appropriately validated for effectiveness and safety (TGA 2018) – in other words, a complete fulfilment of GLP.

All tests manufactured by a laboratory for a therapeutic purpose such as diagnostic, screening, susceptibility or predisposition to disease or monitoring disease progression, regardless of whether or not they attract a Medicare rebate, are still subject to the requirements of the in-house IVD regulatory framework. In-house tests developed by a laboratory for research purposes only are not IVDs.

Both IVD and in-house IVD medical devices are grouped into four categories (Health 2020).

(1) Class 1 IVD medical device or Class 1 in-house IVD medical device that causes no public health risk or contains low personal risk.
(2) Class 2 IVD medical device or Class 2 in-house IVD medical device that poses low public health risk or is a moderate personal risk.
(3) Class 3 IVD medical device or Class 3 in-house IVD medical device that presents a moderate public health risk or high personal risk.
(4) Class 4 IVD medical device or Class 4 in-house IVD medical device that creates a high public health risk.

Figure 2.28 shows IHC assays used within diagnostic pathology to be mostly class 2 or 3. The difference between these two classes is that when the IHC testing has become more specific and the result assists in narrowing down a diagnosis (but not be dependent on it), the category is class 2. It is unlikely that an incorrect result will have a significant impact on patient outcomes. Class 3 tests, however, are reserved for antibodies which dictate treatment decisions such as Her2 and PD-L1 IHC assays. Inaccurate results produce grave consequences for patient safety. General reagents including wash buffers used in IHC testing are generally classified as class 1 because these reagents are not specific to a particular diagnosis. Instruments and analysers are also class 1 medical devices.

Application of Therapeutic Goods Administration Standards

Classifying IHC stains as IVD or in-house IVD medical devices initially brought a high degree of angst and confusion amongst members of the anatomical pathology industry. Adding to this upheaval was the requirement for registration of in-house IVD medical devices with the TGA. As stated before, if a laboratory has elected to use an RUO for patient testing or has modified the manufacturer's recommendations for testing,

	Product Classification:	RUO	Class I	Class II	Class III
	FDA submission	No	No	Yes	**PMA**
Characterization studies performed	Immunoreactivity (ToT ToB)	No	Yes	Yes	Yes
	Robustness	No	Yes	Yes	Yes
	Repeatability	No	Yes	Yes	Yes
	Pre-analytical (fixatives, etc)	No	Yes	Occasionally	Yes
	Stability studies	No	Yes	Yes	Yes
	Design validation	No	Yes	Yes	Yes
	Reader precision	No	No	Yes	Yes
	Inter-laboratory reproducibility or repeatability	No	No	Yes	Yes
	Proof of utility in detecting a disease	No	No	Occasionally	Yes
	Clinical utility proving device performance in relation to drug outcome or potential misdiagnosis	No	No	Occasionally	Yes
	Cut off	No	No	Yes	Yes
	Clinical application:	**None**	**Biomarker detection**	**Aids in treatment decisions**	**Linked to a therapy** (Companion/ Complementary)

Figure 2.28 Classifications of *in vitro* diagnostic devices
Reproduced with permission Ventana Medical Systems Inc.

the TGA must be notified and associated fees paid. In order to register a product or method with the TGA there are accreditation requirements which need to be met (Health 2020):

The laboratory in which the Class 1, 2 or 3 in-house IVD medical device is manufactured must:

(a) Be accredited as a testing laboratory by the NATA, or by a conformity assessment body determined by the secretary, as meeting one of the following standards, as published by the International Organization for Standardization and as amended from time to time:
  (i) ISO 15189. Medical laboratories: Requirements for quality and competence.
  (ii) ISO/IEC 17025. General requirement for the competence of testing and calibration laboratories.

(b) Meet the National Pathology Accreditation Advisory Council standard requirements for the development and use of in-house IVDs, as amended from time to time.

Besides creating more administrative work for IHC laboratories, the shift away from convention and 'the way IHC has always been done' meant a regulated way of ensuring IHC testing for patients was performed against a validated and/or published method. If this was modified in any way, the protocol was acknowledged in the TGA registration. This strategy may be compared to special stains whereby many histology laboratories would have manuals comprising protocols littered with 'modified from' someone's certain technique in their referencing. The same can be said of IHC laboratories modifying a recommended vendor protocol to the requirements of their facility. It may be that the pathologist requests a 'punchier' stain, perhaps due to some of the pre-analytical variables discussed earlier. Although registering in-house IVDs may be perceived as onerous, the TGA has given scope for laboratories to still be able to 'tweak' IHC protocols as the need arises. It just needs to be documented, and this is a good outcome for all parties.

It has meant that for many IHC facilities, the days of random aliquots of antibody concentrate 'x' in freezers have largely disappeared. Many laboratories including the RCH Melbourne have opted to employ IVD-registered, RTU antibodies for as many assays as possible. A 'plug and play' solution, these RTU antibodies have been validated against a vast array of normal and abnormal tissues and require little (if any) modification from the vendor recommendations. For antibodies to which an RTU is not available or whose performance in QA programmes is superior as a concentrate, validation was performed for TGA registration as an in-house IVD medical device.

The RCH Melbourne IHC laboratory utilizes a simple spreadsheet to log all of the in-house IVD antibodies (Figure 2.29). Each RTU vendor protocol was systematically compared against the pathologist-validated method and variations (if any) were noted and tabulated. For antibody concentrates, each protocol step was itemized with future variations noted and submitted to the TGA on a yearly basis.

The Future of Quality Management in Immunohistochemistry

Quality assurance measures must keep pace with the development of new technologies. At the moment, there are possibly three main AQ challenges relating to diagnostic IHC. First is the continuing progress of IHC in providing insights into changes at the molecular level contributing to cancer diagnosis. Immunohistochemistry can be used to demonstrate protein loss in mismatch repair proteins, E-cadherin and INI-1; protein over-expression such as p53, HER2 and Bcl2; or protein transformational changes including ALK, BRAF and IDH1 (Vyberg and Nielsen 2016). The recently adopted TGA regulatory framework labelling IHC as a medical device has thus far adequately addressed the risk to patients, especially the need for class 3 IVDs pertaining to companion diagnostic testing. This important aspect will continue as more markers are discovered to directly influence patient treatments.

Second, the use of digital analysis to provide some standardization in semi-quantification of counts and intensity is already available for markers such as ER, Her2 and Ki67 (Brügmann et al. 2012; Røge et al. 2016). External QA programmes such as the RCPA QAP have been distributing digitized slides for the assessment of diagnostic surveys. It is highly probable that laboratories will soon be able to submit whole scanned images of IHC-stained slides for technical assessment. Reviewers would be able to perform assessments remotely via a virtual multi-header session. This new digital frontier and its associated QA matters need to be addressed. As such, the NPAAC has recently released a draft document available for public consultation about the requirements for digital

In-house IVDs

ANATOMICAL PATHOLOGY

Test / Procedure	Path procedure test code or ID	Department	Variation to standard test	Class of IVD as per TGA classification table	History / first introduced
α-1-fetoprotein	histg/fsg	ANATOMICAL PATHOLOGY	4 mins Ab instead of 16. OV detection instead of UV	2	2007
α-inhibin	histg/fsg	ANATOMICAL PATHOLOGY	CC1 16 mins instead of standard. OV detection used instead of UV	2	2007
Actin (SMA)	histg/fsg	ANATOMICAL PATHOLOGY	28 mins Ab instead of 32. No amp. OV instead of UV	2	2007
ALK-1	histg/fsg	ANATOMICAL PATHOLOGY	Incubation of antibody for 1hr instead of 16min. OV instead of UV	2	2007
Bcl-2	histg/fsg	ANATOMICAL PATHOLOGY	Antigen retrieval CC1 performed for 40 min instead of 64min. OV instead of UV.	2	2007
Ber-EP4	histg/fsg	ANATOMICAL PATHOLOGY	CC1 16 instead of mild, 12 min Ab instead of 16. OV instead of UV.	2	2007
B-catenin	histg/fsg	ANATOMICAL PATHOLOGY	CC1 16 instead of standard. Ab 24 instead of 32. OV instead of UV.	2	2016

Figure 2.29 The Therapeutic Goods Administration spreadsheet used by the Royal Children's Hospital Melbourne

images as an alternative to direct microscopy (NPAAC 2020). Digital whole-slide imaging technologies bring a new set of challenges to overcome. Although the technology has matured to the point of it being a viable technology, quality systems must be set to maximize patient safety. For instance, the laboratory may have the ability to digitize preferential staining of control sections (with included drift) to automatically validate controls on an IHC-stained slide prior to sending it out to the pathologist for reporting. This action is possible, but what are the 'quality' concerns of this practice?

Thirdly, the continued development of multiplex IHC staining on a single tissue section may become more routine in diagnostic settings. Take for example the PIN4 assay for prostate pathology being a dual chromogenic system. It is conceivable that in the near future, consistent and reliable results are achieved for three- and four-chromogen IHC systems. The advent of digital images will assist in this development and will therefore bring about the same QA challenges discussed previously.

These cutting-edge technologies will lead to further requirements for QC and QA in terms of added requirements for validation of the IHC assay as technology progresses and improvements are made in turnaround times and clarity of staining, and as innovations are crafted to detection regimes and novel target epitopes are discovered to improve the efficiency of staining in the future. These advances will always be accompanied by a QA system so as to ensure consistent, accurate and reliable results.

Conclusion

Scientists and technicians at the bench apply quality management principles often without realizing it. Whether this has been ingrained into training or accepted as the nature of the work, it is important to sometimes pause and reflect on why certain practices exist and why a high level of commitment is expended to set up specific processes which ought to be followed day after day. This chapter not only serves as a reminder of the importance of 'quality' matters in IHC, but also allows an appreciation of the huge hurdles that must be overcome in order to guarantee a reliable and accurate IHC stain.

The laboratory's quality management system consists of QC, QA and QI arrangements. These structures are ever present in the background and have a direct impact on IHC staining. The various factors influencing IHC staining have been explored. They are divided into pre-analytic, analytic and post-analytic stages. This compartmentalizing helps the

Appendix 1 Troubleshooting immunohistochemical issues (Lin and Chen 2014)

Immunohistochemical result	Remedy
Strong staining signal/no background	Obtain the highest dilution with the optimal result to save the primary antibody and cut down the cost.
Strong staining signal/weak background	Reduce the primary antibody concentration. Shorten the primary antibody incubation time. Shorten the second antibody incubation time. Further block the background staining.
Strong staining signal/strong background	Reduce the primary antibody concentration. Shorten the primary antibody incubation time. Shorten the second antibody incubation time. Further block the background staining. Try different antigen retrieval (AR) methods.
Weak staining signal/no background	Increase the primary antibody concentration. Increase the incubation time for the primary antibody. Increase the incubation time for the second antibody. Switch to a more sensitive secondary detecting system. Try different AR methods.
Weak staining signal/weak background	Increase the primary antibody concentration and reduce the incubation time. Further block background staining. Increase the incubation time for the second antibody. Switch to a more sensitive secondary detecting system. Try different AR methods. Use a different primary antibody.
Weak staining signal/strong background	Further block background staining. Switch to a more sensitive secondary detecting system. Try different AR methods. Use a different primary antibody.
No staining signal/no background	Follow the general approaches step by step. Increase the primary antibody concentration and incubation time. Try different AR methods. Switch to a more sensitive secondary detecting system. Contact primary antibody supplier for assistance. Use a different primary antibody.
No staining signal/weak background	Follow the general approaches step by step. Increase the primary antibody concentration and incubation time. Try different AR methods. Switch to a more sensitive secondary detecting system. Contact primary antibody supplier for assistance. Use a different primary antibody.
No staining signal/strong background	Follow the general approaches step by step. Try different AR methods. Switch to a more sensitive secondary detecting system. Contact primary antibody supplier for assistance. Use a different primary antibody.

assessment of each parameter in relation to the other variables within the IHC system to warrant good laboratory practices. The use of controls, both internal and external, is as important as the regulatory framework in classifying IHC as a medical device. Ultimately the existence of 'quality' measures ensures the lowest risk to patients. The quality system provides a risk matrix to allow such assessments because at the end of the day it is the safety of patients that matters most.

References

Agilent 2021. Dako proteinase K ready to use package insert (online). Available at www.agilent.com/cs/library/packageinsert/public/301326EN_02.pdf (Accessed 1 June 2021).

Ananthanarayanan V, Pins MR, Meyer RE, Gann PH 2005. Immunohistochemical assays in prostatic biopsies processed in Bouin's fixative. *J Clin Pathol* **58**(3):322–4.

Bogen SA 2019. A root cause analysis into the high error rate in clinical immunohistochemistry. *Appl Immunohistochem Mol Morphol* **27**(5):329–38.

Bromley CM, Palechek PL, Benda JA 1994. Preservation of estrogen receptor in paraffin sections. *Journal of Histotechnology* **17**(2):115–18.

Brügmann A, Eld M, Lelkaitis G, Nielsen S, Grunkin M, Hansen JD, Foged NT, Vyberg M 2012. Digital image analysis of membrane connectivity is a robust measure of HER2 immunostains. *Breast Cancer Res Treat* **132** (1):41–9.

Carson FL, Hladik C 2009. *Histotechnology: A self-instructional text.* American Society of Clinical Pathology Press.

Cates JMM, Troutman KA Jr 2015. Quality management of the immunohistochemistry laboratory: A practical guide. *Appl Immunohistochem Mol Morphol* **23**(7): 471–80.

College of American Pathologists 2009. Definition of quality assurance, quality control, and quality improvement. CAP (online). Available at www.cap.org/apps/cap.portal (Accessed 30 May 2020).

College of American Pathologists 2017. Standards for laboratory accreditation 2017 edition. CAP (online). Available at https://elss.cap.org/elss/ShowProperty?nodePath=/UCMCON/Contribution%20Folders/WebApplications/shared-assets/lap-standards.pdf (Accessed 30 May 2020).

Drew T, Vo MLH, Wolfe JM 2013. The invisible gorilla strikes again: Sustained inattentional blindness in expert observers. *Psychol Sci* **24**(9):1848–53.

Engel KB, Moore HM 2011. Effects of preanalytical variables on the detection of proteins by immunohistochemistry in formalin-fixed, paraffin-embedded tissue. *Arch Pathol Lab Med* **135**(5):537–43.

Evans KK, Birdwell RL, Wolfe JM 2013. If you don't find it often, you often don't find it: Why some cancers are missed in breast cancer screening. *PLoS One* **8**(5):e64366.

Gown AM 2016. Diagnostic immunohistochemistry: What can go wrong and how to prevent it. *Arch Pathol Lab Med* **140**(9):893–8.

Hayat MA 2002. *Microscopy, immunohistochemistry, and antigen retrieval methods: For light and electron microscopy.* Kluwer Academic.

Health 2020. Therapeutic goods (medical devices) regulations 2002. Australian government (online). Available at www.legislation.gov.au/Details/F2020C00112 (Accessed 30 May 2020).

Hewitt SM, Baskin DG, Frevert CW, Stahl WL, Rosa-Molinar E 2014. Controls for immunohistochemistry: The Histochemical Society's standards of practice for validation of immunohistochemical assays. *J Histochem Cytochem* **62** (10):693–7.

Hewitt SM, Lewis FA, Cao Y, Conrad RC, Cronin M, Danenberg KD, Goralski TJ, Langmore JP, Raja RG, Williams PM, Palma JF, Warrington JA 2008. Tissue handling and specimen preparation in surgical pathology: Issues concerning the recovery of nucleic acids from formalin-fixed, paraffin-embedded tissue. *Arch Pathol Lab Med* **132**(12):1929–35.

Jackson P, Blythe D 2008. Immunohistochemical techniques. In Bancroft JD, Gamble M, eds. *Theory and practice of histological techniques.* Churchill Livingstone Elsevier; 433–72.

Jacobs TW, Prioleau JE, Stillman IE, Schnitt SJ 1996. Loss of tumor marker-immunostaining intensity on stored paraffin slides of breast cancer. *J Natl Cancer Inst* **88**(15):1054–9.

Kakimoto K, Takekoshi S, Miyajima K, Osamura RY 2008. Hypothesis for the mechanism for heat-induced antigen retrieval occurring on fresh frozen sections without formalin-fixation in immunohistochemistry. *J Mol Histo* **39** (4):389–99.

Leong AS, Lee ES, Yin H, Kear M, Haffajee Z, Pepperall D 2002. Superheating antigen retrieval. *Appl Immunohistochem Mol Morphol* **10**(3):263–8.

Levenson RM, Krupinski EA, Navarro VM, Wasserman EA 2015. Pigeons (Columba livia) as trainable observers of pathology and radiology breast cancer images. *PLoS One* **10** (11):e0141357.

Lin F, Chen Z 2014. Standardization of diagnostic immunohistochemistry: Literature review and Geisinger experience. *Arch Pathol Lab Med* **138**(12):1564–77.

McCampbell AS, Raghunathan V, Tom-Moy M, Workman, RK, Haven R, Ben-Dor A, Rasmussen OF, Jacobsen L, Lindberg M, Yamada NA, Schembri C 2017. Tissue thickness effects on immunohistochemical staining intensity of markers of cancer. *Appl Immunohistochem Mol Morphol* **27**(5):345–55.

McMahon L 2018. The impact of decalcification on staining. Leica Biosystems (online). Available at www.leicabiosystems.com/knowledge-pathway/the-impact-of-decalcification-on-staining (Accessed 30 May 2020).

Miyatake Y, Ikeda H, Michimata R, Koizumi S, Ishizu A, Nishimura N, Yoshiki T 2004. Differential modulation of gene expression among rat tissues with warm ischemia. *Exp Mol Path* **77**(3):222–30.

NATA 2016. NATA agreements update: Memorandum of understanding with TGA. National Association of Testing Authorities (online). Available at www.nata.com.au/nata-articles/150-nata-agreements-update-memorandum-of-understanding-with-tga (Accessed 30 May 2020).

NATA 2018. Technical circular – General accreditation guidance – Validation and verification of quantitative and qualitative test methods. National Association of Testing

Authorities (online). Available at www.nata.com.au/phocadownload/gen-accreditation-guidance/Validation-and-Verification-of-Quantitative-and-Qualitative-Test-Methods.pdf (Accessed 30 May 2020).

NATA 2019. General accreditation criteria ISO 15189 standard application document, July 2019. National Association of Testing Authorities (online). Available at www.nata.com.au/phocadownload/gen-accreditation-criteria/ISO-15189-Application-Document-Medical-Testing-Supplementary-Requirements-for-Accreditation.pdf (Accessed 30 May 2020).

NCCLS 1999. Quality assurance for immunocytochemistry: Approved guideline. MM4-A **Vol. 19** No. 26. Clinical and Laboratory Standards Institute (formerly NCCLS) (online). Available at http://demo.nextlab.ir/getattachment/50d8822a-bdd5-4f7d-b712-d5f5737d4d76/CLSI-MM4-A.aspx (Accessed 30 May 2020).

NPAAC 2018. Requirements for the development and use of in-house *in vitro* diagnostic medical devices (IVDs) (Fourth edition). Australian Government Department of Health (online). Available at www1.health.gov.au/internet/main/publishing.nsf/Content/health-npaac-dhaivd-2018 (Accessed 30 May 2020).

NPAAC 2020. Requirements for use of digital images as an alternative to direct microscopy (draft). Australian Government Department of Health (online). Available at www1.health.gov.au/internet/main/publishing.nsf/Content/health-npaac-publications-draft.htm (Accessed 30 May 2020).

Prioleau J, Schnitt SJ 1995. p53 antigen loss in stored paraffin slides. *N Engl J Med* **332**(22):1521–2.

Ramos-Vara JA, Beissenherz ME 2000. Optimization of immunohistochemical methods using two different antigen retrieval methods on formalin-fixed paraffin-embedded tissues: Experience with 63 markers. *J Vet Diagn Invest* **12**(4):307–11.

RCPA 2018. Ethical and legal issues in relation to the use of human tissue in Australia and New Zealand. Royal College of Pathologists of Australasia (online). Available at www.rcpa.edu.au/getattachment/ad0d4af1-901a-4056-af05-56bbc06167c1/Ethical-and-Legal-Issues-in-Relation-to-the-Use-of.aspx (Accessed 30 May 2020).

RCPA 2019. Cancer protocols: Published protocols. 2nd edition. Royal College of Pathologists of Australasia (online). Available at www.rcpa.edu.au/Library/Practising-Pathology/Structured-Pathology-Reporting-of-Cancer/Cancer-Protocols (Accessed 1 June 2021).

Roche 2018. Tissue diagnostics product catalog 2019. Roche Diagnostics Corporation (online). Available at https://diagnostics.roche.com/content/dam/diagnostics/us/en/resource-center/Tissue-product-catalog-2019.pdf (Accessed 31 July 2021).

Røge R, Riber-Hansen R, Nielsen S, Vyberg M 2016. Proliferation assessment in breast carcinomas using digital image analysis based on virtual Ki67/cytokeratin double staining. *Breast Cancer Res Treat* **158**(1):11–19.

Rolls G 2013. An introduction to decalcification. Leica Biosystems (online). Available at www.leicabiosystems.com/knowledge-pathway/an-introduction-to-decalcification (Accessed 30 May 2020).

Rolls G 2016. Steps to better grossing. Leica Biosystems (online). Available at www.leicabiosystems.com/knowledge-pathway/steps-to-better-grossing (Accessed 30 May 2020).

Rolls G 2019. An introduction to specimen processing. Leica Biosystems (online). Available at www.leicabiosystems.com/knowledge-pathway/an-introduction-to-specimen-processing (Accessed 30 May 2020).

Sanderson T, Zardin G 2013. Immunohistochemistry quality control. In Suvarna K, Layton C, Bancroft JD, eds. *Bancroft's theory and practice of histological techniques.* Churchill Livingstone Elsevier; 435–54.

Shi SR, Cote RJ, Liu C, Yu MC, Castelao JE, Ross RK, Taylor CR 2002. A modified reduced-temperature antigen retrieval protocol effective for use with a polyclonal antibody to cyclooxygenase-2 (PG 27). *Appl Immunohistochem Mol Morph* **10**(4):368–73.

Shi SR, Cote RJ, Taylor CR 1997. Antigen retrieval immunohistochemistry: Past, present, and future. *J Histochem Cytochem* **45**(3):327–43.

Shi SR, Imam SA, Young L, Cote RJ, Taylor CR 1995. Antigen retrieval immunohistochemistry under the influence of pH using monoclonal antibodies. *J Histochem Cytochem* **43**(2):193–201.

Shi SR, Key ME, Kalra KL 1991. Antigen retrieval in formalin-fixed, paraffin-embedded tissues: an enhancement method for immunohistochemical staining based on microwave oven heating of tissue sections. *J Histochem Cytochem* **39**(6):741–8.

Shi SR, Liu C, Pootrakul L, Tang L, Young A, Chen R, Cote RJ, Taylor CR 2008. Evaluation of the value of frozen tissue section used as 'gold standard' for immunohistochemistry. *Am J Clin Pathol* **129**(3):358–66.

Singh PP, Sood NK 2017. A combination of antigen retrieval methods significantly enhances the unmasking of tedious antigens of lymphangiogenesis and angiogenesis in canine mammary tumour. *Journal of Biosciences and Medicines* **5**(12):44–55.

TGA 2018. Regulatory requirements for in-house IVDs: What is an in-house IVD? Australian Government Department of Health (online). Available at www.tga.gov.au/book-page/what-house-ivd (Accessed 30 May 2020).

Therapeutic Goods Act 1989 Sect 41BD What is a medical device? Commonwealth Consolidated Acts (online). Available at http://classic.austlii.edu.au/au/legis/cth/consol_act/tga1989191/s41bd.html (Accessed 31 May 2020).

Torlakovic EE, Francis G, Garratt J, Gilks B, Hyjek E, Ibrahim M, Miller R, Nielsen S, Petcu EB, Swanson PE, Taylor CR, Vyberg M 2014. Standardization of negative controls in diagnostic immunohistochemistry: Recommendations from the international ad hoc expert panel. *Appl Immunohistochem Mol Morphol* **22** (4):241–52.

Torlakovic EE, Nielsen S, Vyberg M, Taylor CR 2015. Getting controls under control: The time is now for immunohistochemistry. *J Clin Pathol* **68**(11):879–82.

Vyberg M, Nielsen S 2016. Proficiency testing in immunohistochemistry: Experiences from Nordic Immunohistochemical Quality Control (NordiQC). *Virchows Archiv* **468**(1):19–29.

Vyberg M, Torlakovic E, Seidal T, Risberg B, Helin H, Nielsen S 2005. Nordic Immunohistochemical Quality Control. *Croat Med J* **46**(3):368–71.

Williams C, Pontén F, Moberg C, Söderkvist P, Uhlén M, Pontén J, Sitbon G, Lundeberg J 1999. A high frequency of sequence alterations is due to formalin fixation of archival specimens. *Am J Pathol* **155**(5):1467–71.

Williams JH, Mepham BL, Wright DH 1997. Tissue preparation for immunocytochemistry. *J Clin Pathol* **50** (5):422–8.

Yamashita S, Okada Y 2005. Mechanisms of heat-induced antigen retrieval: Analyses in vitro employing SDS-PAGE and immunohistochemistry. *J Histochem Cytochem* **53** (1):13–21.

Chapter 3

Automation and Robotics with the Leica Bond III

Anthony F. Henwood

Overview

In 1950 Coons and Kaplan developed the immunofluorescent technique by conjugating fluorescein to antibodies and applying them to cells and tissue sections. From this development, today's modern immunohistochemistry (IHC) evolved (Henwood 2019a). In 1970, Sternberger and co-workers described an unlabelled antibody enzyme method commonly known as the peroxidase anti-peroxidase (PAP) method. Ten years later, Hsu and colleagues (1981) increased the sensitivity of this technique by utilizing the amplification properties of avidin-biotin systems. At this point in time, these methods were all performed manually utilizing at least 20 manipulations such as dewaxing, buffer rinses, antibody applications and counterstaining, to name a few (Henwood 1981, 1991). Immunohistochemists considered themselves artisans, consistently producing specific brown or sometimes red antigen localization within tissue sections all the while contemplating, 'Can a machine do this better than us?'

In the early 1990s Shi and colleagues (1991) introduced heat-induced epitope retrieval (HIER) to reverse the effect of formalin fixation. This strategy allowed many antibodies previously non-reactive in formalin-fixed tissues to successfully bind to their relevant tissue epitopes. Unfortunately this innovation raised several major problems in the routine histopathology laboratory. Heat-induced epitope retrieval was initially achieved with microwave irradiation. This method has remained the most common technique for antigen retrieval. However, a variety of other means of generating heat have since been developed, including water baths, hotplates, wet autoclaves, pressure cookers and vegetable steamers. All of these processes suffer from the problem of ensuring accurate temperature and time control. These two variables have been shown to be critical to HIER. They are inversely related, meaning antigen retrieval at lower temperatures requires longer time to achieve the same intensity of IHC staining as that obtained with higher temperatures (Leong 2004). Microwave irradiation in particular suffers from uneven staining due to hot and cold spots within the oven chamber (Pileri et al. 1997). In addition, the most frustrating feature of HIER was the regular occurrence of false negative IHC staining due to sections inadvertently drying out during or after HIER (Marsch et al. 2015).

The increasing availability of commercial antibodies that could now be used on formalin-fixed paraffin-embedded (FFPE) sections placed pressure on laboratory workloads. For example, at Children's Hospital Westmead, the number of antigens localized in tissue sections increased from 25 to more than 140 within a few years. The number of slides immunostained daily increased from 20 to nearly 160. Serious consideration had to be given to restructuring the IHC service, increasing staff numbers and expanding laboratory space. Fortuitously, several fully automated IHC platforms available at that time showed the reliability and versatility required whilst promising efficiency gains. For the reasons stated earlier, a Leica Bond Max immunostainer was installed for trial and subsequently purchased in 2005 (serial number 00003) and in 2012 an upgrade to a Bond III immunostainer was successfully employed.

This chapter highlights the nuances of the Leica Bond III IHC platform from a user's perspective. BOND™ is a trademark of Leica Biosystems Melbourne Pty, Ltd. Topics such as proprietary reagents, protocols and detection kits for use are covered as well as a discussion on design, bulk solutions and epitope retrieval programmes. A suggestion on the approach to optimize antibody concentrates is included. Strategies to achieve high-quality IHC are specified with reference to immunofluorescence, double labelling and cytology preparations. Finally a commentary is offered on the maintenance and quality control measures of the instrument along with some suggestions for improvement.

Principle of the Leica Bond III Instrument

The Bond III IHC system consists of a floor-standing processing module driven by a dedicated computer. In comparison to other IHC platforms on the market, it has a reasonable footprint, making it easy to accommodate into existing infrastructure. Figure 3.1 shows the processing module and all the necessary reagents and hardware the staining protocols require to run tissue samples mounted on slides. This module has the capacity to stain 30 slides per batch and contains individual heater pads arranged in three trays of 10 slides. On the right-hand side of the staining trays is the reagent platform area for localization antibodies and demonstration kits. The bulk reagents consisting of buffer wash, retrieval solutions, dewax, alcohol and waste collection containers are connected separately below the staining trays. The unit is self-contained and does not require plumbing into existing pipes. One computer can control up to five processing modules and is also connected to a handheld ID barcode scanner, slide labeller and printer. With dimensions of 775(D) x 1359(H) x 785(W) mm, it would not be difficult for laboratories to accommodate this self-contained floor-standing unit.

Robotics

For fluid transfer the Bond III processing module uses up to four separate robotic systems. Bulk reagents such as dewax and wash buffer are dispensed onto slides via 'bulk fill robots'. Figure 3.2 shows the bulk fill robot in the rest position akin to that of a little mouse ready to come out of a mouse hole. A dedicated bulk fill robot is assigned to each slide-staining assembly in order to help speed up the staining process. This is a major innovation in efficiency over the previous model, the Bond Max. These robots only dispense reagent from bulk containers housed below the three slide-staining assemblies. For antibody transfer, detection kit and chromogen application there is a central aspirating probe to expel fluid onto slides or deployed at the mixing station.

There is only one aspirating probe for the three slide-staining assemblies. Attached to this probe is an ID imager. The camera captures an image of each slide label for the purpose of slide recognition as well as each antibody vial and detection kit loaded onto the module. Lastly, the aspirating probe also contains a liquid-level sensor to detect reagent level in each vial.

Slide Drawers

Slides are loaded and stained in the slide-staining assemblies. Shown in Figure 3.3, each processing

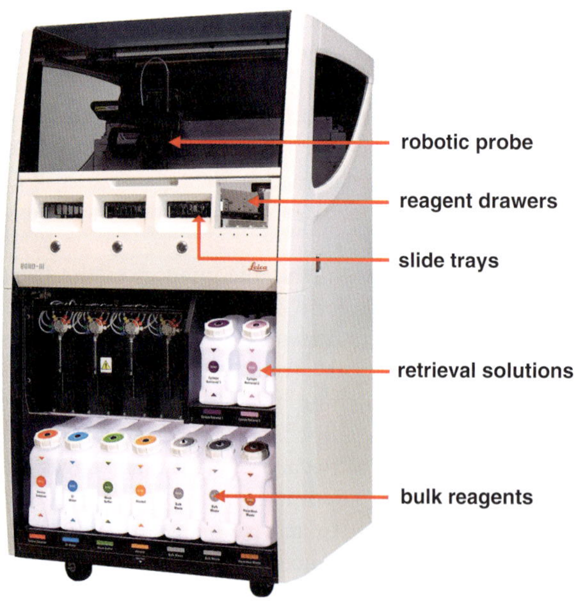

Figure 3.1 The Bond III set-up
Reproduced with permission Leica Biosystems Melbourne, Pty, Ltd.

module contains three slide-staining assemblies that can each accommodate a tray supporting 10 slides. Each slide position has its own heating element which is independently monitored. As the assembly is engineered for each slide to be completely removed from other slides, there is zero chance of crossover or contamination events between patient samples. Precise temperature control is afforded at each slide position and is marked as faulty if a temperature error occurs.

Covertiles

Bond plastic covertiles have been designed to optimize staining and are an essential part of the staining system. It is the technology used in this area that differentiates IHC platforms from different vendors.

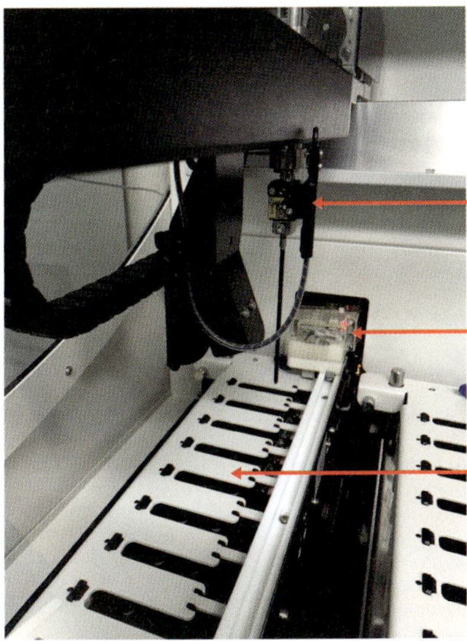

Figure 3.2 Two types of robotic probes

Leica's covertiles must be positioned on top of slides after placing the slides into the slide tray. To ensure correct orientation, the covertile key must fit into the space in the slide tray. They can be reused up to 25 times provided they are not heavily discoloured or damaged. The covertiles are cleaned in 1% bleach overnight and washed in running tap water for five minutes before a rinse in alcohol for five minutes and left to air-dry. Dirty covertiles can contribute to 'bubble artefact' whereby there is a localized circle area of decreased staining. The production of little bubbles prevents the reagents accessing the cells in the area for the full allocated incubation time.

Reagent Drawer

Located next to the slide-staining assembly is an area for antibody vials and detection kits, as shown in Figure 3.4. There is space to accommodate four racks and each rack can hold 10 vials. The light-emitting diode (LED) indicator at the front of each drawer designates when reagents can be loaded and unloaded. A red light specifies the instrument is actively aspirating a reagent located on the rack and locks the drawer. A green light denotes the drawer can be unloaded to add new vials or swap out reagents no longer required.

Chromogens such as diaminobenzidine (DAB) and Fast Red are prepared in the mixing station automatically by the aspirating probe. The mixing station sits in the wash block located behind the antibody reagent area and is replaced weekly with a clean unit. The used unit is cleaned in bleach similarly to the covertiles.

Bulk Reagent Storage

The bottom half of the module contains the bulk containers cavity. Figure 3.5 shows dewax, epitope

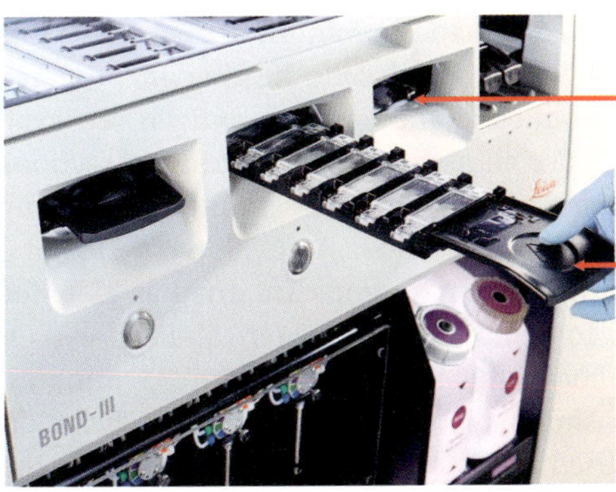

Figure 3.3 Loading slides fitted with covertiles

Reproduced with permission Leica Biosystems Melbourne, Pty, Ltd.

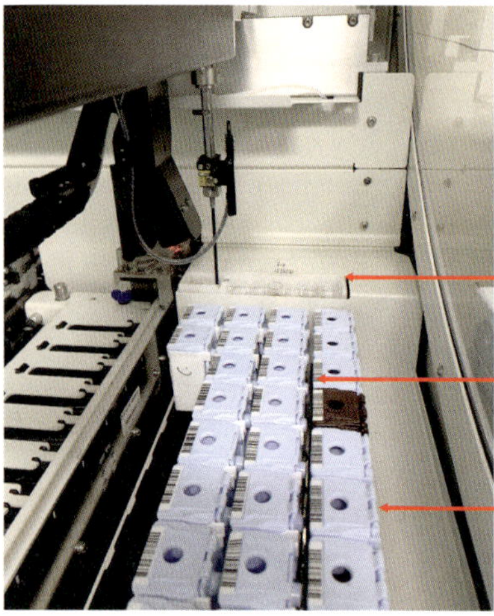

Figure 3.4 Antibody and detection reagent storage

retrieval, buffer wash, alcohol and water are housed in individual packages. For waste management there are separate containers for hazardous (hydrocarbon dewax solution and chromogen waste) and non-hazardous bulk waste (buffer wash, epitope retrieval, alcohol and water waste). For easy identification, these containers are colour coded.

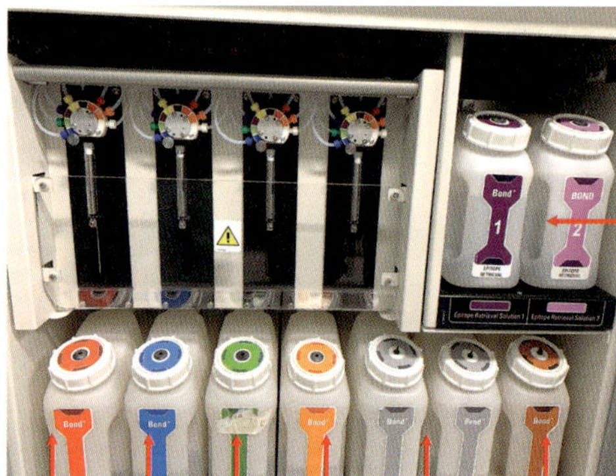

Figure 3.5 Bulk solutions on board the Bond

Pre-staining Processes

Before application of a localization antibody, a range of treatments may be required to tissue and cell preparations. In the case of FFPE sections, slides need to be baked on adhesive slides prior to dewaxing and hydration to water. One source of poor immunostaining is the overheating of tissue sections. Several authors have reported that heated slide drying adversely affects sensitivity in immunohistochemistry. Therefore some have advocated the use of lower-temperature drying using adhesive-coated slides to improve the sensitivity of the test (Williams et al. 1997). In the author's experience, some epitopes were adversely affected by section drying at 80°C, including CK8/18, CMV, S100, HMB45 and CEA (Henwood 2005). Oates (1993) used antisera to EMA from three different vendors and found that staining of slides dried at 58°C was often paler than that of slides dried at room temperature or at 37°C.

Laboratory ovens can be variable in their ability to maintain a constant temperature, the implication being that it is possible to either 'overcook' sections thus adversely affecting epitopes or 'under-heat' them, compromising subsequent dewaxing. There is also the human element. Oven doors are opened and closed numerous times during the day, and how often are slides removed from the oven at the required time? Modern IHC automatic immunostainers have excellent controlled on-board slide heating in order to achieve reproducible and accurate antigen retrieval. This feature also allows controlled 'baking' of sections and being able to programme a set time removes the possibility of human error. At Children's Hospital Westmead, freshly cut sections are dried at 37°C for 5 minutes to remove excess water. Slides are then baked on board the Bond at 63°C for 35 minutes. Figure 3.6 shows the immunostaining for Bcl-6 on a section dried at 70°C for one hour compared to the

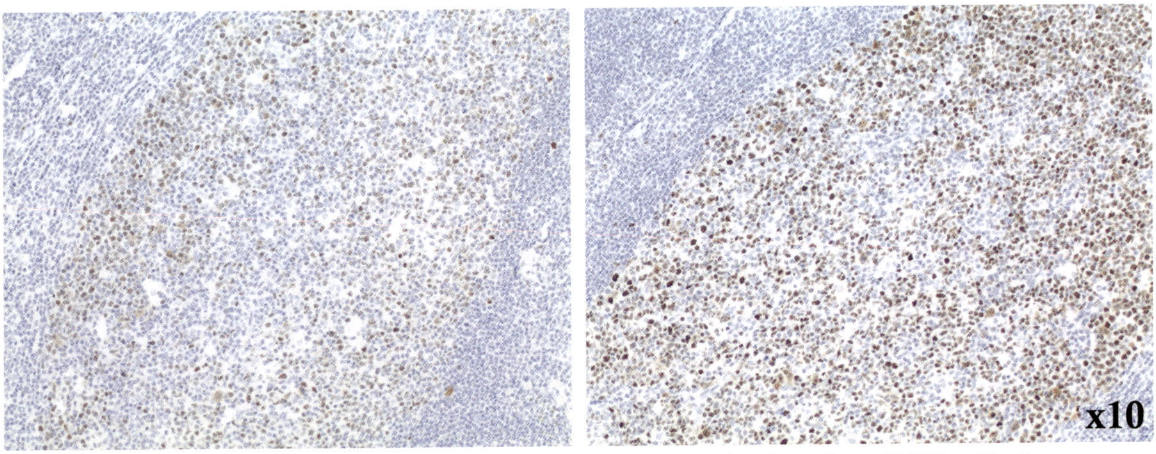

Figure 3.6 Tonsil Bcl-6 immunohistochemical (IHC) staining results from different baking protocols

Bond baking protocol described previously. Using the same stain protocol for each situation, note the difference in IHC staining intensity achieved from the Bond III onboard baking system. As this is an all-in-one IHC solution, dewaxing and hydration of FFPE sections prior to staining is done on the instrument.

Tray Allocation

With some forethought to logistics, the Bond III immunostainer can be judiciously loaded to complete runs in the minimum of time. As mentioned previously, each Bond III has the capacity to stain 30 slides concurrently. There are three staining assemblies with each assembly holding 10 slides. This capacity is in line with other IHC platforms and seems to be the sweet spot in IHC automation. An increase in capacity may lead to increased complexity, which may result in longer staining turnaround times. It is far easier to add additional modules if the workload demands it.

To gain an efficiency advantage on the Bond III, the only requirement is that each staining tray assembly uses one protocol only at any given time. For example, slides for IHC on FFPE tissue are incompatible with *in situ* hybridization slides and therefore cannot be loaded onto the same staining assembly tray. For instances when a staining tray requires enzyme retrieval on some slides and HIER on others, the pretreatments are performed sequentially (not simultaneously). It is therefore preferable to allocate slides with different pretreatment parameters on separate trays. Grouping 'like with like' has been shown to save approximately 30 minutes in staining time.

Antibodies requiring no retrieval such as S100 and SMA will process faster if they are arranged on their own tray. However, since the amount of demonstration reagents are prepared per tray (for 10 slides) each time, then this advice may not be efficient for small batches of slides. In other words, frequently having empty spots on the staining assembly can be wasteful in terms of detection reagents as well as space since additional slides cannot be added to a tray that has been committed for staining. The empty spots on the assembly tray are not available once the 'start' button is pressed. Sometimes it may be better to place all of the slides on the one tray even if they have different pretreatments. On the other hand, if there are urgent slides to stain, then waiting for a full tray can delay a diagnosis. These conundrums are faced by the Bond user on a daily basis and require a delicate balancing act with good judgement to maximize the efficiency.

Bond Bulk Solutions

Several proprietary bulk solutions are used on the Bond. These Bond ancillary products are designed and optimized for use exclusively on the Leica Bond IHC platform. For bulk reagents, they include the Bond Dewax Solution, Bond Epitope Retrieval Solutions (1&2) and Bond Wash Solution (which needs to be diluted 1:9 before use). User-supplied bulk solutions include ethanol (denatured alcohol works well) and distilled water.

The Bond dewax solution contains isoalkanes approximately 11 to 13 carbon atoms long. Less than 2% are aromatics. Alkanes, also known as paraffins, are saturated hydrocarbons with a general formula C_nH_{2n+2}. Aromatic hydrocarbons are considered more toxic and more resistant to microbial degradation than the corresponding normal alkanes, isoalkanes, cycloalkanes and the unsaturated aliphatic hydrocarbons (Adeniji et al. 2017).

The Bond wash solution is supplied as a 10x concentrate. To make 1 L, add 100 mL of Bond wash solution to 900 mL of deionized water. The wash buffer primarily consists of TRIS buffer saline with some surfactant and antimicrobial agent. All bulk reagents are colourless, which means there is a potential source of human error when replenishing the bulk containers. To assist in ensuring the correct reagent is filled to the corresponding bulk container, Leica has used colour-coded labels with their ancillary reagents. The onus ultimately lies with the end user to ensure the ER2 container is not filled with dewax, for example.

It is important to monitor the quality of the distilled water (Henwood 2019b). Unfortunately, corruption of laboratory-distilled water supply is a common occurrence which may lead to bacterial contamination of tubes and bulk containers. This impurity can be quite difficult to remove. Microscopic collections of brown-stained bacteria are scattered over the stained section, as seen in Figure 3.7. To prevent this unwanted artefact from happening again, exclusive use of one-litre bottles of sterile water for irrigation is employed on the Bond instrument at Children's Hospital Westmead.

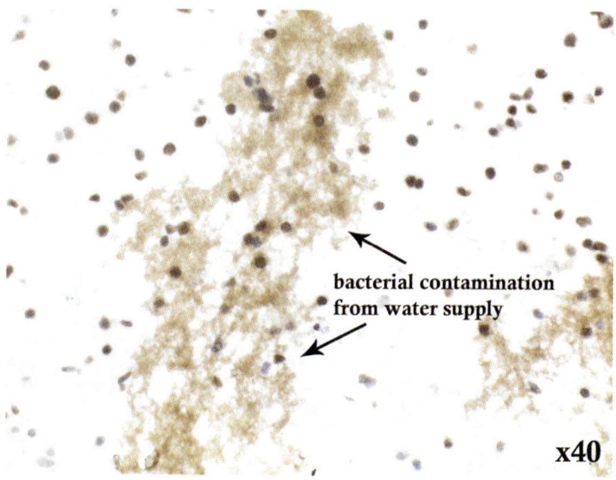

Figure 3.7 Immunohistochemical staining artefact due to contaminated water used in wash buffer preparation

Antigen Retrieval on the Bond

Historically many epitopes were successfully localized in tissue without the need for prior treatment. Examples include S100 protein, prostatic acid phosphatase, insulin and growth hormone. There are antigens, however, which require a retrieval treatment to render the antigens recognizable by their relevant antibodies. Success was achieved using enzymes trypsin and pronase for cytokeratins AE1/AE3, CD68, and factor VIII. Since the early 1990s HIER has become commonplace and allowed the successful demonstration of many more antigens that were unable to be demonstrated in FFPE sections. Shi and colleagues (1991) described the novel method of using a microwave oven to heat slides in a saturated lead thiocyanate solution. The retrieval of certain antigens is pH and solution component dependent. For example, the optimal HIER regimen for factor 13a is citrate buffer pH 6 since EDTA pH 9 buffer will not work.

The Bond offers two types of buffers for HIER. Epitope retrieval 1 (ER1) is a pH 6.0 citrate-based buffer and epitope retrieval 2 (ER2) is a pH 9.0 EDTA-based solution for HIER. The programmable temperature range is 35°C to 100°C and the time limit for incubation can be set for between 5 and 45 minutes. Along with the enzyme pretreatment kit containing proteinase K, these are the three main reagents available for antigen retrieval on the Bond instrument. Epitope retrievals 1 and 2 are ready to use and require direct transfer to their corresponding bulk containers. The enzyme, however, requires prior mixing of the proteinase K with TRIS buffer into a Bond open container included with the kit. The enzyme kit supplies a choice of three different working strengths.

With many tissues, excessive microwaving during epitope retrieval can destroy antigenicity and morphology. It may result in HIER lipofuscin pigment artefacts. Yaziji and Barry (2006) identified a 'microwave burn' pattern in loose connective tissue and fat. The degree of deterioration is possibly related to the fixation time, being more pronounced in minimally fixed tissues. Children's Hospital Westmead uses a routine 20-minute retrieval setting at 100°C in either ER1 or ER2 (depending on the antibody) for small

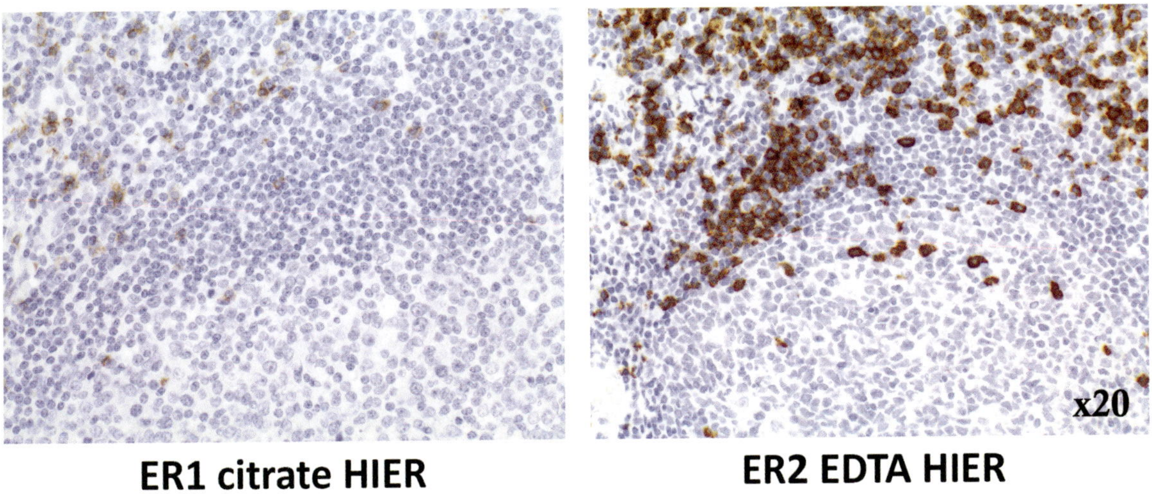

Figure 3.8 Tonsil CD8 immunohistochemistry at citrate-low pH and EDTA high-pH heat-induced epitope retrieval

biopsies that have been fixed for 6 to 8 hours. For larger blocks fixed for 24 hours or more, the retrieval time is often extended to 30 minutes or more.

The appropriate antigen retrieval is different from antigen to antigen and therefore antibody to antibody. These parameters are established at the antibody validation stage and should be determined individually for each antigen and antibody. Figure 3.8 demonstrates the improved immunolocalization for CD8 with pH 9.0 EDTA HIER (ER2) compared to pH 6.0 citrate HIER (ER1). Kim and colleagues (2016) recommended that enzymatic retrieval or no retrieval in addition to HIER be trialled initially during antibody optimization.

Localization Antibodies

Localization antibodies are commonly referred to as primary antibodies. These antibodies direct the precise position of epitope site within tissue sections and are accessed in several ways on the Bond III. Leica have a range of ready-to-use (RTU) antibodies in packaged containers. These reagents are provided in concentrations optimized by the vendor for the Bond system. The RTU antibodies only require registration into the Bond software before use. Lot numbers, expiry dates and other important parameters are recorded upon registration, contributing to the overall laboratory quality system.

Leica also supply 'open containers' for when the user opts to titre from an antibody concentrate. User-supplied concentrates are necessary for when an RTU of a localization antibody is not available from Leica. These open containers are available in 7 mL and 30 mL varieties and can be refilled until a total maximum of 40 mL of reagent has been delivered. Only one reagent can be used for each container.

The last container type available is the titration container, and each houses a 6 mL removal test tube. They are available within the Bond titration kit, which consists of 10 empty containers and 50 (6 mL) inserts. These containers are designed to be used in the validation of new antibodies from concentrates for determination of optimum titre as well as for research testing where limited antibody is available. Small volumes of each primary antibody concentration can be prepared and placed into the inserts. Each container may be used for a total of 40 mL of reagent.

The aspiration probe cannot reach the bottom of the container. There is always a residual volume in each container that the probe is unable to reach. This volume is referred to as 'dead volume', and it is different for each type of container. Dead volume for a 7 mL open container is 555 μL. For 30 mL vials, it is 1,618 μL vial and for titration tubes, it is 200 μL. In practical terms, the Bond III logs that these containers are empty even though some reagent is still present.

Localization Antibody Optimum Titre on the Bond

To keep things simple, titration of concentrated antibodies can be achieved using serial twofold dilutions. The containers of the titration kit can be programmed into the Bond system with the titles: OT A, OT B, OT C etc. Alternatively, a set of titration containers labelled with 1:50, 1:100, 1:200, 1:400 etc. may also be utilized. These containers require specific conditions as to dewax, retrieval settings, detection kit incubation time, temperature parameters etc., when setting up to titre a new primary antibody. A 6 mL insert is placed in each container labelled A onwards to cover all dilutions used. Label each tube with the container ID (e.g. A), titre and antibody name.

There is no definitive set approach when validating new antibodies and it depends on a variety of factors. Using RTU antibodies certified for *in vitro* diagnostic (IVD) use as opposed to concentrates for research use only (RUO) will influence the end protocol. The quality of information contained within the manufacturer's specification sheet can also impact the validation process. The validation strategy itself can range from simple to more complicated affairs. For instance, some laboratories run validation studies testing the new antibody with both low- and high-pH buffers as well as enzyme pretreatments at varying antibody dilutions all at once. Others take a two-stage approach, finding the suitable retrieval parameters first and then refining the antibody dilution until the final protocol is decided. The Bond software is capable of accommodating a range of validation methods the end user specifies.

Table 3.1 specifies a twofold or double-dilution strategy. Starting off with the recommended immunohistochemistry dilution given by the manufacturer, continue doubling the dilution until a final titre is reached. For example, if a 1:100 dilution is recommended, place 1 mL of diluent in tube A and 500 μL in each of the remaining tubes. Add 10 μL of antibody concentrate into tube A, mix using the vortex mixer, remove 500 μL from tube A and add to tube B, mix and continue until the last tube is reached. The last tube should contain 1 mL of solution. Remember there is 200 μL of dead volume in each tube, which leaves 300 μL reagent in each tube (except the last tube) available. The Bond uses 150 μL per slide.

At Children's Hospital Westmead, initially all of the localization antibodies were prepared in house from concentrates with dilution and assay conditions chosen from validated manual methods. Integrating the Bond platform into the laboratory meant that for each antibody, selected tissues initially used for optimization and verification were used again to obtain equivalent staining between manual and automated systems. The two major findings from the Bond trial were that validation antibodies could be used at a higher dilution and the Bond demonstration system afforded improved consistency of IHC staining.

When clinical need required the introduction of new antibodies, the department soon realized there was an advantage in using Bond RTU antibodies when available. The RTUs are optimized and certified *in vitro* diagnostic (IVD) for use by Leica, conferring consistent and accurate staining. There is now greater emphasis from laboratories on standardizing pre-analytical factors such as tissue fixation and processing such that equivalent inter-institutional staining results are achievable with RTU antibodies. Leica promotes these preparations worldwide, confident that these antibodies are fit for purpose on the Bond IHC platform. Using identical clones but switching from concentrates to RTUs was a valuable exercise. Again, the advantages of inter-laboratory consistency, accurate titre and the notification of expiry dates goes a long way to providing continuous quality staining. There is also the fact that these RTUs help the laboratory meet quality assurance requirements.

Bond Polymer Detection Kits

Several detection kits are available for the Bond. Recommended for routine diagnostic IHC are kits based on the enzyme conjugated polymer system. These polymer-based detection systems are designed to work on unlabelled localization antibodies, otherwise known as primary antibodies. Depending on the species the primary antibody is derived from, a post-primary linker antibody may be employed before introducing a dextran polymer to which are bound large numbers

Table 3.1 Twofold dilution strategy

Tube	A	B	C	D	E	F	...
Diluent	1 mL	0.5 mL	0.5 mL	0.5 mL	0.5 mL	0.5 mL	...
Antibody	10 μL	0.5 mL (from A)	0.5 mL (from B)	0.5 mL (from C)	0.5 mL (from D)	0.5 mL (from E)	...
Titre	1:100	1:200	1:400	1:800	1:1600	1:3200	...

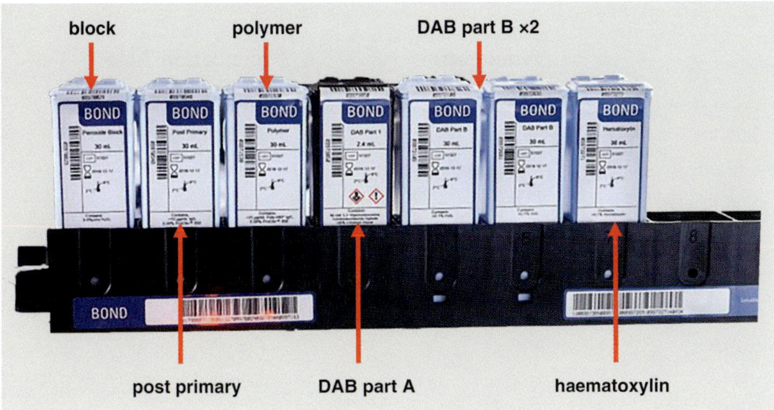

Figure 3.9 Leica's polymer detection kit for the diaminobenzidine tetrahydrochloride hydrate chromogen

Reproduced with permission Leica Biosystems Melbourne, Pty, Ltd.

of peroxidase and antibody molecules to bind to the unlabelled primary or linker antibody (Yaziji and Barry 2006).

A major component of the Bond Polymer Refine kit is a rabbit anti-mouse IgG linker called the post primary. This is for detection of mouse (and rat) localization antibodies. Figure 3.9 shows the complete kit with the protein polymer linked to multiple enzyme molecules and multiple anti-rabbit IgG molecules. The anti-rabbit antibodies located on the polymer bind to rabbit localization antibodies as well as any rabbit anti-mouse linker antibodies bound to the mouse primary antibodies used. To summarize, for IHC assays using a mouse primary antibody, there is a three-layer approach – the mouse localization antibody, the post-primary rabbit anti-mouse linker and the polymer with the peroxidase and anti-rabbit antibodies. For assays using a rabbit primary antibody, there are only two layers – the rabbit localization antibody and the polymer with peroxidase and anti-rabbit antibodies. At present, polymer-based IHC solutions are preferred over avidin-biotin systems because biotin blocking is unnecessary and negative reagent controls are no longer required if using polymer-based detection systems according to the College of American Pathologists (Marsch et al. 2015).

Leica have two enzyme systems available for chromogenic IHC labelling. They include peroxidase matched with 3,3'-diaminobenzidine tetrahydrochloride hydrate (DAB) and alkaline phosphatase using Fast Red. Rounding out the refine kit is an appropriate endogenous enzyme-blocking reagent (for peroxidase) as well as a haematoxylin nuclear counterstain. Blocking for endogenous alkaline phosphatase activity is not required for FFPE tissue since the enzyme is rendered inactive after tissue processing.

Bond-Staining Protocols

In the Bond software, protocols are the series of steps performed to stain tissue samples. Protocols are divided into pre-staining and staining sections. The stages of bake and dewax, HIER and enzyme pretreatment are the pre-staining steps. For *in situ* hybridization, it is the denaturation and hybridization process. Staining protocol section includes the localization antibody and the detection steps for both single and double sequential staining as well as *in situ* hybridization detection.

When a new antibody is registered to be used on the Bond III, a preferred protocol (both pre-staining and staining) is nominated and chosen for the antibody. This covers all the necessary steps (bake and dewax, enzyme pretreatment, HIER and staining) to produce the IHC stain. The emphasis here is to select the correct protocol with the most appropriate parameter settings for each localization antibody.

Each staining protocol is designed to be used on a particular Bond detection system. The Bond has a selection of protocol templates, each prefixed with a star (*) character. For example, the *IHC Protocol F is designed to use the Bond Polymer Refine Detection kit (DS9800), whereas the *IHC Protocol H is for the Oracle HER2 IHC system. Each staining protocol includes appropriate blocking steps, localization antibody incubation time and temperature and counterstains. The software allows users to copy

Table 3.2 *IHC Protocol F at Children's Hospital Westmead

Step	Reagent	Temperature	Incubation Time
1	Peroxide block	Ambient	5 min
2	Bond wash solution	Ambient	3 rinses
3	Localization antibody	Ambient	15 min
4	Bond wash solution	Ambient	3 rinses
5	Post primary	Ambient	8 min
6	Bond wash solution	Ambient	3 rinses 6 min total
7	Polymer	Ambient	8 min
8	Bond wash solution	Ambient	4 rinses 6 min total
9	Deionized water	Ambient	Rinse
10	Mixed DAB refine	Ambient	10 min
11	Deionized water	Ambient	3 rinses
12	Hematoxylin	Ambient	5 min
13	Deionized water	Ambient	Rinse
14	Bond wash solution	Ambient	Rinse
15	Deionized water	Ambient	Rinse

protocol templates and rename them to local conventions. For example, *IHC Protocol F (Bond Polymer Refine IHC) can be copied and renamed DAB Polymer FFPE. The protocol steps can then be modified to suit local conditions as defined by the end user after appropriate validation. Table 3.2 shows the routine IHC protocol based on *IHC Protocol F for FFPE tissue at Children's Hospital Westmead.

This protocol, specific for mouse primary antibodies, includes 35 minutes slide drying, dewaxing and 20 minutes antigen retrieval. The combined staining time from start to finish is approximately 2.5 hours. For routine diagnostic IHC on FFPE tissue, this staining time is acceptable. It becomes even more advantageous when a tray of 10 slides can be batched and stained in 2.5–3 hours. Loading a full 30 slides at once may prolong the overall staining times but still be within acceptable limits. The exact amount of time depends on the different protocols being run concurrently. This gain in efficiency over manual methods also makes IHC assays easier to manage.

The versatility of the Bond IHC platform allows logical modification of the protocols. The following are variations that have been used in some laboratories.

Flippin Protocol

For most antibodies, blocking of endogenous enzyme activity should generally be performed after HIER and before primary antibody incubation. Marsch and colleagues (2015) found that antibodies with membranous staining patterns such as CD3 and CD31 are very sensitive to endogenous blocking procedures. And in these cases, the investigators suggest the blocking step be relocated to after the primary antibody incubation.

The Flippin Protocol addresses this issue and is an edited version of *IHC Protocol F. The peroxidase block step before the antibody has been deleted and is inserted after the localization antibody application step. Pax-5 clone 1EW and AMACR are two specific antibodies that require the Flippin Protocol. This strategy has also been used to clean up background staining that commonly occurs with antibodies to Helicobacter pylori.

Immunofluorescence Protocol

Matt Collier from New Zealand has shared an ingenious way to use the Bond to perform direct immunofluorescence (DIF). First, a used kit is required and obtained from another Bond laboratory. Any kit will suffice because an empty used kit from another laboratory will be recognized as a new kit by the Bond software in your facility. This is the critical point. The other key aspect is that for any protocol created, at least one step from the original kit must be used. Table 3.3 highlights a protocol obtained from a donated used kit. Note the Bond software thinks the original peroxide block step (which contains buffer

Table 3.3 Direct immunofluorescence protocol

Step	Reagent	Supplier	Incubation (min)
1	Peroxide block	Leica Microsystems	1.00
2	Bond wash solution	Leica Microsystems	0:00
3	Bond wash solution	Leica Microsystems	0:00
4	Bond wash solution	Leica Microsystems	0:00
5	MARKER	Leica Microsystems	25:00
6	MARKER	Leica Microsystems	20:00
7	Bond wash solution	Leica Microsystems	0:00
8	Bond wash solution	Leica Microsystems	0:00
9	Bond wash solution	Leica Microsystems	0:00

wash) from the donated kit is used. It has been 'tricked' into making this step another buffer wash process. In practical terms, each container must be thoroughly rinsed and filled with Bond wash solution.

As is standard for DIF on frozen sections, the dewax and retrieval steps are unnecessary. A choice of titration or open containers can be employed for each FITC-conjugated antibody. Figure 3.10 illustrates IgG immunological deposit seen in bullous skin lesions demonstrated with DIF.

It is interesting to consider the appropriate optimum dilution of the FITC-labelled antibodies. A common across-the-board dilution is 1:10, and this has often been quoted in the literature. Dilutions up to 1:50 have also been used, although dilutions are often not recorded in many publications. One wonders whether many of the dilutions have been determined empirically and were based on historical data (Henwood 2019a).

Immunostaining Cytology Preparations Using the Bond

Immunohistochemistry on cytology specimens are common and have been successfully achieved using the Bond platform. Cytology smears occur when cellular material is smeared or deposited directly onto slides. Each smear is unique and non-reproducible whereas cell blocks aggregate fixed cytology material into a medium such as agar or thrombin clot and routinely processed to a wax block. Similar to FFPE tissue blocks, multiple sections can be obtained for IHC.

Cytology Smears

Applying cells onto glass slides can be done in a number of ways. A direct smear is the simplest method often performed manually and can be either air-dried or ethanol fixed. The yield of diagnostic cells may be low. To increase the chances of obtaining adequate cell populations, cytocentrifugation of the sample is employed in order to concentrate cells into a 'cytospin'. A suitable alternative to cytospun samples is the liquid-based thin-layer preparations marketed as 'ThinPrep' or 'SurePath'. Although the Bond IHC platform can be used to immunostain these preparations, there are issues with appropriate positive controls and acceptable validations of these procedures (Fischer et al. 2014). It is advisable to target a small number of diagnostically useful antibodies and validate them on cases as they appear in the department and record the results as an ongoing verification study. A reliance on accumulated experience to support the validation of these antibodies for cytology smears is the best approach.

Care needs to be taken with preparation paying attention to thickness of the material and fixation. Cytocentrifuge preparations work well using adhesive slides. Avoid slides with a raised circle that is used to mark the area of the centrifuged cells since this raised circle disrupts the flow of reagent during the staining procedure. Successful IHC stains have been achieved with 95% ethanol fixed smears and cytospins particularly with intermediate filaments such as desmin and cytokeratins (Anderson et al. 2007). Figure 3.11 shows a rhabdomyosarcoma labelled with desmin.

Happerfield and colleagues (2008) optimized antibodies to haemopoietic antigens on air-dried smears and cytospins. They found that fixation at room temperature in an acetone/methanol/formalin mixture (19:19:2 for 90 seconds) gave the best combination of morphological and antigenic preservation for a large range of antibodies. These investigators also

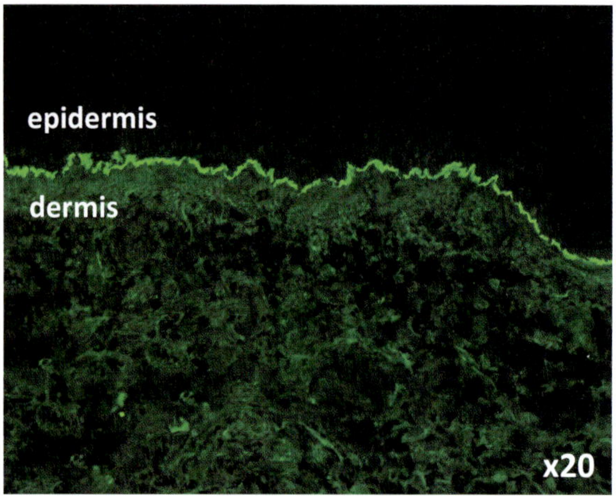

Figure 3.10 Immunoglobulin deposit within the epidermal/dermal junction in a bullous skin lesion

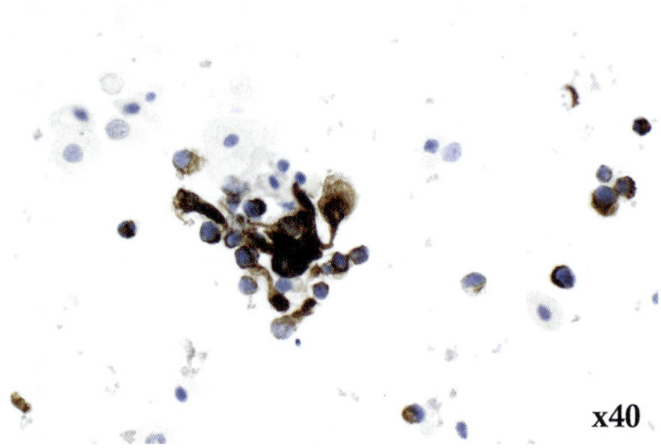

Figure 3.11 Desmin immunohistochemistry showing rhabdomyosarcoma in urine cytospin and fixed with 95% ethanol

recommended the use of alkaline phosphatase labelling since peroxidase labelling gave a high background due to the high level of endogenous peroxidase found in red blood cells and granulocytes.

Cell Blocks

This type of preparation closely mimics the routine FFPE samples usually immunostained on the Bond and other automated platforms. These are commonly known as 'cell blocks' or 'cell buttons' and are centrifuged preparations of liquid samples such as pleural fluids and bronchial washings. A cell pellet is produced that is formalin fixed and routinely processed to wax. These cell pellets can also be incorporated into a clot with plasma and thromboplastin or dispersed in molten agar and allowed to cool and set before processing to paraffin wax. A known issue with plasma-thrombin preparations is increased background staining caused by the unmasking of rabbit immunoglobulins present in the rabbit brain thromboplastin used in the preparation of the cell blocks. Another source of spurious staining is the possible antigen degradation due to excessive heat used to melt the agar. Figure 3.12 shows decreased staining intensity due to overheating agar in cell block preparations. There are also commercial systems such as Cellient that produce cell blocks. When using commercial kits, it is important to note the fixative type since many of these commercial systems use an alcohol-based fixative that may require adjustments to the immunohistochemical staining protocol (Gomes et al. 2008; Kruger et al. 2014; Sauter et al. 2016).

Double Labelling with the Bond

Multiple IHC staining requires careful analysis and considerable knowledge to obtain true, robust and reliable results. You can't go at it like a bull at a gate. As Chan and colleagues (2011) have implied, double staining using standard IHC needs histotechnologists who possess significant expertise and who are capable of undertaking complex histological laboratory techniques.

Chris van de Loos and Peter Teeling (2008) remarked: 'a truly generally applicable double chromogenic staining method that allows for the visualization of co-localization (two markers present at one cellular location, yielding a mixed colour) does not exist'. There is more chance of success if the two targets exist in different compartments of the cell (i.e. nuclear, cytoplasm, cell membrane or extracellular). Each attempt at double (multiplex) IHC staining must be done on a case-by-case basis. The nature of the antibodies, the proposed combination, FFPE or fresh frozen sections and chromogenic or fluorescent labels all need to be considered as these factors determine the overall strategy. In general terms, there are two main approaches: classified as either simultaneous or sequential techniques for double IHC staining.

Simultaneous (Parallel) Double Immunohistochemical Staining

Simultaneous multiple labelling immunohistochemistry, also known as parallel IHC staining, requires the two localization antibodies to be raised in different species or at least to be of different immunoglobulin

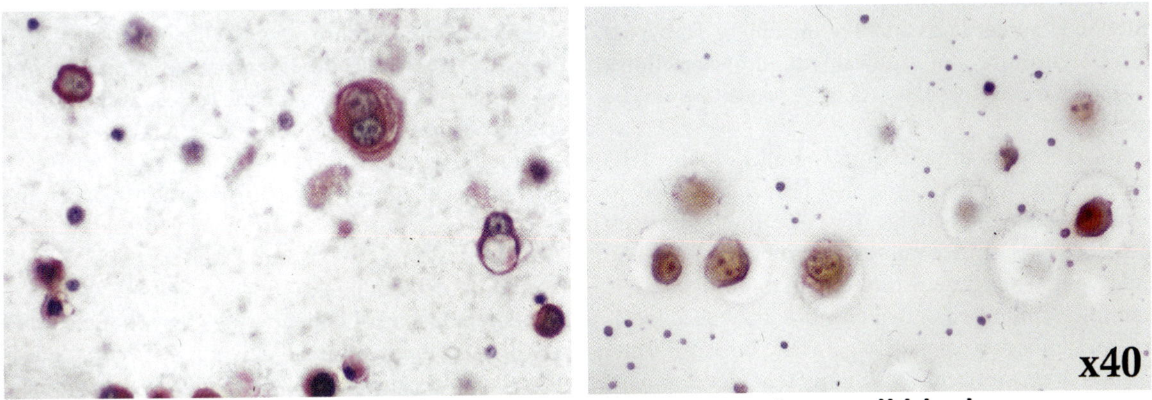

Figure 3.12 CEA immunohistochemistry (alkaline phosphatase) cell block preparations of adenocarcinoma in pleural fluid

isotypes if developed in the same species. This is to avoid cross-reactivity between the detection systems used to visualize the signals (Pirici et al. 2009). Usually, fewer problems occur if the bridging (linker) antibodies are of the same species. One such example would be a mouse anti-CD20 with peroxidase labelled goat anti-mouse, combined with a rabbit anti-CD3 with phosphatase labelled goat anti-rabbit. A common diagnostic application based on this theory is the IHC double stain to differentiate prostate carcinoma from prostate intraepithelial neoplasia and benign mimic lesions. An antibody cocktail containing monoclonal mouse anti-human CK 34ßE12 and monoclonal mouse anti-human CK 5/6 along with monoclonal rabbit anti-human AMACR is commonly applied.

For simultaneous double IHC staining, the Bond III system uses *IHC protocol K and the 'chromoplex 1 dual detection' kit. Essentially the end user provides the antibody cocktail which must contain one mouse and one rabbit origin. Pre-staining parameters for the antibody cocktail such as HIER must be determined. The kit is centred on the mouse localization (primary) antibody being matched to peroxidase-based DAB chromogen and the rabbit localization antibody paired to alkaline phosphatase-based Fast Red chromogen. The order of chromogenic development is DAB chromogen first followed by Fast Red. The main reason for this is DAB chromogen, when used to label peroxidase activity for the first staining sequence has been found quite effective in 'shielding' the first staining sequence. The brown DAB reaction product covers the first localization and labelling antibodies so well that reagents from the second detection system can no longer react with components from the first staining sequence (Sternberger and Joseph 1979). This shielding has been found effective only if the first localizing antibody is optimally titrated. To date, DAB is the only known enzymatic reaction product that shows this unique sheltering characteristic (Van der Loos and Teeling 2008; Pirici et al. 2009).

The DAB can also mask antigens close to the first antigen, causing binding failure of the second localization antibody. This is the reason it is best to target different tissue compartments when using double-staining applications that use DAB as a chromogen. The DAB prevents the binding of a second antibody at the same site. For example, take two nuclear antibodies such as Ki67 and oestrogen receptor in a double IHC stain on the same tissue section. If the Ki67 was detected using DAB and oestrogen receptor with alkaline phosphatase, the oestrogen receptor positive nuclei could be underrepresented. Another important note to highlight is that mountants such as DPX and Entellan will cause the Fast Red to fade. Leica CV Ultra-mount and some others do not affect the Fast Red chromogen as outlined in the Leica documentation for the dual detection kit.

Sequential Double Immunohistochemical Staining

During simultaneous double IHC staining, it is obvious that in the case of two localization antibodies from the same species, the detection system is able to develop and visualize both localization antibodies, leading to false co-localization attributable to cross-reaction (Van der Loos and Teeling 2008). To bypass this occurrence of unwanted cross-reactions, a sequential multiple IHC staining procedure can be undertaken.

In addition to simultaneous (parallel) double IHC staining, the Bond III can also be programmed to perform sequential double IHC staining. Although the protocol is more complex, it can be a worthwhile endeavour. The strategy of sequential multiplex IHC staining is composed of two or more unlabelled localization antibodies applied separately, one at a time, including chromogenic or fluorescent development independent of each other. That is, the chromogenic reaction or fluorescent label is developed for the first antibody before the assay proceeds with the second antibody and so on.

Proteins, including immunoglobulins, are denatured at high temperatures. As such, antibodies will lose the subtle forces responsible for specific antigen–antibody binding (Kolodziejczyk and Baertschi 1986). This phenomenon is deployed during the intervening heating step to remove the first localization antibody and first linking antibody completely, thus preventing false cross-reaction with the second detection system (Van der Loos and Teeling 2008). The HIER methods with citrate effectively elute bound antibodies from sections and leave behind the bound DAB product (Lan et al. 1995; Ikeda et al. 2011). One further advantage of HIER treatment is the ability to permanently destroy enzymatic activity within peroxidase and alkaline phosphatase complexes (Lan et al. 1995).

Tornehave and colleagues (2000) suggested the use of microwave for double sequential labelling and reported that moderate microwaving does not elute bound antibodies but rather prevents them from binding to subsequent applied reagents. Ikeda and colleagues (2011) though, showed that the heat inactivation time differed among localization antibodies, whereas the bridging antibodies and labelled enzymes were inactivated after heating for 10 minutes. They recommend localization antibodies needing a longer inactivation time should be used second in double-immunoenzyme assays in order to avoid a high background. Examples include cytokeratins, CD15, CD20, CD45 and CD68.

Recognizing and differentiating two antigens present at the same site can be used to clarify dilemmas. For example, CD34 stains both vascular and lymphatic endothelial cells whereas D2-40 (Podoplanin) labels lymphatic endothelium only (Williams et al. 2007). Both CD34 and D2-40 clones are of mouse origin. Therefore, to separate lymphatic vessels from vascular vessels within the one tissue section, a sequential double IHC stain can be employed. Using DAB and Fast Red chromogen, the main issue to overcome is matching the correct chromogen to the localization antibody. That is, for each epitope, which antibody detection–chromogen method will give the best result? Remembering that polymerized DAB is quite effective in 'shielding' the first staining sequence and that D2-40 only labels lymphatics, stain for D2-40 using peroxidase first, followed by CD34 and alkaline phosphatase labelling. Figure 3.13 shows the result of this strategy with brown lymphatic vessels and red capillaries. Reversing the antibody–chromogen combination will result in the DAB brown developed for both capillary and lymphatics with little (if any) red D2-40 labelling.

For situations when one epitope requires retrieval (HIER or enzyme) whereas the other antigen does not, label and stain for the non-pretreatment antigen first. Ikeda and colleagues (2011) recommend labelling nuclear antigens before attempting cytoplasmic epitopes in order to obtain good contrast images. In these settings, a brown nuclear stain using the peroxidase kit first followed with a red cytoplasmic stain from the alkaline phosphatase kit strategy is endorsed. Other considerations which may help include performing the HIER once only if both antibodies require it. A second short five-minute heat retrieval with ER1 is useful after the DAB reaction in order to aid the removing of unbound antibodies. Also, consider using HIER rather than enzyme digestion for antibodies, since this will be less deleterious on morphology. For *in situ* hybridization, consider using ER1 antigen retrieval rather than enzyme digestion reactions. This works well for EBER, and kappa and lambda mRNA *in situ* hybridizations and should work well for other probes.

Bond Quality Control

The Bond system uses a database to record all Bond data including case and slide details, reagents and protocols. These data are critical for the correct operation of the system. All slide and case histories, as well as set protocols, reagent inventories etc., will be lost if

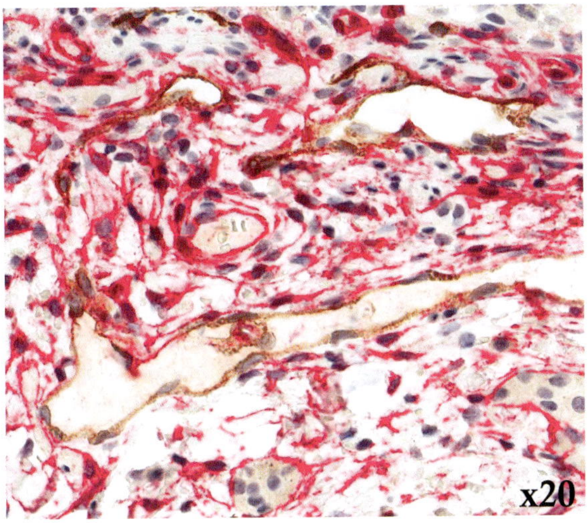

Figure 3.13 Double immunohistochemical staining for D2-40 (brown) and CD34 (red) in appendix tissue

for any reason the database is lost or corrupted. It is thus critically important that the database be well maintained and be backed up regularly. An external USB drive for routine database backup as scheduled by the Bond software is all that is required. By default, a reminder window appears every two weeks.

Ultimate quality control monitoring relies on microscopic assessment of each IHC-stained slide. In line with accepted convention, control sections are placed on the same slide as the test section usually close to the slide label. The quality of IHC performed on FFPE slides is highly dependent on antigen preservation. While antigenicity of tissue within FFPE blocks stored at room temperature is maintained for decades, many studies have demonstrated a loss of antigenicity, or epitope instability, when tissue is sectioned and stored as unstained paraffin slides. The reason for antigenicity loss of stored paraffin sections is unknown; however, multiple sources have been proposed. A rapid decline in antigenicity is seen with slide storage at high temperatures. Blind and colleagues (2008) demonstrated photo-oxidation, secondary to ultraviolet exposure and dry heat increased the rate of stored slide antigenicity decline. Xie and colleagues (2011) suggested hydrolysis of proteins due to inadequate dehydration of the tissue during tissue processing may be an important source of reduced immunoreactivity over time. Personal observations at Children's Hospital Westmead have found the following antigens give weaker reactions in aged sections: BCOR, BOB1, PAX5, CD4, c-MYC, CD30, Bombesin and Parvovirus. Figure 3.14 shows the difference in IHC staining using an identical parvovirus protocol on freshly cut and pre-cut sections.

There have been anecdotal comments within the IHC community about 'capillary artefact' caused by the cover plate technology as used by the Bond and other vendors such as Shandon's 'Sequenza' IHC platform. Essentially, there is a subtle staining gradient observed on the tissue section by way of more intense staining towards the top of the slide and fading near the bottom of the slide that is only noticeable when performing IHC on tissue sections covering most of the glass slide. Although this phenomenon can be visually observed, it doesn't detract from the interpretation of results. At Children's Hospital Westmead, this artefact has not been observed. In addition, we experience a very low error rate from the Bond III. Repeat staining attributed to machine failure is about two slides per year. Repeat staining due to human error and other pre-analytical issues makes up the majority of cases. We have found the Bond a very reliable instrument with few emergency unscheduled repairs (less than one per year).

Maintenance on the Bond

Routine maintenance on the Bond is a relatively straightforward affair and the manual covers this in extensive detail. An important warning is to not use cotton-tipped applicators to clean inside the wash block holes or the slide staining assembly wicking posts, as the cotton tip can come off and cause a blockage which needs an engineer to remove.

When the Bond is turned off and then on, it goes through a priming cycle where liquid from each bulk container is pumped through the instrument. This can use a significant volume of reagent. In light of this, it is recommended that the Bond (including the software) be shut down weekly. This will clear accumulated buffers and lead to better long-term operation of the software and to better system performance. The shutdown process on the Bond is quite easy: turn off the processing module (red switch on right side), close down the Bond software and finally turn off the computer.

In order to protect the instrument from unexpected power surges, it is advisable to use a surge protector and for added protection an uninterrupted power supply (UPS). If power is cut to the hospital during staining, the Bond won't be able to resume

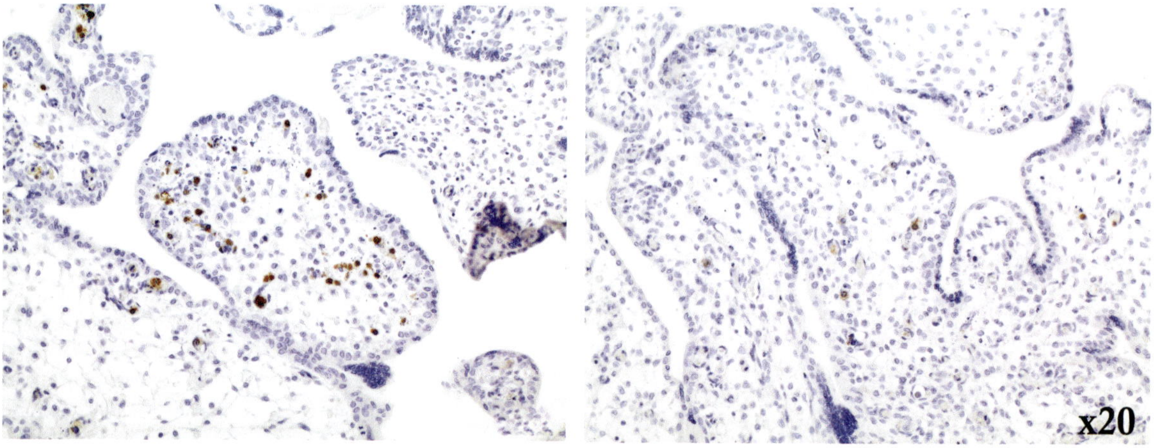

Figure 3.14 Parvovirus immunohistochemistry on fresh cut and pre-cut placental tissue

staining the slides when power is restored. All slides will be lost if there is no UPS backup.

Prior to each run bulk solutions are checked and refilled if needed and bulk waste containers emptied. Try to fill bulk reagents while the bottles are still connected to the machine. Removing the bulk solutions from the instrument will trigger a fluidics prime when they are returned to the instrument.

Conclusion

The Bond III is a reliable, efficient and fully automated instrument for IHC. However, a few enhancements would be useful in future models. Some suggestions that will elevate the Bond platform further include the use of a more environmentally friendly and faster dewax system by using heated detergent; the availability of improved and flexible programs for *in situ* hybridization using user-supplied probes; and the development of a broader range of Leica-validated TGA- and FDA-approved companion diagnostic predictive tests such as BRAF and PD-L1 assays.

The best things about the Bond III when compared to other available IHC platforms include excellent heat control of the heater pads and the fact that the Leica Bond RTU range of antibodies are supported by Novocastra, a highly reputable antibody manufacturer. Other strong points include the relative ease of optimizing new antibodies with programmable titration containers, enzyme retrieval and both EDTA and citrate HIER at differing times and temperatures. The user-friendly and user-intuitive software allows ease of slide programming and routine operations. The quality control of reagents and record of run events is excellent. Finally, Leica offers excellent post-acquisition assistance in terms of service maintenance and applications support. BOND™ is a trademark of Leica Biosystems Melbourne Pty, Ltd.

References

Adeniji AO, Okoh OO, Okoh AI 2017. Analytical methods for the determination of the distribution of total petroleum hydrocarbons in the water and sediment of aquatic systems: A review. *Journal of Chemistry*. Article ID 5178937.

Anderson L, Henwood A, Graf N, Arbuckle S 2007. Diagnosis of pediatric genitourinary embryonal rhabdomyosarcoma by urine cytology. *Acta cytologica*. **51** (3):437–9.

Blind C, Koepenik A, Pacyna-Gengelbach M, Fernahl G, Deutschmann N, Dietel M, Krenn V, Petersen I 2008. Antigenicity testing by immunohistochemistry after tissue oxidation. *J Clin Pathol*. **61**(1):79–83.

Chan A, Matias MAT, Farah CS 2011. A novel and practical method using HRP-polymer conjugate and microwave treatment for visualization of 2 antigens raised from the same or different species in paraffin-embedded tissues. *Appl Immunohistochem Mol Morphol* **19**(4):376–83.

Fischer AH, Schwartz MR, Moriarty AT, Wilbur DC, Souers R, Fatheree L, Booth CN, Clayton AC, Kurtyz DFI, Padmanabhan V, Crothers BA 2014. Immunohistochemistry practices of cytopathology laboratories: A survey of participants in the College of American Pathologists Nongynecologic Cytopathology Education Program. *Arch Pathol Lab Med* **138**(9):1167–72.

Gomes L, Mackie N, Catchpoole D, Henwood T 2008. Test and teach: Immunohistochemistry on 60 year old tissue blocks. *J Histotechnol* **31**(4):183–4.

Happerfield LC, Saward R, Grimwade L, Bloxham D, Erber WN 2008. Automated immunostaining of cell smears: An alternative to flow cytometry. *J Clin Pathol* **61**(6):740–3.

Henwood AF 1981. The localisation of hepatitis B surface antigen by the immunoperoxidase technique. *Aust J Med Lab Sc* **2**:55–60.

Henwood AF 1982. The importance of optimum titre in immunoperoxidase techniques. *Aust J Med Lab Sc* **3** (1):21–7.

Henwood AF 1991. A rapid immunohistochemical stain for Pneumocystis carinii using the Lipshaw Stain Plate. *Aust J Med Lab Sc* **12**:59–61.

Henwood AF 2005. Effect of slide drying at 80°C on immunohistochemistry. *Journal of Histotechnology* **28** (1)45–6.

Henwood AF 2019a. Immunofluorescence. In Cox G, ed. *Fundamentals of fluorescence imaging.* Jenny Stanford; 81–116.

Henwood AF 2019b. *A survival guide for laboratory professionals.* Amazon Create Space Independent Publishing Platform.

Henwood AF, Charlton A 2014. Extraneous epithelial cells from thromboplastin in cell blocks *Cytopathology* **25** (6):412–13.

Hsu SM, Raine L, Fanger H 1981. Use of avidin-biotin-peroxidase complex (ABC) in immunoperoxidase techniques: A comparison between ABC and unlabeled antibody (PAP) procedures. *J Histochem Cytochem* **29**:577–80.

Ikeda K, Suzuki T, Tate G, Mitsuya T 2011. Multiple immunoenzyme labeling using heat treatment combined with the polymer method: An analysis of the appropriate inactivation conditions of primary antibodies. *Acta histochemica* **113**:117–24.

Kim SW, Roh J, Park CS 2016. Immunohistochemistry for pathologists: Protocols, pitfalls, and tips. *J Pathol Transl Med* **50**(6):411–18.

Kolodziejczyk ERIC, Baertschi AJ 1986. Multiple immunolabeling in histology: A new method using thermo-inactivation of immunoglobulins. *J Histochem Cytochem* **34**(12):1725–9.

Kruger AM, Stevens MW, Kerley KJ, Carter CD 2014. Comparison of the Cellient™ automated cell block system and agar cell block method. *Cytopathology* **25**(6):381–8.

Lan HY, Mu W, Nikolic-Paterson DJ, Atkins RC 1995. A novel, simple, reliable, and sensitive method for multiple immunoenzyme staining: Use of microwave oven heating to block antibody Crossreactivity and retrieve antigens. *J Histochem Cytochem* **43**:97–102.

Leong AS 2004. Pitfalls in diagnostic immunohistology. *Adv Anat Pathol* **11**(2):86–93.

Marsch AF, Truong JN, McPherson MM, Junkins-Hopkins JM, Elston DM 2015. A dermatopathologist's guide to troubleshooting immunohistochemistry. Part 2: Troubleshooting immunohistochemical tests in the laboratory. *Am J Dermatopathol* **37**(9):665–79.

Oates J 1993. The effect of temperature on immunostaining. *Br J Biomed Sci* **50**:157–8.

Pileri SA, Roncador G, Ceccarelli C, Piccioli M, Briskomatis A, Sabattini E, Ascani S, Santini D, Piccaluga PP, Leone O, Damiani S, Ercolessi C, Sandri F, Pieri F, Leoncini L, Falini B 1997. Antigen retrieval techniques in immunohistochemistry: Comparison of different methods. *J Pathol* **183**(1):116–23.

Pirici D, Mogoanta L, Kumar-Singh S, Pirici I, Margaritescu C, Simionescu C, Stanescu R 2009. Antibody elution method for multiple immunohistochemistry on primary antibodies raised in the same species and of the same subtype. *J Histochem Cytochem* **57**(6):567–75.

Sauter JL, Grogg KL, Vrana JA, Law ME, Halvorson JL, Henry MR 2016. Young investigator challenge: Validation and optimization of immunohistochemistry protocols for use on cellient cell block specimens. *Cancer Cytopathol* **124** (2):89–100.

Shi SR, Key ME, Kaira KL 1991. Antigen retrieval in formalin-fixed, paraffin-embedded tissues: An enhancement method for immunohistochemical staining based on microwave oven heating of tissue sections. *J Histochem Cytochem* **39**:741–8.

Sternberger LA, Hardy P Jr, Cuculis JJ, Meyer HG 1970. The unlabeled antibody enzyme method of immunohistochemistry: Preparation and properties of soluble antigen-antibody complex (horseradish peroxidase-antihorseradish peroxidase) and its use in identification of spirochetes. *J Histochem Cytochem* **18**:315–33.

Sternberger LA, Joseph SA 1979. The unlabeled antibody method. Contrasting color staining of paired pituitary hormones without antibody removal. *J Histochem Cytochem* **27**(11):1424–9.

Tornehave D, Hougaard DM, Larsson LI 2000. Microwaving for double indirect immunofluorescence with primary antibodies from the same species and for staining of mouse tissues with mouse monoclonal antibodies. *Histochemistry* **113**(1):19–23.

Van der Loos CM, Teeling P 2008. A generally applicable sequential alkaline phosphatase immunohistochemical double staining. *Journal of Histotechnology* **31**(3):119–27.

Williams JH, Mepham BL, Wright DH 1997. Tissue preparation for immunocytochemistry. *J Clin Pathol* **50** (5):422–8.

Williams K, Flanagan A, Folpe A, Thakker R, Athanasou NA 2007. Lymphatic vessels are present in phosphaturic mesenchymal tumours. *Virchows Archiv* **451** (5):871–5.

Xie R, Chung JY, Ylaya K, Williams RL, Guerrero N, Nakatsuka N, Badie C, Hewitt SM 2011. Factors influencing the degradation of archival formalin-fixed paraffin-embedded tissue sections. *J Histochem Cytochem* **59** (4):356–65.

Yaziji H, Barry T 2006. Diagnostic immunohistochemistry: What can go wrong? *Adv Anat Pathol* **13**(5):238–46.

Chapter 4

Automation and Robotics with the Roche Ventana BenchMark ULTRA

Ahida Batrouney

Overview

Immunohistochemistry (IHC) is the process of employing antibodies to recognize epitopes within tissue sections and visualizing the reaction. Automation is the process of programming a machine to perform tasks, thereby reducing human intervention or keeping human operations to a minimum. Contrasted to traditional manual methods, automating IHC provides a higher degree of consistent and reproducible results. Many devices are currently available to automate the IHC process. The level of automation, however, may differ from instrument to instrument even though most IHC machines are centred around reagent placement in sequence onto tissue sections. Robotics of the current generation are 'self-contained all-in-one platforms' that can also execute dewax and epitope retrieval duties whilst monitoring accurate temperature and reagent volumes.

The ability to be 'fully automated' provides numerous advantages. These platforms generate faster turnaround times, permit protocol flexibility and reduce the risk of errors. The Roche Ventana BenchMark ULTRA is one example of a fully automated floor-standing IHC and *in situ* hybridization (ISH) system primarily designed for diagnostic histopathology purposes. Although the BenchMark XT, GX and Discovery systems are also available from Roche, the BenchMark ULTRA seen in Figure 4.1 is the focus of this chapter. Its technology, principle of staining, proprietary reagents, inventory management and system maintenance are explored. Practical aspects of maximizing the number of reagents on board for staining efficiency are outlined whilst covering slide, reagent and waste administration. Other highlights include individual slide drawers, reagent access points (RAPs), liquid coverslip technology and reagent delivery methods. Suggestions are provided to tackle validation procedures for both ready-to-use (RTU) antibodies and concentrates.

The central theme of standardization within IHC and ISH assays has been explored in other chapters. Unsurprisingly, it is also a major consideration here, especially in the future direction of computer-assisted quantitative test evaluation (Cartun et al. 2019). Automation promotes good laboratory practice and helps the IHC facility achieve its quality assurance commitments through system tracking and recording of staining attributes. Parameters such as slide identification, logged reagent lot numbers and temperature errors are examples of important indices because of the increasing diagnostic companion IHC and ISH assays for personalized medicine.

This review is from a user's practical perspective utilizing the BenchMark ULTRA at the Royal Melbourne Hospital (RMH) and is intended to provide valuable information for histology technicians/scientists and laboratory managers considering a viable solution in automating IHC within their diagnostic histology facilities.

Principle of the BenchMark ULTRA

A variety of automation methods are available to detect, localize and visualize epitopes within tissue sections. All forms of instrumentation must deliver specified reagents to tissue sections at a specific time in the protocol with a definite volume in controlled incubation parameters. Roche has employed a few innovative technologies when compared to other vendors. While some manufacturers base reagent utility on cover-plate or dynamic gap expertise, the BenchMark ULTRA employs liquid coverslip (LCS) technology to achieve a strong and specific IHC stain with minimal non-specific background. Other points of difference include the use of a 'hammer' system for reagent delivery instead of conventional aspiration probes, individual slide drawers for complete separation of slide assays and the ability to manually apply primary antibodies.

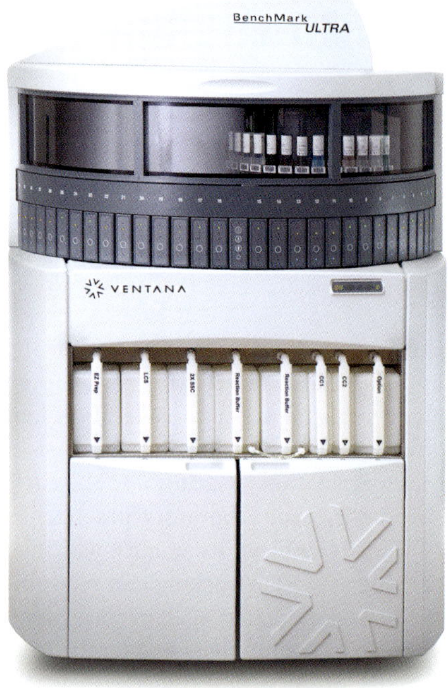

Figure 4.1 Roche Ventana BenchMark ULTRA
Reproduced with permission Ventana Medical Systems Inc.

Apart from the differences highlighted, the BenchMark ULTRA does share common themes with other automated platforms for detecting specific antigens in tissues. The obligatory proprietary reagents for antigen retrieval, buffer wash and detection kits must be used with the instrument. A software package developed by the vendor to execute protocols and monitor IHC performance metrics is also a must, and *in vitro* diagnostic (IVD) companion diagnostic assays approved and certified by the US Food and Drug Administration (FDA) are specifically verified by Roche for the BenchMark ULTRA.

Formalin-fixed paraffin-embedded (FFPE) tissue or cytology cell block preparations on charged 'sticky' slides are the main samples stained on the BenchMark ULTRA. The slides are appropriately labelled with sample identification and stain protocol tracked by the instrument via barcode technology. External control tissue mounted on the same slide as test tissue is standard practice. Cytology smears and frozen tissue sections can also be used, but caution is advised in these situations because these IHC assays have difficult control measures. For instance, using FFPE tissue as control tissue whilst the test is a fresh frozen section is not best practice in a diagnostic setting.

From here on, the basic principles of IHC staining are adhered to with pretreatments for antigen retrieval, application of primary antibodies, blocking endogenous signals, activation of detection kits and counterstain all administered on the instrument. The protocol also includes buffer rinsing steps in between so as to wash residual active reagent off the slide. DNA and RNA probes are used instead of antibodies for ISH assays. Enhancement of the signal is possible using amplification kits. The slides are loaded individually, all required reagents are placed onboard, bulk reagent levels are checked and the instrument is started. The stainer sequentially follows the selected protocol steps, applying the incubation conditions by reading barcoded information on the slide and reagent vials. At the completion of the run, slides are manually removed and coverslipped using post-staining methods appropriate to the protocol detection system used. A personal computer (PC) with Ventana Software System (VSS) drives manages and maintains the system (Ventana 2012).

To a certain degree, the BenchMark ULTRA can also be utilized for research activities staining FFPE sections, cytological preparations or fresh frozen sections. Flexible protocols are achieved with on-board baking, dewaxing, epitope retrieval and a plethora of staining techniques. Methods range from single chromogenic IHC, multiplex IHC, immunofluorescence and ISH techniques. Single and dual hybridization probes are labelled with silver or chromogenically developed for optical light microscopy. The research capabilities are enhanced further with the BenchMark GX and Discovery systems.

The instrument does not generate excessive heat. Any noise generated is for the purpose of prompting action from the operator, certain to get attention when an error message alarm is triggered. It is recommended that the system is connected to an uninterrupted power supply (UPS). A backup battery may be connected to the instrument, providing four to six hours of power in case of an outage, which is enough time for most IHC staining protocols to be finished. Once the BenchMark ULTRA is operating and a protocol is being run, the PC may be shut down or restarted. It is best to exit the Ventana system software before shutting down the computer.

BenchMark ULTRA Components

This IHC and ISH platform is self-contained and floor standing. There is no need for external plumbing to the system. However, adequate floor space is needed to accommodate the physical footprint along with adequate clearance above as the hood opens up 38 cm. The slide drawers open out 10 cm towards the operator and 15 cm is required at the back of the instrument for ventilation. The overall dimensions as given from the manufacturer are 111.76 cm wide x 84.07 cm deep x 158.50 cm high. It weighs just under 300 kg. The BenchMark ULTRA system is comprised of five main parts (Ventana 2012):

(1) Reagent dispensing system and carousel housed under the reagent hood.
(2) Thirty individual slide drawers.
(3) Bulk reagents section located just below the slide drawers.
(4) Two waste containers below the bulk reagents.
(5) Computer, label printer setup and system software.

Reagent Hood and Dispensers

At the top of the instrument is a reagent hood that can be opened to access reagents required for IHC or ISH assays. Figure 4.2 shows the hood opened to expose vials arranged in a circular fashion. There are a total of 35 dispenser positions on the carousel which can quickly fill up as detection kits, enzyme, counterstain and antibodies all need to be housed here. For example, using three different detection systems at the same time will require 16 spots in the carousel, as shown in Table 4.1. Adding enzyme (if required), counterstain, bluing reagent and the three antibodies will use well over half of the spots available. This doesn't leave many places for other antibodies as the capacity of the instrument is 30 slides.

The dispensers containing primary antibodies, enzymes and reagents for detection sit in black trays. Figure 4.3 shows dispensers clipped into position (A) and one being loaded into place (B). Each tray holds up to seven dispensers and five of these trays fit on the carousel, giving a total of 35 spots. The vendor supplies pre-filled dispensers containing antibodies, enzymes, detection kits and counterstains. They are available in volumes ranging from 50 to 250 tests.

The hood can only be opened at certain times as the lid locks automatically when staining protocols are in progress. Access to the carousel to add or remove dispensers as the need arises can be 'booked' as RAPs. The reagent vials are plastic disposable syringe-like dispensers and they clip securely into trays on the carousel. The carousel rotates to align the required reagent dispenser directly above the slide needing the component at the given time. A robotic 'hammer' plunges the dispenser to apply a fixed volume of 100 μl of reagent onto the slide below.

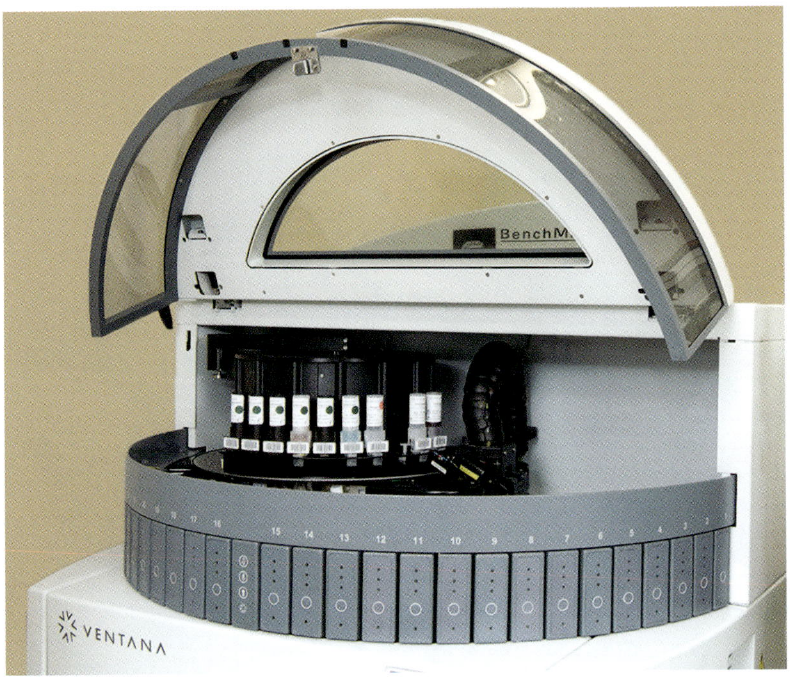

Figure 4.2 Reagent hood opened to reveal dispensers

If two of a particular dispenser or detection kit are on board, they are used in order of their expiry date and number of tests available, respectively. Take for example when there are only 10 tests left in an OptiView detection kit. To run more than 10 IHC assays a new kit is needed. To get the instrument to deplete the old kit before starting the new one, ensure the expiry date of the new one is earlier than the old kit. Otherwise, load 10 slides to use up the low-volume kit and request access to add a new detection kit before loading more slides on the ULTRA. It can be quite tricky to utilize the spaces available in the most efficient way. There must be some planning beforehand, taken on as a challenge by many ULTRA operators. In a busy diagnostic laboratory, batching may not always be an option. One approach employed by laboratories with multiple instruments is to dedicate a number of common antibodies or panels to one instrument, enabling continuous loading of slides. As the RMH offers up to 200 IHC and ISH assays and employs multiple detection systems, the reagent dispenser trays fill up rapidly. The most common panels are for respiratory cases, renal biopsies, breast pathology, brain biopsies and lymphoma investigations. In addition, immunofluorescence panels are available for fresh frozen tissue of mainly renal and skin biopsies. Grouping antibodies into panels may assist with logistics in the dispenser allocation under the reagent hood. Reagent access points are incredibly

Table 4.1 Tray allocation of commonly used reagents on the ULTRA

Reagent vial	Spots required in carousel
OptiView DAB detection kit	6
UltraView Universal DAB detection kit	5
UltraView Universal Alkaline Phosphatase Red detection kit	5
OptiView Amplification kit	3
Enzyme	1
Counterstain	1
Bluing reagent	1
Antibodies – unconjugated	1+
Antibodies – FITC conjugated	1+
ISH iVIEW Blue detection kit + ISH enzyme + counterstain + probe	7+
HER2/Chromosome 17 Dual ISH detection kits + probe + ISH enzyme + Hybready buffer + counterstain	16
Dual IHC detection kits + antibodies + counterstain	15+

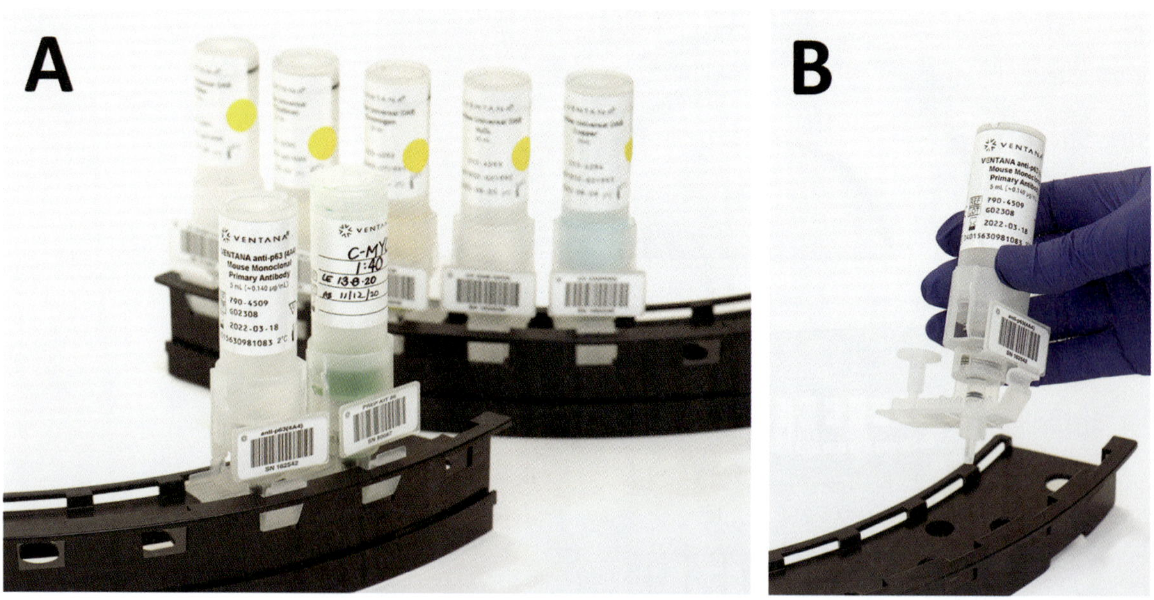

Figure 4.3 Reagent dispensers positioned into trays to be loaded onto the instrument

useful for on-demand loading of slides but they are not always conveniently available.

Reagent delivery to the slide is a rotary automated system via a hammer action. The dispensers resemble a syringe with a spring-loaded nozzle at the bottom for expulsion of solution. The top of the dispenser is flat, facilitating the hammer action as it is brought down to activate the spring, dispensing 100 µl of reagent each time over a slide. This system is vastly different to the conventional aspirating probes commonly employed by other vendors. This mechanism is reliable; however, a couple of limitations have been observed. Dispenser quality and user-related factors are involved in the limitations of this reagent delivery method. As each 'plunge' is a spring-loaded mechanical action from the hammer, the spring mechanism may jam and get stuck, resulting in low or no reagent being expelled whilst some dispensers may expel too much volume. This may occur sporadically, especially with high-volume (250 tests) dispensers. To compensate, Ventana deliberately provides a little extra reagent in each of their RTU dispensers in order to allow for this margin of error. There are instances where a dispenser may be physically exhausted, but the instrument still registers two to three tests left. The operator may accidently press the spring whilst handling the dispenser. A few drops are lost but the instrument does not know this and therefore does not register the volume change. Similarly, there is no mechanism to inspect whether 100 µl has been actually delivered. The instrument registers that the hammer has been engaged and assumes the correct volume has been delivered. It cannot differentiate if the dispenser is faulty or has a sticky spring or if solution is expelled too freely. These are the reasons why it is essential that each dispenser is visually checked before loading onto the instrument carousel.

Fortunately, most of the dispensers are made of clear plastic, allowing the operator to physically observe the remaining volume of solution. It would be easier if all of the reagents in the vials were coloured instead of some being a clear liquid. Light-sensitive reagents are contained in brown opaque dispensers. This includes detection kits and fluorochrome-conjugated antibodies. In this situation, the only way to ascertain if liquid is left in the vial is to gently shake it, listen for the sound of the liquid and prime the dispenser nozzle. Keeping the nozzle of the dispensers clean by removing debris from the tip is also done prior to loading. This is to ensure an accurate volume is dispensed onto the slide. When not in use, reagent dispensers are best stored in the refrigerator with their lids capped so as to prevent evaporation.

Each dispenser has a unique barcode, so the instrument knows the exact location of each dispenser by scanning them individually. At the exact moment, the carousel spins to position the required dispenser over the slide. As no sensors are involved in the reagent delivery system, the instrument performs a physical countdown each time the dispenser is used. For example, when using an RTU antibody dispenser manufactured for 50 tests, the instrument records the first IHC test and acknowledges 49 tests remaining. The countdown continues until zero tests are left or when the antibody has expired, indicating end of life for the reagent.

All reagents, whether they are RTU antibodies, prep kits or bulk fluids, have an expiry date. When this date is reached, the reagent dispenser cannot be used. The instrument will not allow expired dispensers to be loaded even if volume is left in the vial. Some operators would happily use an antibody past its expiration date because they are using appropriate controls, mainly via manual primary antibody application directly onto the slide. Ventana does not recommend this and programmes the instrument accordingly. From the manufacturer's point of view, they can only guarantee their products will work until the expiry date.

User-fillable dispenser prep kits are available in 50, 100 and 250 test volumes. They expire 18 months after container registration and are primarily used for automating RTU antibodies purchased from other manufacturers or antibody concentrates diluted in house with Ventana antibody diluent. A prep kit number is registered via its data button and its corresponding barcode is stuck to the dispenser in order to identify the antibody. These user-fillable prep kits are not necessary if RTU reagents are purchased from Ventana or if the operator wants to manually titrate the primary antibody directly onto the slide.

Slide Drawers

Located below the carousel are 30 separate slide drawers lined up next to each other in a semicircle arrangement. Each slide is housed individually in its own drawer which can be opened independent of the other drawers. Slides can be loaded and placed in

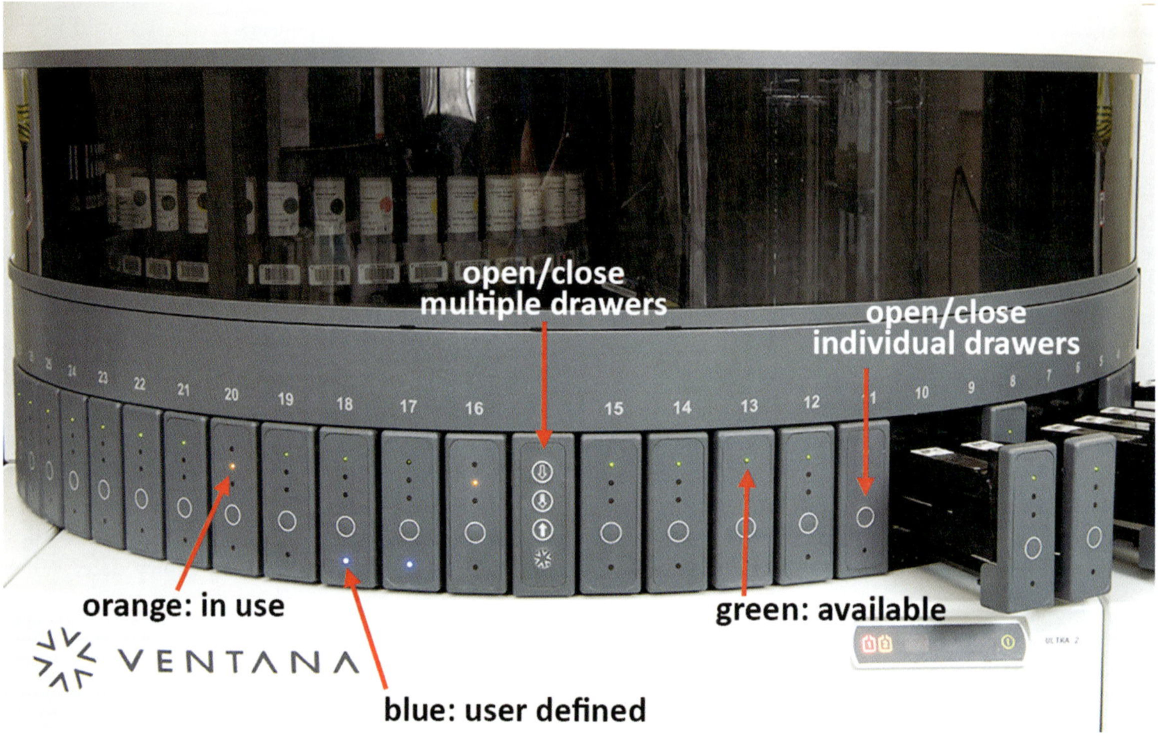

Figure 4.4 The slide drawer with indicating LED colours

any position in any order. This arrangement allows for quick, ready access to slides and for either batch staining or individual on-demand continuous loading. Each drawer has an individual thermo pad and PC board, which allows precise temperature control during protocols. It takes three minutes for the heater pads to increase from room temperature to 98°C. Light-emitting diodes (LEDs) on each drawer indicate activity and drawer availability (Ventana 2012). Figure 4.4 shows a green LED to indicate an available drawer. Orange means it is occupied. The user can direct a blue light to indicate something special about that position. Perhaps the slide is urgent and needs to be unloaded as soon as it is finished.

There is also a slide control panel in the centre situated between slide positions 15 and 16. This is used to open or close slide drawers to add or remove slides which can also be done using a similar panel on the VSS. Rounding out this section is an instrument panel located on the right side below the slide drawers, displaying instrument status with lit icons.

The slide drawers open out to the front of the instrument for loading with the section face up and label end towards the centre of the instrument as shown in Figure 4.5. Posts are positioned at the foot and top of the slide pad to guide the slide edge against and centre the slide in the drawer. The bottom edge of the slide sits against the posts at the foot of the slide pad. When the slide moves off the slide pad due to a broken post, the drawer is effectively faulty and needs to be replaced. The slide is detected with a sensor followed by a barcode reader to initiate staining protocols, only if the instrument has all the necessary reagents loaded. The same sensor can also detect if a slide moves off the heater pad or was positioned incorrectly and will pause as an alarm is registered for operator intervention. This requires opening of the drawer, repositioning of the slide between the posts and closing the drawer to continue staining. It is possible to add more slides on demand without disturbing any of the other slides already loaded. A slide should be added only when all required reagents for the protocol have been loaded.

As there are no 'trays' to contend with, each slide submitted is its own assay independent of other slides on the same machine. Individual slide staining prevents physical cross-contamination from one slide to another. If a piece of tissue floats off, it will be simply

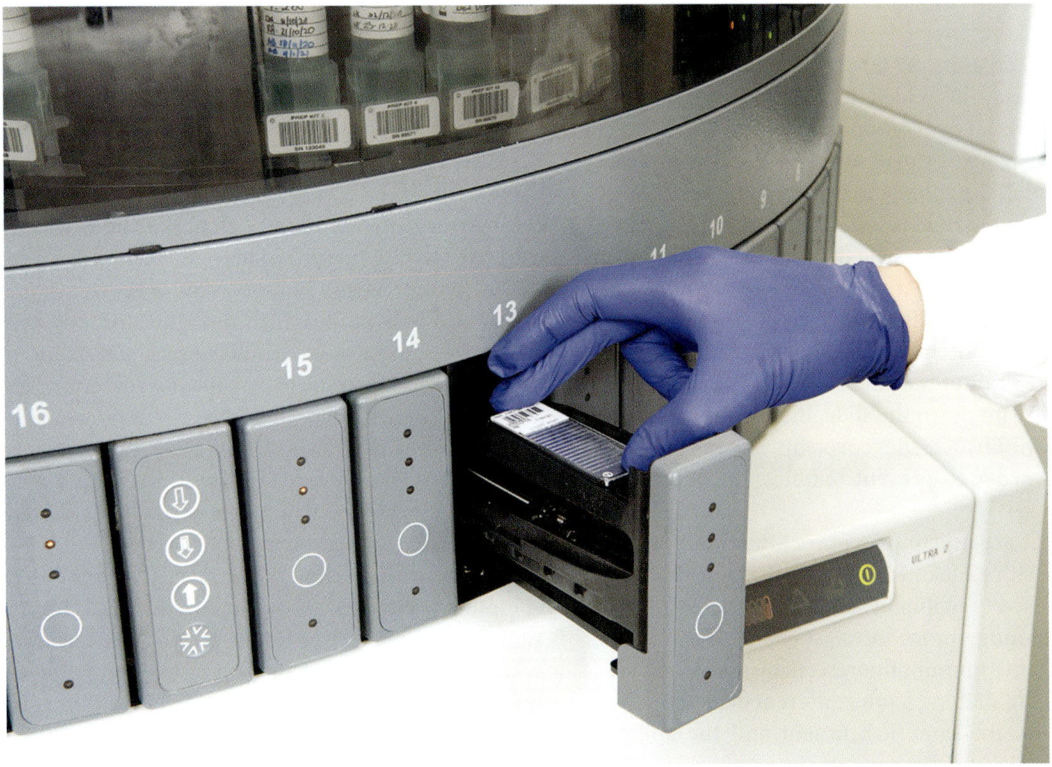

Figure 4.5 Loading slide into the drawer

drained away. Thus there is an elimination of contamination risk during this analytical stage. However, it doesn't guarantee a risk-free environment as 'floaters' may manifest during the pre-analytical stage. Areas such as 'macro cutup' (grossing), embedding and microtomy are common sites for 'carry-over' contaminants reaching the tissue block or tissue section.

Slides recommended for the BenchMark ULTRA are 'standard' 25 x 75 mm or 26 x 76 mm positively charged 'sticky' slides. Commercially available slides for IHC include Superfrost Plus, Matsunami or Trajan series 2 or 3. Slide properties such as cleanliness, date of expiry and appropriate storage conditions are attributes which affect the staining quality. An often forgotten parameter when troubleshooting IHC problems, factors which help the even distribution of the staining reagents and slide surface chemistry are equally important as the quality of the antibodies. Best practice is to freshly cut 3 µm test sections on new charged slides and to use pre-cut control slides as quickly as possible. Avoid double-dipping slides into the water bath or double baking slides in the 60°C oven. Slide baking temperature and duration prior to staining may also affect the staining results. Rapidly rubbing charged slides onto a laboratory coat sleeve in an attempt to clean them may effectively 'discharge' them, losing the 'sticky' properties required for IHC protocols. Optimal slides to use for IHC purposes ensure tissue adhesion during antigen retrieval procedures and even distribution of reagent volume and efficient mixing on the slide surface.

Ventana have the EBAR system for printing slide labels. One label kit contains 2,700 labels (5 rolls, 520 labels per roll) whilst the print ribbon is used for 8,100 labels. The label can be described as a regular slide label with the addition of a transparent plastic flap affixed to the label after the printing is completed. This overlay renders the labels solvent resistant by repelling oil- and water-based solutions. The barcode labels contain the protocol information and identification details. The label also has a special function of acting as a border for the LCS and staining reagents to flow to. This maintains accurate reagent volume and staining on the slide. Great care must be taken with placement of the label onto the slide; it should be applied to the frosted end of the slide. The transparent flap needs to be pressed down, perfectly smooth, without any creases or air bubbles. Handwritten information may be added to the label before the clear protective layer is smoothed down. The lifting of the label edge will cause solutions to flow underneath, changing the volume dynamics on the slide and thus impacting the final result. This may appear trivial, but suboptimally applying the slide label can cause many issues such as patchy staining and loss of time and money. Care is also taken with post-staining procedures. Do not leave labelled slides in xylene longer than 15 minutes as the label will lift, directing the glue to stream down the slide, interfering with the coverslipping. Ensure the coverslip edge is below the label in order to prevent bubbles and lifting as the slide dries.

Slides that are urgent or require attention may be highlighted with a blue LED light on the slide drawer. This is also used to highlight slides that require different post-staining procedures such as Fast Red chromogen and immunofluorescence-stained slides. Individual slide staining allows different detection kits to be used on the same instrument and the ability to add urgent slides or late sample arrivals can be accommodated, improving workflow flexibility if all required reagents have been preloaded on the instrument.

Bulk Reagents

The bulk reagents are found below the slides within a cabinet. Highlighted in Figure 4.6, there are seven different bulk reagents housed in internal reservoirs and external bulk bottles. Including the antibody and detection kits, these bulks are all the reagents required to run IHC and ISH tests. Facing the instrument, from left to right, there is EZ prep, ULTRA LCS (with a fail-safe connection to prevent mixing oil with aqueous solutions), SSC buffer for ISH assays, reaction buffer x2 with a connecting balance tube that allows shared buffer between two carboys, ULTRA CC1, ULTRA CC2 or filled with reaction buffer if CC2 is not needed and Option bulk for SISH or fill with buffer if Option is not needed. The use of Roche proprietary reagents is compulsory as they are optimized by the manufacturer for use on the BenchMark ULTRA. This also gives the manufacturer a chance to confer distinctive

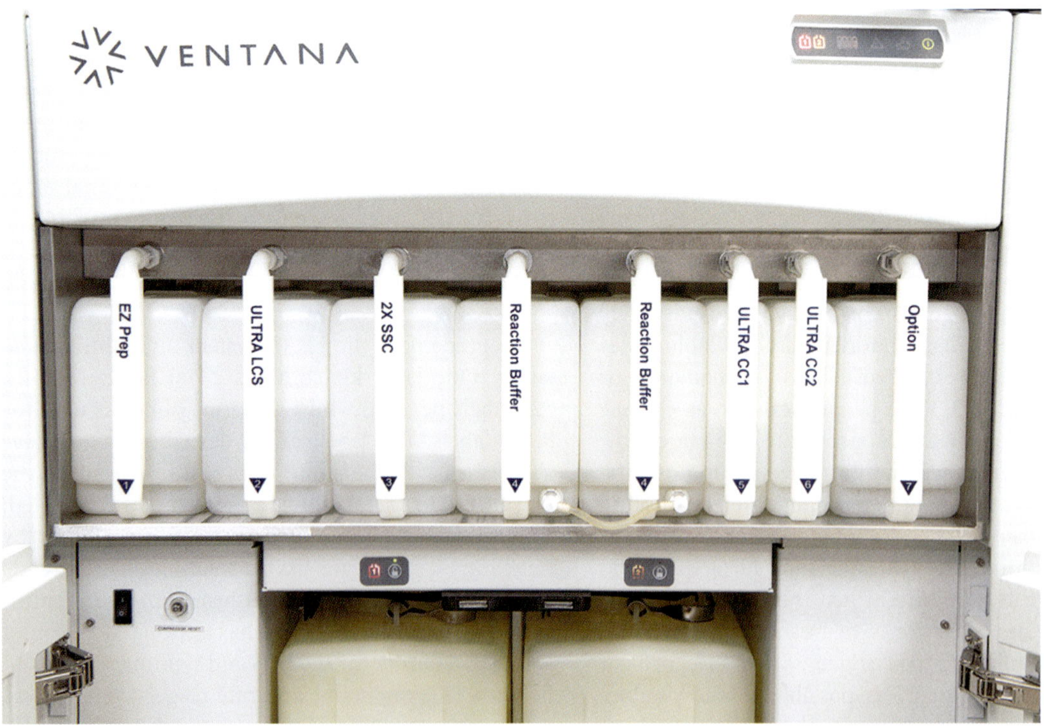

Figure 4.6 Bulk reagent housing

names for each reagent. Appendices 1, 2 and 3 list all of the Roche reagents with the translation in normal histology terms. For example, EZ prep is known to histology technicians simply as dewax reagent. The Ventana product document library website can be accessed via eLabsDoc (https://pim-eservices.roche .com/eLD/web/gb/en/home).

Each bulk reagent can be refilled independently as the instrument is running without disruption to staining. The only requirement is that all bulk reagents have to be connected to the instrument at the start of each batch run. As the BenchMark ULTRA is operating, bulk containers can be removed, refilled or topped up. This is possible as there are internal reservoirs for each bulk reagent within the instrument. These internal tanks get replenished at the start of each batch run. The instrument feeds the internal tanks from the bulk bottles so protocols may continue even if the external bottles are empty. The internal reservoirs hold enough volume to process 30 IHC assays. If the reagent level is too low, the instrument will alert the operator. The level of bulk reagents is easy to observe through the semi-clear plastic, but adding some colour to these reagents would assist in identifying the correct reagents for refilling. Inadvertently adding reaction buffer to the dewax station can be avoided if the two reagents are of differing colour. The external bulk fluid carboys are continually monitored, refilled and maintained by the operator. Quality of these reagents depends on careful refills, accurate preparation of bulks in deionized or distilled water, correct pH of the reagent and adequate maintenance of the carboys. Deionized or distilled water is recommended for use on the BenchMark ULTRA. It helps to reduce build-up of water contaminants in the tubing and to ensure correct pH of the reagent, which affects stain quality (Ventana 2012).

Waste Containers

Beneath the bulk fluids and behind the front doors of the instrument are located two 20 L waste containers. Shown in Figure 4.7, they sit on low trolleys for easy removal when full. As there are two separate containers, a full waste container may be changed without disruption to the processing. The instrument waste valve clicks over from the full waste container to the empty one, alerting the operator that one container is full. The full waste container is unlocked by the operator and carefully wheeled out for safe disposal. The

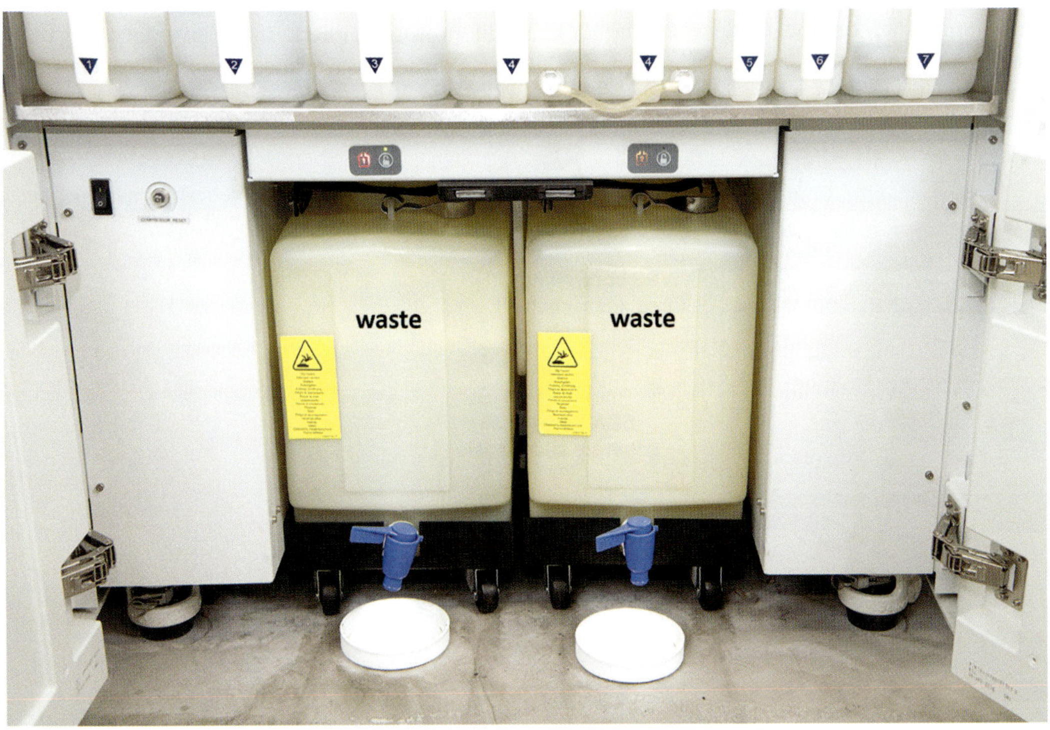

Figure 4.7 Two waste containers need to be manually emptied when full.

instrument calculates the amount of waste to be produced from a run and the amount of space required in the waste container. There is minimum risk of spillage because the waste container is locked into place during use. Diaminobenzidine (DAB) is the most common chromogen used in IHC assays, but it is also hazardous and requires safe disposal as directed by local regulations.

When a full waste container is removed, an empty container is locked into position in the instrument. Ensure the empty waste container spigot tap handle is closed (in the OFF position) or the oily waste will spill onto the floor, creating a slippery safety hazard. Due to the fact that LCS is oil based, the waste volume is physically separated into two layers. The water-based waste is isolated towards the bottom with the oil-based layer at the top. Depending on local regulations, the aqueous waste may be neutralized before disposal down the sink with running tap water and the oil-based waste may be stored in labelled containers for safe disposal by a chemical disposal company.

The VSS allows the operator to nominate when the bulk waste level is at full capacity. With occupational health and safety issues involving heavy objects at the forefront of this design, programming the waste container to be 'full' when in reality it is only half full means less exertion required to lift the container to empty it. Adjusting the volume level can be done when the instrument is not in running mode. A waste level slider is used to set the maximum level to a value between 25% and 100%. Set the level at a volume that suits the personnel in the laboratory. The waste needs to be disposed more often if the set value is too low.

Personal Computers and Peripherals

The BenchMark ULTRA is driven by a PC (LCD monitor, central processing unit, mouse, keyboard), printer, EBAR slide labelling system (barcode printer), a box for communication between the PC and the instruments (HASP key and USB back-up device) and iButton product registration wand. The software is based on the Microsoft Windows platform, allowing up to eight BenchMark ULTRAs operating from one PC station. Figure 4.8 shows the VSS controlling three instruments. This allows the operator to monitor and manage all instruments from a single workstation (Ventana 2012). There is continuous communication between the software and the stainer. Slides and reagents are scanned and monitored and individual protocols followed. The staining will not start until all required reagents are loaded on the instrument. The system alerts the operator with error messages of sub-optimal heating and insufficient or incorrect reagents which the operator must acknowledge. All information is recorded from workload and individual stain reports to reagent lists and lot numbers used during a staining protocol. The software program is also used to create and edit protocols, check stock inventory, organize IHC tests, order assay panels, print slide labels and run the stain. It is very user friendly, allowing the operator to check finishing times on the slides that

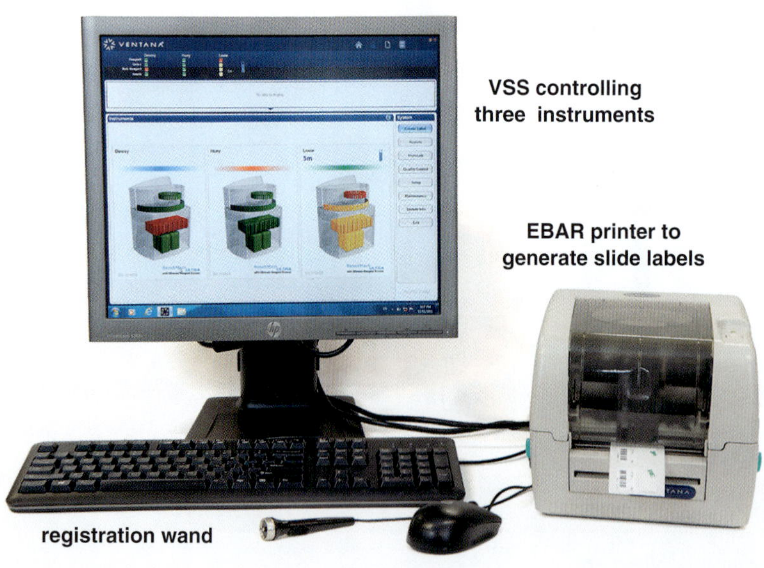

Figure 4.8 The Ventana Software System personal computer controls the BenchMark ULTRA.

are currently staining and inspect the antibodies and reagents loaded onto the instrument. This enhances the laboratory's quality system.

The VSS accommodates different levels of users. The system administrator has the ability to restrict operators from performing certain functions such as editing protocols. Roche offers an advanced training workshop introducing the operator to all aspects of the instrument which is highly recommended. Advanced users are expected to understand most of the software features, train staff, monitor stain quality and troubleshoot problems. They are also involved in creating, editing and managing protocols as well as optimizing, validating and implementing new assays. A Roche Ventana application specialist is available to assist with set-up, training and ongoing technical support.

The BenchMark ULTRA may be connected to the laboratory information system for automatic test orders. To register products onto the VSS inventory, metal buttons are used instead of conventional barcodes. Each purchased reagent is packaged with this data button. A registration wand is pressed on top of the button to register the product into the system. This allows registration and tracking of reagent lot, serial number and expiration dates. If this button is missing, the reagent cannot be used as it cannot be loaded onto the instrument. If the button does not register properly, cleaning the button with an alcohol wipe or placing the button on a flat surface may resolve this issue. Roche may be notified to replace a faulty button. All registered products can be shared among the connected instruments. Once a reagent is registered to a particular Ventana PC, it cannot be unregistered and reregistered to another. For instance, it is not possible to give another laboratory a reagent if it has already been registered but is still unopened to your instrument. Best practice is to register products as they are needed, just prior to use. Careful monitoring of stock inventory is therefore critical. Roche Tissue Diagnostics is moving towards using a 2D barcode product registration technology, replacing the current iButton wand registration for BenchMark and DISCOVERY system consumables. A barcode scanner and an updated device driver will be provided for each host PC. This transition is planned to commence with bulk fluids containing 2D barcodes being received in late December 2021, followed by dispenser/ancillary products in early 2022.

The VSS also tracks what the instrument has done, keeps data for statistical analysis, tracks individual slides, prints run reports, records RAPs, adverse effects or errors, and checks when the next maintenance task is due. The instrument knows the number of tests left in the dispensers and calculates the reagents and their volumes needed to complete a staining run. After the staining batch is completed, inventory records are updated by subtracting the volume used from the amount present at the start of the run. The number of tests left in any registered dispenser or detection kit can be checked at any time. This may not be accurate as the instrument counts down every time the dispenser is used. There are no sensors or probes to measure the remaining volume at any given time. For example, if the instrument inventory states five tests are left but the container is physically empty, the instrument will still accept the run and continue as normal, leading to a failed IHC stained slide.

Once the slide is accepted for staining and is committed, the instrument can operate independent of the PC. That is, the PC can be switched off or restarted as the BenchMark ULTRA continues staining. Disruption of power supply to the instrument will cause all slide assays to be aborted by the system, however. Therefore the instrument is best connected to a back-up power supply.

Liquid Coverslip Technology

In essence the technology behind the BenchMark ULTRA is the ULTRA liquid coverslip (LCS). It is Ventana's interpretation of how reagents are placed on a glass slide for the purpose of staining. The LCS is best described as an oil-based solution that sits on top of the reagent directly in contact with tissue on the slide (Ventana 2021a). Its purpose is to prevent reagent evaporation and thus drying artefact whilst allowing incubations with heat and high temperature denaturation steps. For this to work, a precisely level instrument is essential for the success of the stain. True for every stain, an even spread of reagent over the entire section is required. As there is no glass or plastic to act as a physical barrier, the reagent can easily flow to one side, causing patchy staining, or drain off the slide altogether, causing total lack of staining.

The reagents such as antibodies or detection kits dispensed onto the slides are in contact with the tissue section protected by the LCS layer on top. As the LCS is oil based, there is a distinct separation of the two liquids with no mixing involved. In addition, an air vortex mixing feature is available to distribute the reagent and enables full edge-to-edge coverage of the slide. This feature makes it possible to only use 100 μl of fluid to cover the entire surface of the glass slide. Another advantage of LCS technology is the ability to perform manual primary antibody application on the BenchMark ULTRA. When the primary antibody step is reached, the instrument beeps, prompting the operator to manually dispense 100 μl of antibody onto the slide before the staining run is resumed. Disadvantages include the cost of safe disposal of 'oily' waste generated from the LCS and the instrument needs to be 'dead' level for the liquid coverslip to work. It doesn't take much for things to go wrong. A slide label may be placed suboptimally, creating a channel for reagent to flow away from the tissue section, resulting in patchy or failed staining. If all slide, label, maintenance and reagent preloading checks are adhered to, the LCS technology is very efficient.

Reagent Access Points

Continuous loading slides on demand is made possible by the individual slide drawers and the ability to access the reagent carousel to add or remove reagent dispensers without disrupting the staining of slides. This sounds simple in theory but can be logistically challenging in practice. During operation, the instrument hood is locked to protect the slides, reagents and operator. To address potential bottlenecks, the BenchMark ULTRA provides ultimate RAPs. Access is usually granted when the slides are either rinsing or incubating during a protocol. When an RAP is scheduled, the instrument looks at all tests currently running and tries to find a suitable gap to pause for four minutes. This could mean waiting a couple of minutes to more than an hour, depending on what has been loaded and the protocol times of individual stains.

When an RAP is granted, the software directs the instrument to unlock the reagent hood and alerts the operator with audible beeps and flashing blue lights on the slide drawers. At this stage, the instrument gives the operator one minute to open the hood. If the lid is not opened, a new RAP needs to be scheduled. Be prepared with the dispensers to be loaded and pre-plan where to load them on the carousel before the lid is opened as the ULTRA only gives a four-minute window of opportunity. When an RAP is requested, a 'pick list' is generated listing all the reagents needed for the new slides as well as the reagents that may be safely removed. Care is taken not to touch the hammer mechanism. Staining resumes when the reagent hood is closed. Staff need to stay close to the instrument until staining resumes in case any issues arise and intervention is needed to prevent slides from being aborted.

Manual Antibody Titrations

Although the BenchMark ULTRA offers full automation from dewax to counterstain, there is the option to manually apply primary antibody to the tissue section during a staining protocol. Individual slide drawers and LCS technology make it possible to manually titrate primary antibodies for some slides while staining other slides in full automatic mode. The decision to titrate manually must be made prior to slide loading as the appropriate protocol including titration step needs to be selected. The instrument still automates all other processes and prompts the operator to apply 100 μl primary antibody at a designated time during the protocol.

Manual titration is selected in the protocol editor instead of automated antibody application. The instrument will alert the operator when the slide is ready for the primary antibody titration via a software message, audible beeping and flashing yellow light on the slide draw. At this moment, the slide drawer is opened and 100 μl is manually dispensed by holding the pipette at a 45° angle with the tip just under the LCS (Ventana 2012). Care is taken not to spill reagents over the edge of slide. The slide drawer is closed and the close button held down for two seconds until the light stops flashing to resume the protocol run.

The ability to do this is advantageous when no more spots are left on the reagent carousel. It also improves efficiency via continuous loading of slides. For instance, in times when the instrument is operating and several IHC assays are in progress, adding another antibody to the machine may mean scheduling a RAP, but the earliest opportunity may be an hour away. The slide can be programmed as a titration and as long as required detection kits and counterstain are on board the instrument, the slide can be loaded immediately. Another advantage is when staining infrequent antibodies. As there are no 'dead volumes' inside a vial, only 100 μl is required for the assay so there is no wastage of antibody. This is particularly useful for researchers as they will only use the quantity required from their 'home-made' antibody. Manual titrations may introduce human error, however. The instrument does not have the ability to check that the operator has applied the correct antibody to the assay. The laboratory worker may have applied CK20 instead of CD20, for example, and the machine would still log the assay as a success, recording no errors. Once the operator applies the primary antibody, the instrument resumes the staining protocol.

As mentioned before, manual antibody titration is useful when optimizing new antibody concentrates. Small volumes of antibody diluted at recommended concentrations or serial dilutions are tested on known positive and negative tissue sections to find optimal antibody concentration for a protocol.

Antigen Retrieval on the BenchMark ULTRA

The introduction of epitope retrieval techniques in the early 1990s (Shi et al. 1991) revolutionized diagnostic IHC, enhancing the staining by placing tissue in buffer and heating it in a microwave. Excessive microwaving produced loss of antigenicity and 'microwave burn pattern' (Yaziji and Barry 2006). The ULTRA has fully automated antigen retrieval methods with heat. The most common antigen (epitope) retrieval methods performed on FFPE tissue are heat-induced epitope retrieval (HIER), enzyme retrieval or a combination of both. Essentially the antigen retrieval breaks the bonds created by fixation, allowing antibodies better access to antigens, increased antibody binding and reduced background. Automated heating on the instrument is useful for on-board baking, antigen retrieval protocols and DNA target denaturation. Each slide holder has its own thermo pad and circuit, allowing individual slide retrieval protocol and temperature control. There is zero chance of cross-contamination of tissue because any floaters generated are simply washed away. Slide drawers can be opened individually independent of other drawers and slides can be placed in any position and in any order. Temperature increase from ambient to 98° C occurs in three minutes on the thermo pad. Protocol temperature selection options include ambient room temperature, 37°C and up to 100°C (Ventana 2012). Heating buffer solution at low or high pH and enzyme digestion may be combined and used in the same protocol. Antigen retrieval needs to be optimized for each antibody. Equally important is the capacity of automated IHC and ISH platforms to consistently apply these retrieval parameters on each occasion for every assay. This is the main advantage instruments have over manual operations.

Retrieval protocols can be switched off for antibodies that do not require it. The RMH stains adrenocorticotrophic hormone and follicular stimulation hormone IHC assays on FFPE tissue without the need for retrieval activities. Direct immunofluorescence staining on frozen tissue also does not require antigen retrieval.

Pretreatment solutions supplied by Roche include high- and low-pH buffers as well as enzymatic reagents. ULTRA Cell Conditioning solution 1 (ULTRA CC1) is a Tris-based buffer at pH 8–8.5 (Ventana 2014a). At high temperature, this solution can hydrolyse the covalent bonds formed by formalin fixation. ULTRA Cell Conditioning solution 2 (ULTRA CC2) is a citrate buffer at pH 6.0, also used at high temperature for antigen retrieval (Ventana 2014b). The majority of antibodies today favour high-pH retrieval systems. Enzymes can be used for both IHC antigen retrieval methods and ISH pretreatments. Three strengths of protease are available from Roche. Protease 1 is the strongest at 0.38 mg/mL alkaline protease enzyme suspended in a stabilizing solution (Ventana 2011a). Protease 2 is 0.1 mg/mL enzyme and Protease 3 is the weakest at 0.24 casein U/mL (Ventana 2011b; Ventana 2015a). ISH-protease 3 is commonly used for ISH pretreatments to cleave peptide bonds and digest proteins surrounding the DNA or RNA target sequence (Ventana 2015b).

Localization Antibodies

Antibodies are available in RTU and concentrate forms. Automation has improved the standardization of staining protocols within and between IHC laboratories, especially where the instrument has a closed system for particular protocols (Myers 2004). For instance, the availability of RTU antibodies optimized for a certain platform by the manufacturer eliminates one big parameter from the IHC protocol. Decisions about optimal working antibody titres are abolished. Efforts to 'standardize' IHC are actually conscious attempts to reduce variation in reagents, protocol options and incubation times on board the instrument. The compulsory use of proprietary reagents on the instrument and 'locking' certain aspects of the method have greatly contributed to this endeavour. The term 'locked' may also refer to the on-board HIER system being under a closed lid (Prichard and Biting 2015), but in this context it is the lack of freedom for the operator to 'tweak' conditions within IHC protocols for individual preferences. Closed systems provide less flexibility but more consistency in staining results. Conversely, 'open' platforms allow more flexibility in choice of reagents, incubation times and detection kits from other manufacturers, but this freedom can become troublesome because there are so many variables to account for. The BenchMark ULTRA leans towards being a 'closed' system when compared to the GX and Discovery systems but still has enough flexibility for operator preferences. One such example is the ability for the laboratory to use RTU antibodies available from the vendor as well as specific antibody clones diluted from concentrates sourced from other companies.

The RTUs are pre-diluted antibodies for IVD use, verified for use by the manufacturer on their IHC instrument and proprietary reagents. The antibodies enhance standardization and quality control in the IHC laboratory. The instructions for use (IFU) for each antibody have invaluable information for antibody validation and recommended external tissue controls. All manufacturers of RTU antibodies impose an expiry date on each product and the instrument will not accept the expired antibody dispenser. There is a definite shift to RTU antibodies as they are more readily available compared to 20 years ago. The biggest advantage is convenience and their costs are also weighed against the uncertainty and time associated with manual preparation of antibodies from concentrates. Roche supplies RTU antibodies for the BenchMark ULTRA and if a specific RTU is not available, the option to purchase concentrates from other vendors comes in handy. Therefore, optimization of RTUs on the instrument is limited to antigen retrieval and primary antibody incubation times and temperatures, localized using a Roche detection kit. All lot numbers and other parameters are recorded on Ventana software as part of quality system.

Antibody concentrates can be sourced from any provider supplying a particular clone of interest to the laboratory. A literature review is commonly performed in consultation with the pathologist or investigator requesting the new antibody. Reference articles are a good source of information about antibody clones. Quality assurance programme data records of antibody protocols also may be helpful – for example, NordiQC. Antibody data sheets may provide a starting point with recommended working dilution range. Using Roche's OptiView detection system as an example, the choice of polyclonal and monoclonal concentrates raised in mouse or rabbit is recommended since they have been proven to work with this kit. The secondary 'linker' in this detection kit is raised in goat, so theoretically antibodies raised in other animals (except goat) should also react. Ultimately the most suitable choice of concentrates depends on price, availability and consistency of performance. Reputable vendors will have adequate documentation accompanying the concentrate with data sheets listing positive and negative tissue types and recommended protocol guidelines.

Serial antibody dilutions (1:50, 1:100, 1:200 etc.) are very useful for validation of new antibody concentrates. Finding the 'sweet spot' for an optimal working antibody titre is possible on the BenchMark ULTRA using the manual antibody application protocol. Start by referring to the product package insert IFU. Choose positive and negative tissue controls from archives of routinely processed FFPE blocks and start with the antibody dilution recommended in the data sheet or found in the literature. If the recommended range is 1:50 to 1:200, start with 1:50. The VSS can be programmed to trial several 'testing' protocols, keeping retrieval times the same on each occasion and allowing a variety of different antibody dilutions to test the staining. Only 100 μl volume of diluted antibody is required per slide, so the double dilutions can be planned with this in mind. If done correctly, there is no wastage of antibody since no 'dead volumes' are generated in a vial. Details of the antigen retrieval, antibody dilution and incubation times/temperatures may be printed on the slide label to differentiate one protocol from another. There is great protocol flexibility for running many slides using antigen retrieval in different cell conditioning solutions (low and high pH) with heat, with or without enzyme pretreatment and different antibody incubation times. For example, run the antibody on known positive and negative tissue using Ultra CC1 at 100°C for 32 minutes, with antibody incubation for 32 minutes, along with second slide for Ultra CC1 at 100°C for 64 minutes, with antibody incubation for 32 minutes. The aim is to achieve a strong staining signal with little or no background.

When the parameters for antibody dilution, antigen retrieval, detection kit and counterstain have all been optimized, the protocol is ready to be validated on a minimum of 10 positive and 10 negative cases

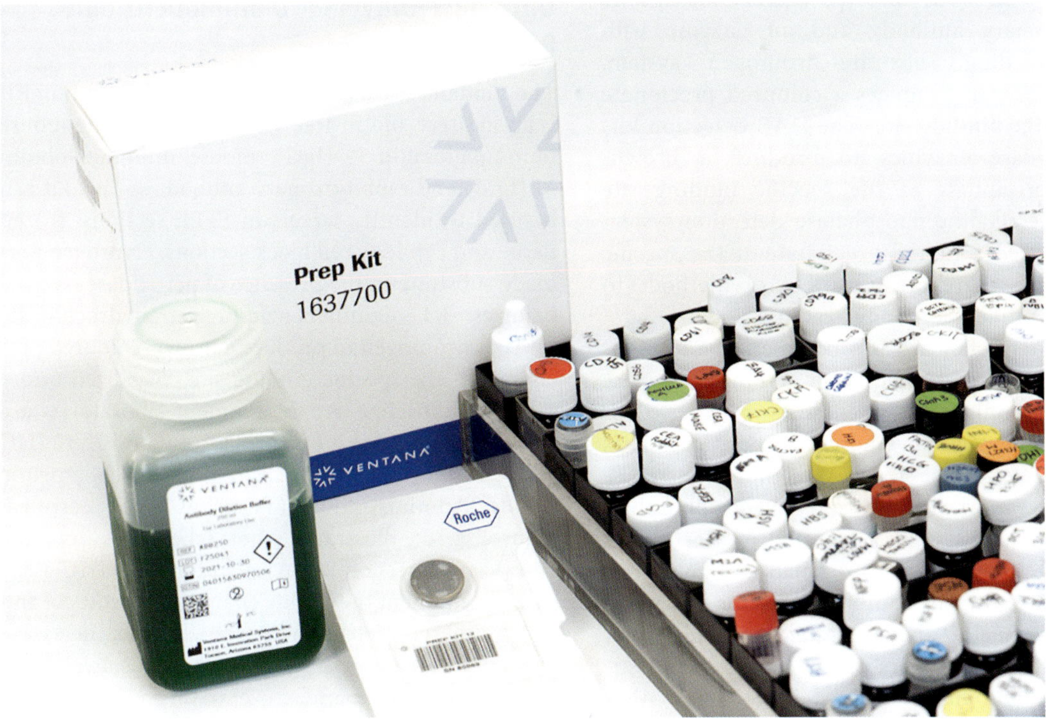

Figure 4.9 Ventana prep kits are used to dilute antibody concentrates for use on the BenchMark ULTRA.

from the laboratory archives (Lin and Shi 2015). At this stage the recommendation to use Roche user-fillable dispenser prep kits instead of continuation of antibody manual applications should be adhered to. Shown in Figure 4.9, these prep kits are essentially empty vials in which the optimal diluted working concentrate resides. The VSS records a new, empty prep kit number, associating it with a stain protocol, allowing the operator to effectively become the manufacturer of this 'pre-dilute' antibody. This strategy allows the facility to determine the specificity and sensitivity of the new antibody. Results about its performance on real cases are documented and reviewed by a pathologist, head of department and scientist in charge of IHC. When the new IHC assay is deemed fit for purpose, it is implemented into the routine laboratory inventory along with appropriate quality assurance measures. Lot numbers, expiry dates and protein concentration are all recorded. Similar to every other antibody within the laboratory's register, ongoing monitoring of the stain is required along with daily equipment and reagent maintenance, tissue processing and controls. New batches of reagent or any change to a validated protocol require testing on known positive and negative tissue to confirm staining quality is maintained. Staining checks are important, including failed slides, mislabelling, an incorrect block being sectioned, presence of artefact, lifting of tissue and coverslipping issues. Monitor all aspects of the stain results and troubleshoot accordingly, with quality issues communicated to the reporting pathologist and BenchMark ULTRA operators.

Ventana Detection Kits

Roche base their detection kits upon multimer technology which is their answer to other manufacturers' polymer technology. Before this is explored further, perhaps it is a good opportunity to review the basic IHC concepts.

Remember IHC is a laboratory assay using primary antibodies to localize and bind to antigens in FFPE, frozen tissue and cytology preparations. In this context, to keep things simple, only chromogenic development for optical light microscopy is outlined. The binding of the antibody is visualized with a direct or indirect detection method. The techniques for indirect methods use a secondary antibody directed against the species of the primary antibody and an enzyme with a corresponding substrate-chromogen system. This combination produces a coloured precipitate at the specific binding site. The DAB detection kits use peroxidase enzymes to produce a brown-coloured precipitate at the specific binding site whereas the alkaline phosphatase detection system produces a red-coloured precipitate at the specific binding site. There are a variety of methods to detect the antigen–antibody reaction.

The current standard is a polymer-type technology where the secondary antibody and the peroxidase enzyme are conjugated to an inert polymer. This polymer can deliver many more secondary antibodies and enzymes to the one signal. As a point of difference from other vendors, the DAB and Alkaline phosphatase red detection systems advocated by Roche uses multimer technology. They are small molecules with the secondary antibody combined with the enzyme in a single molecule. At about half the size of a polymer molecule, these multimers can penetrate into tissue more easily and thus reduce staining times. Also, multiplying the number of sites for chromogen development increases the intensity of the signal. In these systems, enzymes are attached by long arm linkers to a secondary or tertiary antibody depending on the type of detection kit. Three common Roche detection kits include UltraView DAB, OptiView DAB and UltraView Fast Red kits, and these are now explored further.

UltraView Universal Diaminobenzidine Detection Kit

The Ventana UltraView Universal DAB Detection Kit is an indirect, biotin-free system for detecting mouse immunoglobulin G (IgG), mouse immunoglobulin M (IgM) and rabbit primary antibodies. This kit can be used to identify targets in FFPE sections, frozen tissue and cytology cell block sections. Hydrogen peroxide substrate in the presence of peroxidase enzyme oxidizes 3,3 diaminobenzidine tetrahydrochloride (DAB) chromogen to produce a brown-coloured precipitate at the specific binding site, visualized under a light microscope. At the moment laboratories are obliged to use this kit for their ER, PR and Her2 IHC assays as they have been cleared by the Therapeutic Goods Administration (TGA) as IVD certified. Figure 4.10 illustrates the schematics of the UltraView detection kit (A) used for Her2 IHC assay (B). The moment the facility changes the protocol and uses a different detection kit, for example, the assays become in-house IVDs, shifting the onus away from the vendor as the manufacturer of this medical device and nominating the laboratory as the 'manufacturer'. The UltraView Universal DAB Detection Kit contains sufficient reagent for 250 tests. The kit is comprised of five 25 mL containers (Ventana 2021b):

(1) The UltraView Universal DAB Inhibitor contains 3% hydrogen peroxide solution.
(2) The UltraView Universal HRP Multimer contains a cocktail of horseradish peroxidase

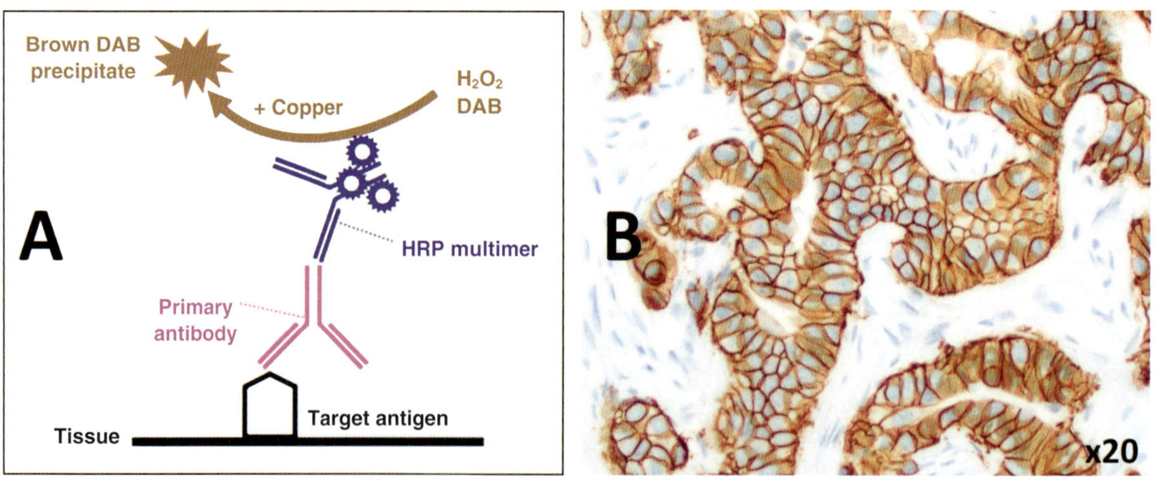

Figure 4.10 Schematic of the UltraView universal DAB detection kit (A) demonstrated by Her2 IHC (B).
Image A reproduced with permission Ventana Medical Systems Inc.

(HRP)–labelled antibodies (goat anti-mouse IgG, goat anti-mouse IgM, and goat anti-rabbit) (5.5 g/mL) in a buffer containing protein with ProClin 300, a preservative.

(3) The UltraView Universal DAB Chromogen contains 0.2% 3, 3 diaminobenzidine tetrahydrochloride in a proprietary stabilizer solution with a proprietary preservative.

(4) The UltraView Universal DAB H_2O_2 contains 0.04% hydrogen peroxide in a phosphate buffer solution.

(5) The UltraView Universal Copper contains copper sulphate (5 g/L) in an acetate buffer with proprietary preservative.

OptiView Diaminobenzidine

This IHC detection kit is also an indirect, biotin-free method designed for 250 tests. Slightly different to the UltraView kit, OptiView employs hydroxyquinoxaline (HQ) haptens conjugated to a linker secondary antibody containing 12–15 haptens per antibody. Roche chose HQ molecules because they are synthetic and non-endogenous to mammals, reducing the risk of unwanted background staining. A tertiary antibody layer comprising horseradish peroxidase (HRP) multimer binds to the HQ haptens. This form of IHC detection enhances the visualization of low-expressing antigens in a cleaner background. Figure 4.11 outlines the schematics of the OptiView detection kit (A) used for a CD3 IHC assay (B). Similar to the UltraView kit, DAB chromogen reacts with HRP and H_2O_2 to produce a brown signal. Blocking endogenous peroxidase may be performed before or after the primary antibody incubation step. The ability to decide for each antibody is a useful feature as Cartun and colleagues (2019) found some antibodies such as CD4 are damaged by H_2O_2, resulting in decreased staining intensity.

The kit is comprised of six 25 mL containers (Ventana 2021c):

(1) The peroxidase inhibitor contains 3.0% hydrogen peroxide solution.

(2) The HQ universal linker contains a cocktail of HQ-labelled (HQ is a proprietary hapten covalently attached to the goat antibodies) antibodies (goat anti-mouse IgG, goat anti-mouse IgM, and goat anti-rabbit) (~50 μg/mL) in a buffer containing protein with ProClin 300, a preservative.

(3) The HRP multimer contains a mouse monoclonal anti-HQ-labelled HRP tertiary antibody (~40 μg/mL) in a buffer containing protein with ProClin 300, a preservative.

(4) The H_2O_2 contains 0.04% hydrogen peroxide in a phosphate buffer solution.

(5) The DAB contains 0.2% DAB in a proprietary stabilizer solution with a proprietary preservative.

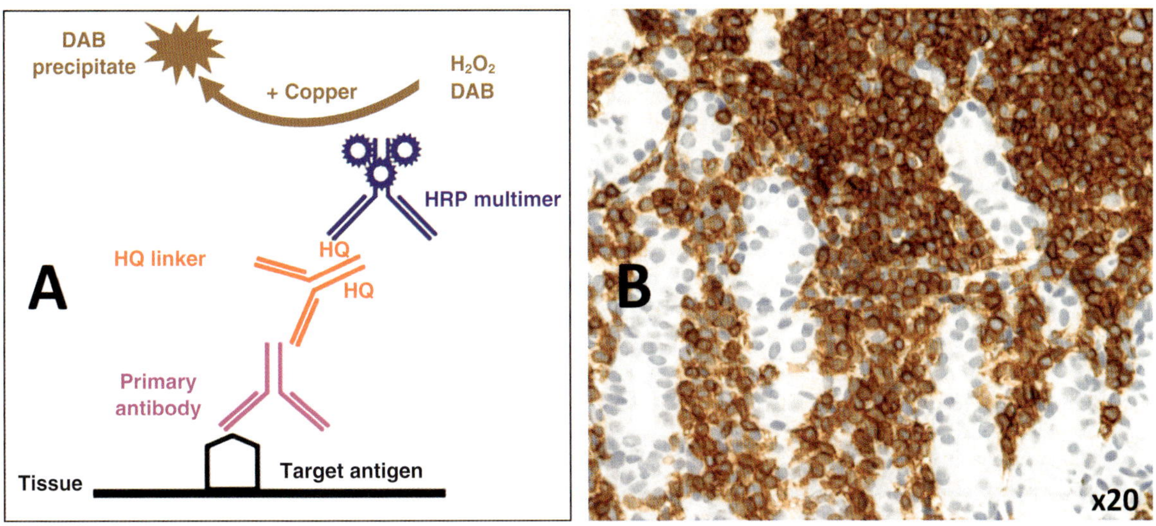

Figure 4.11 Schematic of the OptiView diaminobenzidine immunohistochemical detection kit (A) demonstrated by CD3 immunohistochemistry (B)

Image A reproduced with permission Ventana Medical Systems Inc.

(6) Copper contains copper sulphate (5.0 g/L) in an acetate buffer with a proprietary preservative.

UltraView Fast Red

The 250-test 'red' kit supplied by Roche is based on the enzyme alkaline phosphatase and is an indirect, biotin-free system for detecting mouse IgG, mouse IgM and rabbit primary antibodies. Although the choice of chromogen is decided from laboratory preferences, the red chromogen is actually handy in certain situations. Tissue with high endogenous peroxidase activity such as haematological granulocytes is notorious for interfering with DAB chromogens showing unwanted positive brown staining. In other circumstances, endogenous pigments such as melanin mimicking the brown DAB may render false positive results. Switching from peroxidase to alkaline phosphatase and changing the brown chromogen to red chromogen eliminates these conundrums. Figure 4.12 summarizes the schematic of the enzyme alkaline phosphatase facilitating the reaction of the azo dye Fast Red with Naphthol substrate (A) along with $MgCl_2$ to render a bright red chromogen at the antigen–antibody site under optical light microscopy (Ventana 2021d). An example is shown for the AMACR antibody-staining prostate adenocarcinoma (B).

The kit is comprised of five 25 mL containers:

(1) Universal AP Red Multimer contains a cocktail of alkaline phosphatase (AP)–labelled antibodies (< 50 µg/mL) in a buffer with ProClin 300 solution, a preservative.

(2) Universal AP Red Fast Red A contains ≤ 1.0% (w/v) Fast Red in acetate buffer with ProClin 300 solution, a preservative.

(3) Universal AP Red Fast Red B contains ≤ 1.0% (w/v) Fast Red in acetate buffer with ProClin 300 solution, a preservative.

(4) Universal AP Red Naphthol contains ≤ 1.0% (w/v) Naphthol in Tris buffer with ProClin 300 solution, a preservative.

(5) Universal AP Red Enhancer contains ≤ 3.0% (v/v) $MgCl_2$ in a Tris buffer with ProClin 300 solution, a preservative.

Amplification Kits

If further enhancement is required, amplification kits are available to increase the intensity of IHC staining. A note of caution must be highlighted as these kits artificially inflate the signal which can be helpful to visualize those low-expressing antigens. However, they can be detrimental for quantitative analyses where counts are required, especially when grouping cell populations into categories based on staining intensities. In addition, there is an increase in the cost of the test and the staining time.

An amplification kit is produced for the Ventana detection kit and is applied between the primary antibody and multimer steps to increase the number of antibodies bound at the antigen site. The theory is

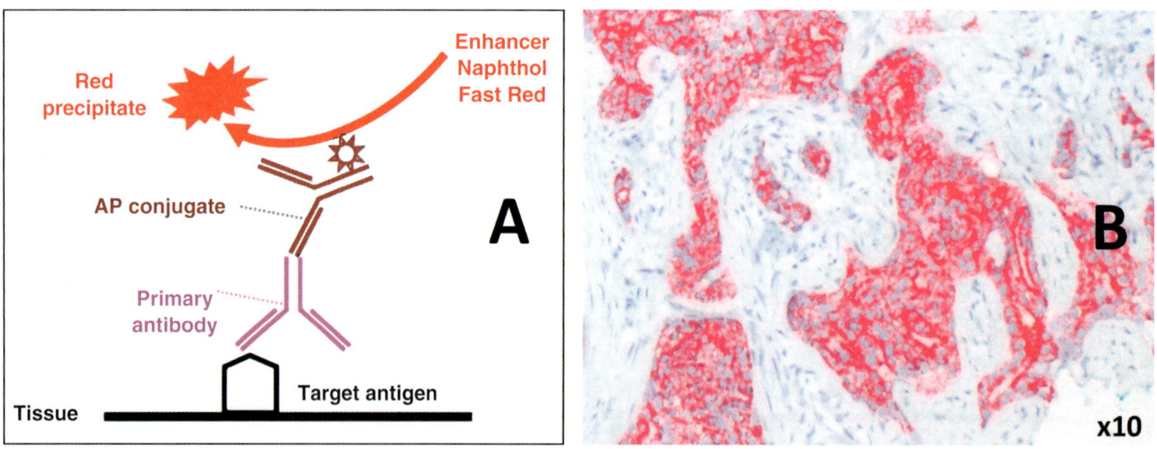

Figure 4.12 Schematic of the UltraView Universal Alkaline Phosphatase Red Detection Kit (A) demonstrated by AMACR immunohistochemistry (B)

Image A reproduced with permission Ventana Medical Systems Inc.

to impart more enzymes into the system to enhance the DAB chromogen development. The OptiView amplification kit is used with the OptiView DAB kit, applied after the multimer to enhance intensity of staining. The RMH utilizes amplification for the ALK IHC assay clone D5F3 for non-small cell lung cancer investigations; the protocol step is locked in by the manufacturer. Amplification kits do increase the signal. However, they add another level of complexity, increase staining time and costs to the protocol.

Ventana Staining Protocols

The BenchMark ULTRA can perform chromogenic IHC, fluorescence IHC, and *in situ* hybridization assays. All of the required reagents are supplied by Roche and it comes down to user preference to decide on the type of protocol to employ in a given situation. Figure 4.13 illustrates a Kappa light chain immunoglobulin IHC assay in both fluorescence and chromogenic forms. In this instance fresh frozen tissue was prepared for direct immunofluorescence using fluorescein isothiocyanate (FITC) as the fluorochrome (A). Formalin-fixed paraffin-embedded tissue was used for immunoperoxidase staining with DAB chromogen (B). Both techniques provide the same outcome of demonstrating deposits in the kidney glomerulus. Each method, however, has its advantages and disadvantages and this is for the user to decide on the merits of choosing a suitable protocol.

Chromogenic Protocol

The general protocol for chromogenic IHC consisting of dewax, antigen retrieval, primary antibody, enzyme block, detection and counterstain steps is replicated on the BenchMark ULTRA. Routinely, tissue sections are cut, mounted on positively charged slides, drained, dried, labelled and loaded onto the instrument. Slide baking may be selected for FFPE sections before dewax procedures in order to ensure good attachment of the tissue section to the slide. All required reagents are loaded on board. The bulk fluids and waste containers are checked and the staining run started. At the completion, slides are removed and coverslipped, ready for quality control assessments, and then analysed by the pathologist.

The IHC, ISH and multiplex staining procedures are automated by defining a set protocol. The staining method may be customized for the laboratory and edited as required. The protocols consist of many steps in which reagents are incubated at predetermined times and set temperatures. After each incubation step, the instrument washes the slides with reaction buffer wash. The application of LCS on top of incubating reagents prevents evaporation and promotes even distribution of solutions on the slide aided by air vortex mixing and bulk solutions that are optimized specifically for use on the BenchMark ULTRA.

Using the VSS, specific protocols are created or edited by firstly selecting the detection kit to be used. A previous protocol for an existing antibody can be used as a template for the new antibody.

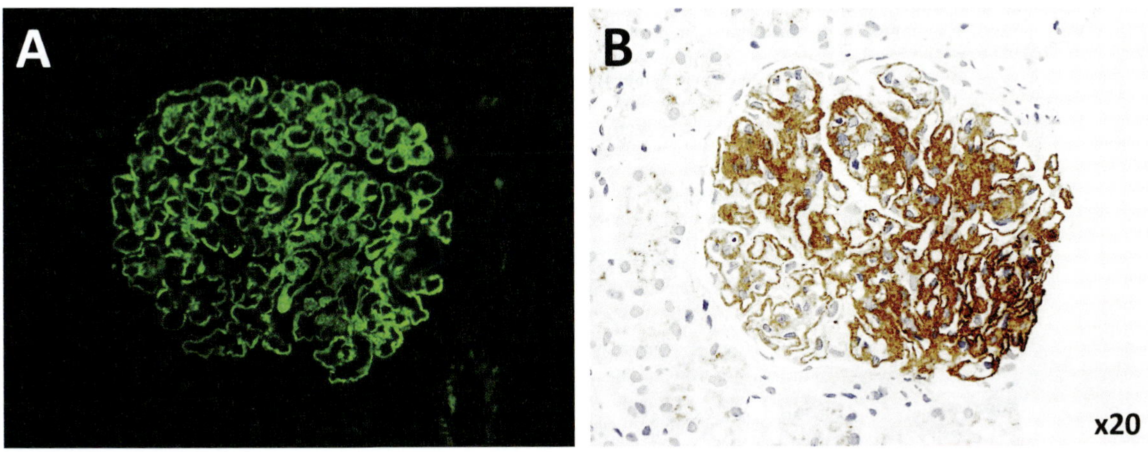

Figure 4.13 Compilation of Kappa light chain immunoglobulin in direct immunofluorescence fresh frozen (A) and diaminobenzidine formalin-fixed paraffin-embedded tissue (B). Image courtesy of Dr. Moira Finlay, Anatomical Pathologist, The Royal Melbourne Hospital

A sample IHC protocol for SATB2 antibody based on OptiView detection is found in Appendix 4. Note that LCS is also applied for each reagent excluding the reaction buffer rinses. When applied to an aqueous buffer pool the surface tension causes the lighter oil to spread out over the surface of the buffer, forming a chamber (Ventana 2021a). Although there is the option to bake slides on the instrument, this selection may be omitted as the slides are dried in a 60°C laboratory oven whilst preparations are made to accommodate the loading of the antibody assay on the instrument. At the RMH on-board baking is selected in addition to time in the 60°C laboratory oven in many of the protocols. The VSS offers the ability to print the protocol, either in summary form or full procedure.

After completion of the staining run, slides are removed from the BenchMark ULTRA and washed in warm soapy water to remove the LCS followed by distilled water or clean tap water to wash the residual soap away. Dehydrate with absolute alcohol and then xylene and coverslip in a permanent mountant such as CV Mount. Change the dehydration and clearing solutions frequently for optimal post-staining treatment of slides. For the Fast Red chromogen, the same soapy water rinse followed by distilled water is applied, but dehydration is via oven drying instead of the routine alcohols. The red chromogen is soluble in alcohol and acetone so will wash out in these reagents. Once completely dried, the slide is dipped in xylene and coverslipped.

Immunofluorescence Protocol

Fluorescence was the main detection signal (Coons et al. 1941) until the 1970s, when horseradish peroxidase and anti-horseradish peroxidase were used (Sternberger et al. 1970). The ULTRA offers a simple one-step direct immunofluorescence (DIF) procedure on predominantly fresh frozen tissue sections. Fluorescein isothiocyanate–conjugated antibodies are used to directly detect antigens in fresh frozen tissue. The primary antibody binds specifically to the target antigen and is then visualized using a fluorescence microscope with appropriate filter set. Figure 4.14 is an example of DIF performed on a salt split skin test. The hematoxylin and eosin (H&E) is from a frozen section, highlighting the separation of the epidermis from the dermis of the blister (A). The corresponding DIF confirms IgG linear deposition on the blister roof and floor (B). Roche provides a range of RTU FITC–conjugated antibodies in a 50-test dispenser for dermatopathology and renal pathology investigations.

Fresh frozen tissue is routinely cut at 4 μm onto positively charged slides. The back of the slide is etched with a diamond pen circling around the sections for easy location of macroscopically colourless stain. No antigen retrieval is required. At the RMH, the protocol is very simple, requiring only the fluorescently labelled antibody incubation time of 16 minutes to be selected. The steps include reaction buffer rinse, LCS application and FITC-labelled antibody incubated at 36°C, and the run is completed with

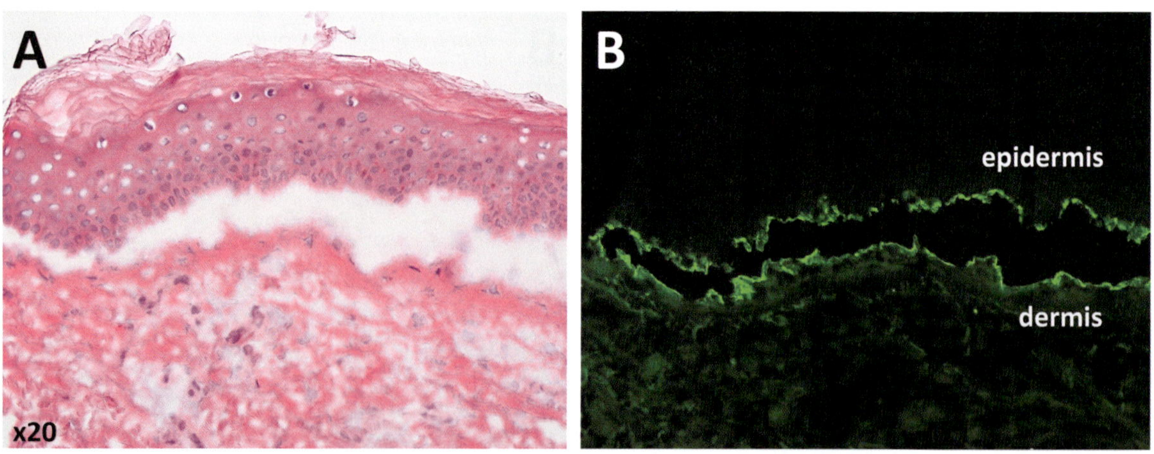

Figure 4.14 Salt split skin test hematoxylin and eosin (A) and direct immunofluorescence showing immunoglobulin G deposition at the roof and floor of the blister (B)

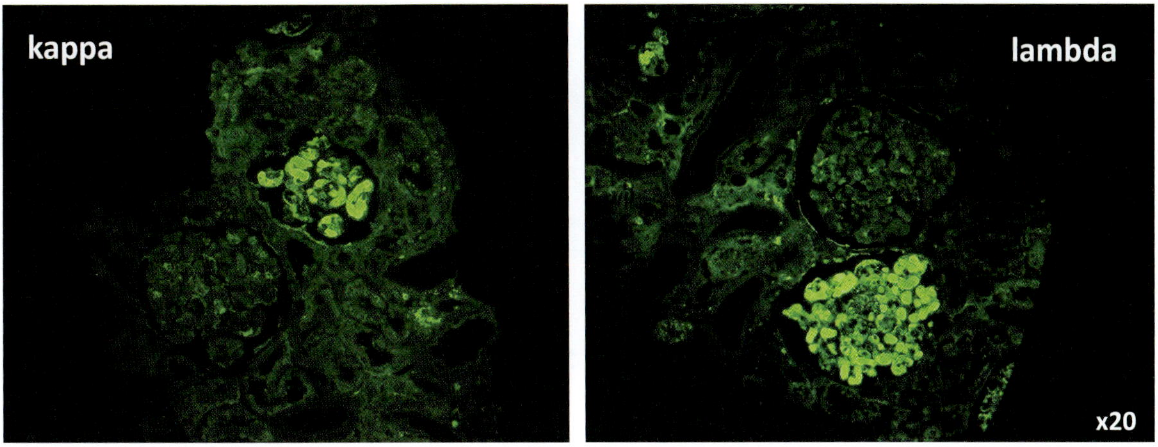

Figure 4.15 Direct immunofluorescence on formalin-fixed paraffin-embedded tissue showing kappa and lambda light chain deposits in kidney glomerulus. Image courtesy of Dr. Moira Finlay, Anatomical Pathologist, The Royal Melbourne Hospital

another rinse in reaction buffer. The blue LED light on the slide drawers is used to identify DIF slides so appropriate post-staining procedures are executed.

Direct immunofluorescence can also be performed on FFPE tissue. In this situation sections must be baked, dewaxed and enzyme antigen retrieval performed before starting the immunofluorescence protocol. Figure 4.15 demonstrates both kappa and lambda light chain deposits within kidney glomerulus using FFPE tissue.

On completion of a staining run, DIF-stained slides are washed in cool soapy water or in reaction buffer to remove residual LCS followed by distilled water and coverslipped using an aqueous mountant with anti-fade properties. Avoid exposure of stained slides to light and store at 4°C until ready to view under a fluorescence microscope, preferably within 24 hours of staining.

In Situ Hybridization

Roche favours chromogenically labelled ISH assays for the BenchMark ULTRA on FFPE tissue or cytology cell block preparations. Instead of antibodies, ISH techniques employ labelled probes to detect specific DNA or RNA target sequences within cells. To summarize, proteins surrounding the target sequences are digested away so as to enable better access. The nucleic target sequences are exposed by heating the tissue and probe solutions to denature them. Under appropriate stringency conditions, the labelled nucleic acid probe hybridizes to its complementary nucleic acid sequence in the tissue and then visualized with a detection kit.

The RMH uses three Roche ISH kits. They are chromogenic in nature for optical microscopy. An Epstein-Barr Virus Early RNA (EBER) ISH probe is labelled with fluorescein and matched to a blue detection kit. The HER2 dual ISH assay for breast and gastric pathology utilizes black (reduced silver ions) and red detection kits in combination. No fluorescently labelled ISH (FISH) assays are currently available for use on the BenchMark ULTRA.

Ventana's iView blue detection kit for EBER ISH is manufactured for 200 tests and has six 20 mL dispensers (Ventana 2021e):

(1) Anti-fluorescein mouse monoclonal antibody in phosphate buffered saline with protein stabilizer and preservative.
(2) Biotinylated immunoglobulins containing affinity purified goat anti-mouse IgG in phosphate buffered saline with protein stabilizer and preservative.
(3) Streptavidin alkaline phosphatase in Tris buffer with $MgCl_2$ and $ZnCl_2$.
(4) Enhancer containing $MgCl_2$ solution with preservative.
(5) Nitro blue tetrazolium (NBT) in 1% dimethylformamide (DMF).
(6) 5-bromo-4-chloro-3-indolyl phosphate (BCIP) in a Tris buffer.

Highlighted in Figure 4.16, the fluorescein-labelled EBER probe binds to a mouse anti-fluorescein antibody that when followed by an indirect biotin streptavidin system allows the visualization of the hybridization via

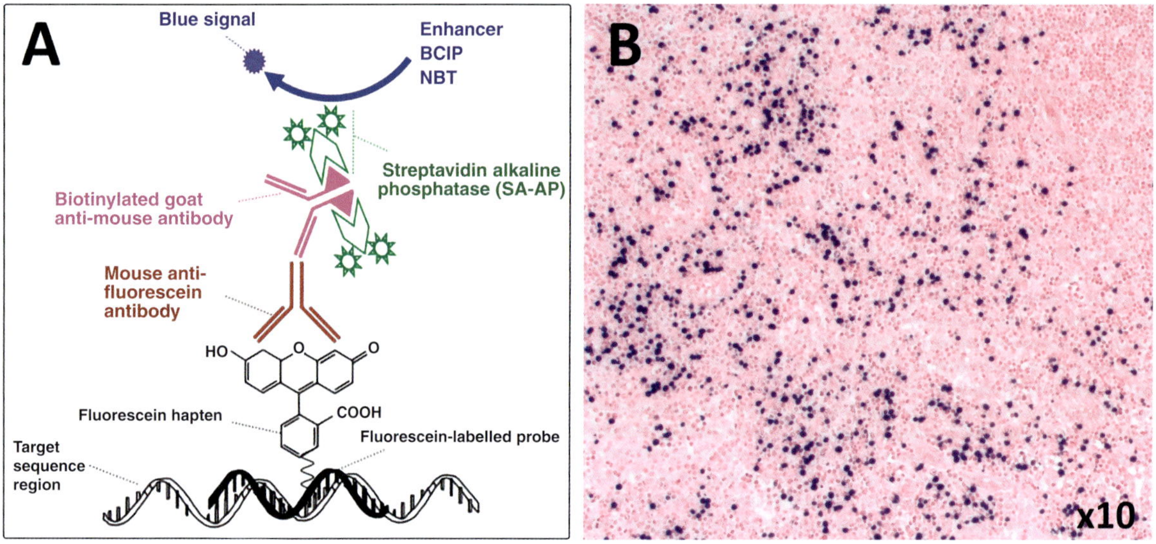

Figure 4.16 Schematic of the Roche iView blue *in situ* hybridization detection system (A) demonstrated by Epstein-Barr Virus Early RNA *in situ* hybridization (B)

Image A reproduced with permission Ventana Medical Systems Inc.

BCIP-NBT chromogen (A). To expand and summarize the assay, the mouse anti-fluorescein antibody is attached to a biotinylated secondary antibody of goat anti-mouse. This step is followed by the addition of a streptavidin alkaline phosphatase enzyme conjugate binding to the biotin present on the secondary antibody. The complex is then visualized with 5-Bromo-4-chloro-3-indolyl phosphate (BCIP) and nitro blue tetrazolium (NBT) chromogen thus produces a blue precipitate readily detected by light microscopy. The counterstain is Red II as seen in Figure 4.16B labelling EBER in lymph node. Post counterstain, the slide is dehydrated in clean absolute alcohols to remove LCS and water before clearing in xylene and coverslip. Alcohol solutions need to be changed frequently.

Similar to all IHC assays, pre-analytic factors including specimen preparation and tissue processing affect stain quality for ISH iView blue procedures. Fixation time and section thickness may impact ISH results. As with all IHC/ISH tests, mounting both test and control sections on the same slide is recommended. Specific traps to avoid include incomplete dewaxing of sections leading to a 'bubbling' artefact, and incomplete dehydration before coverslipping, which can lead to chromogen deposit artefact seen as blue crystals.

The Roche Her2 dual ISH DNA probe cocktail is used to determine if the Her2 gene is amplified in invasive breast carcinoma tissue specimens, for example. Patients with overexpression of Her2 are prime candidates for Herceptin therapy. In order to calculate the ratio of Her2 gene numbers to chromosome 17 (Ch17), two probes are required. One probe is for the Her2 gene and this is detected using a dinitrophenyl (DNP)–labelled probe paired to a peroxidase-based detection system that oxidizes silver ions to a black precipitate as shown in Figure 4.17A. The other is a digoxigenin (DIG)–labelled probe to the centromeric region of chromosome 17 (where the Her2 gene resides) and is detected via an alkaline phosphatase-based detection system with a Fast Red chromogen as highlighted in Figure 4.17B. Although the two probes exist as a cocktail and are applied simultaneously, the chromogens are developed sequentially with the silver established first before the red chromogen. Essentially, black and red dots (signals) are seen microscopically and counted within invasive cancer cell nuclei as illustrated in Figure 4.17C. Quality control of the stained sections includes checking normal cells (such as stromal fibroblasts and endothelial cells showing one to two HER2 and Ch17 signals) adjacent to invasive breast cancer cells in external control tissue. Twenty malignant cell nuclei are assessed and the sum

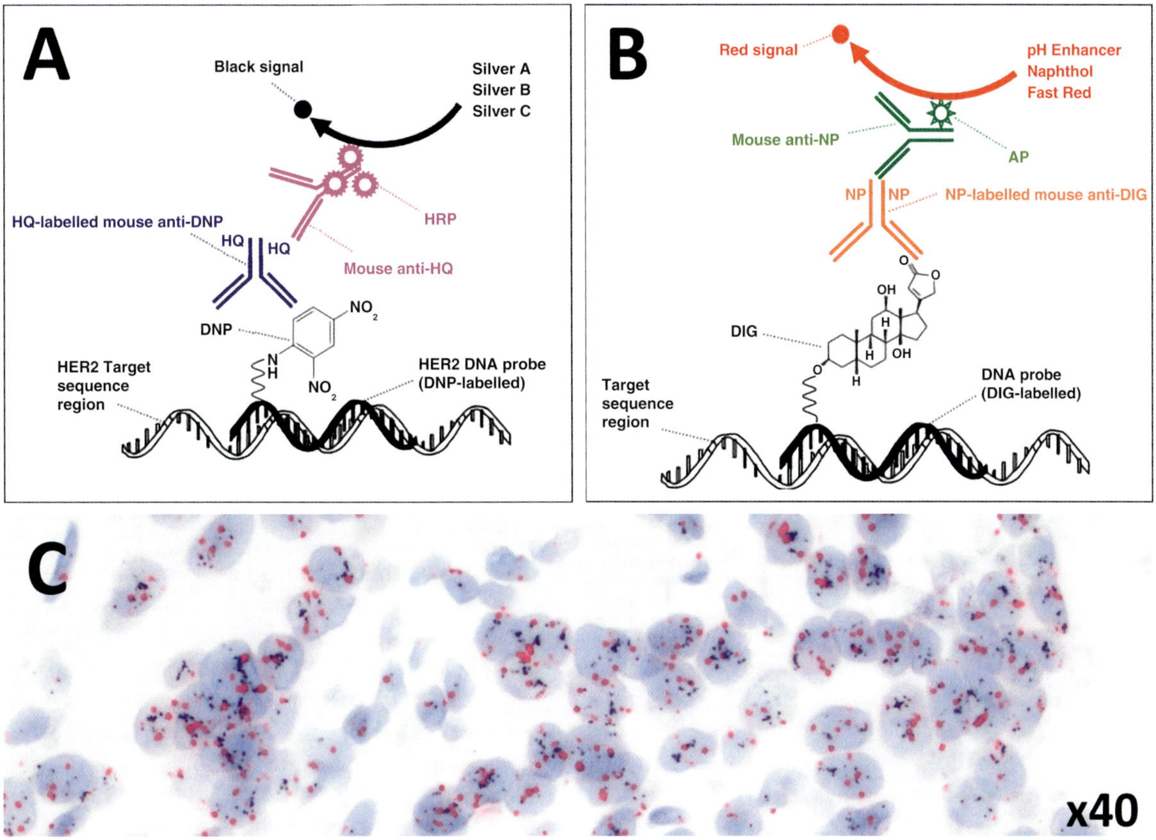

Figure 4.17 Schematics for Ventana silver *in situ* hybridization dinitrophenyl (A) and red *in situ* hybridization digoxigenin (B) assays demonstrated by a combined Her2 dual *in situ* hybridization amplified in breast carcinoma (C). Image A and B reproduced with permission Ventana Medical Systems Inc.

of Her2 (black dots) is divided by the sum of chromosome 17 (red dots) for all twenty nuclei. A Her2-to-chromosome 17 ratio of ≥ 2 means amplified while a ratio of < 2 is not amplified (Ventana 2020).

This assay is used on routinely processed FFPE tissue preferably fixed in 10% NBF for 8 to 72 hours. The importance of standardization of pre-analytical factors such as fixation time, tissue processing, section thickness and quality and the freshness of the cut section is highlighted as these variables may impact the quality of the ISH assay (Cartun et al. 2019). Sections are routinely cut at 4 μm and mounted on recommended charged slides. Slides are drained and baked in a 60°C laboratory oven for 30–45 minutes before loading on the ULTRA. Preloading checks including prime ULTRA function and careful cleaning and priming of the probe, detection kit and ancillary dispensers are essential to optimize stain quality and reduce potential repeats of the stain. Tissue digestion times and stringency wash temperature may be varied; however, the rest of the staining protocol is locked by the manufacturer (Ventana 2020).

The Ventana Her2 dual ISH detection kit is manufactured for 60 tests and is composed of two separate detection systems. The Ventana ISH kit for Her2 gene contains five dispensers (Ventana 2021f):

(1) Anti-DNP hapten-labelled antibody (~12.5 μg/mL) in a protein and phosphate containing buffer with ProClin solution, a preservative.
(2) Anti-HQ horseradish peroxidase (HRP) enzyme conjugate antibody (~25 μg/mL) solution in a protein and phosphate containing buffer including ProClin solution, a preservative.
(3) Chromogen A reagent contains < 1% CH_3COOAg (silver acetate) in an aqueous solution.

(4) Chromogen B reagent contains < 1% C6H6O2 (hydroquinone) in an aqueous solution.
(5) Chromogen C reagent contains < 0.2% H_2O_2 in an aqueous solution.
The Ventana red ISH kit for chromosome 17 contains five dispensers (Ventana 2021g):
(a) Anti-DIG hapten-labelled antibody (~7.5 μg/mL) in a protein and phosphate containing buffer with ProClin solution, a preservative. The hapten in this kit is nitropyrazole (NP).
(b) Anti-NP alkaline phosphatase enzyme conjugate (~10 μg/mL) solution in a protein containing buffer including ProClin solution, a preservative.
(c) Enhancer reagent contains < 3% $MgCl_2$ in a tris buffer solution.
(d) Naphthol reagent contains < 8 g/L Naphthol in a tris buffer solution.
(e) Fast Red Chromogen reagent contains < 3 g/L Fast Red salt in acetate buffer solution.

The post-staining procedure for the HER2/Ch17 dual ISH assay is similar to the alkaline phosphatase Red IHC protocol outlined previously. Since the Fast Red chromogen is soluble in alcohol and acetone, stained slides that are exposed to these solvents show reduced or loss of specific signal. The recommendation is for stained slides to be washed in warm soapy water in order to remove residual LCS followed by fresh water wash before completely drying them in an oven (45–60°C) or at ambient temperature. Slides must be completely dry before dipping in xylene and coverslip with an approved permanent mountant. Care is required with choice of mountant as some may cause the silver stain to oxidize further, producing a yellow artefact. The probe data sheet has a list of approved mounting media (Ventana 2020).

Companion Diagnostics

The FDA defines a companion diagnostic as one that provides essential information related to the safety and efficacy of use for a therapeutic in patients (FDA 2021). These diagnostic tests must be confirmed to be reliable, accurate and clinically meaningful and provide clinical utility Hence, there is now a shift in the importance of IHC in anatomical pathology from the role of tumour differentiation to include predictive markers guiding the use of specific therapies. One of the pioneering companion diagnostic IHC assays arrived in the late 1980s when the FDA gave approval for Dako's Hercep Test to select breast cancer patients identified as suitable for the drug Herceptin marketed by Roche formally Genentech. The drug and the test were developed together in a combined clinical study (Cartun et al. 2019).

Roche Ventana offers a range of companion diagnostic assays. Some of these are listed next. All of these assays have protocols that are mostly 'locked'. Efforts to 'standardize' IHC are actually conscious attempts to reduce variation in reagents, protocol options and incubation times on board the instrument. Quality control and careful monitoring of the results are essential. Digital pathology and image analysis will play an increasing role in providing consistent, reproducible and quantitative IHC results, especially for double staining and counting nuclear staining signals and comparing intensity of stain with a control material (Lin and Shi 2015).

Ventana PD-L1 (SP263), programmed death-ligand B7 homolog is a membranous stain with or without cytoplasmic staining. The staining is expressed in immune cells and tumour cells. This helps to identify patients who benefit from PD-1-directed therapy (Patel and Kurzrock 2015). Recommended controls are tonsil, with positive and negative lung non-small cell lung cancer tissue. Fixation should be in 10% neutral buffered formalin (NBF) for 6–72 hours and 3–4 μm sections are most suitable. Roche advise the running of a negative reagent control with each sample (Ventana 2017).

Ventana PD-L1 (SP142) assay is used for triple negative breast cancer (TNBC) FFPE tissue sections to identify patients eligible for treatment with TECENTRIQ (atezolizumab). Tumour-infiltrating immune cells (IC) are assessed as a proportion of tumour area, including intra-tumoural and contiguous peritumeral stroma occupied by PD-L1 staining IC of any intensity. Normal tonsil is recommended as a control. This assay is not validated for use with cytology samples or decalcified bone specimens. Recommended fixative is 10% NBF, with loss of specific PD-L1 protein observed with alcohol-based fixatives such as alcohol formalin acetic acid (AFA). Roche advise the running of a negative reagent control with each sample (Ventana 2018).

Ventana ROS1 SP384 Rabbit Monoclonal Primary Antibody IHC is used as a screening test for ROS1 gene rearrangements to predict eligibility for crizotinib and entrectinib, a tyrosine kinase inhibitor for treatment of ROS1-positive advanced NSCLC cases. Immunohistochemistry detects cytoplasmic ROS1 protein expression in FFPE NSCLC tissue or cytology cell block samples, identified in 1–2% of NSCLCs. ROS1-rearranged NSCLC usually shows homogenous, diffuse moderate to strong positivity. Focal weak to moderate staining may be seen in ROS1-negative cases (Conde et al. 2021). There's frequent staining of non-neoplastic type II pneumocytes with ROS1 IHC. As with all IHC assays, same-slide external positive and negative tissue controls are required. Fluorescence *in situ* hybridization (FISH) is the genetic testing method for confirming ROS1 rearrangement. A molecular test such as reverse transcription PCR (RT-PCR) or next-generation sequencing (NGS) may also be used to confirm ROS1 IHC positive cases. Roche advise the running of a negative reagent control with each sample to show non-specific background staining (Ventana 2019).

Ventana ALK D5F3 Rabbit monoclonal primary antibody is an assay for the detection of anaplastic lymphoma kinase (ALK) protein in FFPE NSCLC. This is used to identify patients eligible for treatment with crizotinib, ceritinib, alectinib or lorlatinib (Ventana 2014c). Expression of the protein may be cytoplasmic in FFPE NSCLC tissue. The assay is run with same-slide external positive and negative controls. Roche advise the running of a negative reagent control with each sample. The detection of the ALK D5F3 protein in NSCLC is confirmed by FISH staining.

Cytology Preparations

Cytology preparations, in particular FFPE cell block sections and cytospin slides, can also be stained on the Ventana ULTRA. Cell blocks are prepared in agar or plasma-thrombin, depending on the amount of material available.

Cell blocks are routinely prepared from cell suspensions, centrifuged pellets, natural clots and tissue fragments that are fixed in 10% NBF. Needles from fine needle aspirate (FNA) procedures are routinely rinsed in 10% NBF. Cells from fresh material such as effusions and brush tips are fixed for a minimum of 30 minutes before being spun into pellets and agar is added, allowed to solidify, fixed and finally processed to paraffin block. Care is taken not to overheat the agar as it may damage the cells.

The plasma-thrombin clot method is used for unfixed sparsely cellular samples and effusions. The clots are prepared and fixed in 10% NBF, followed by processing to paraffin block. Immunohistochemistry is performed on FFPE cell block preparations, similar to FFPE tissue blocks. Figure 4.18A is an example of a FNA taken from a lymph node of a patient, establishing metastatic lung adenocarcinoma. The marker is ALK D5F3 and it is a positive result, so the patient is a potential candidate for tyrosine kinase inhibitor treatment.

Urine cytology preparations may be cytospun directly onto charged slides for immunohistochemistry. Figure 4.18B displays pap-stained urine containing cytopathic changes consistent with polyomavirus infection. The corresponding IHC for SV40/BK virus is indicated in Figure 4.18C and confirms detection of polyomavirus infection. Standardization of smear thickness, fixation and the challenge of appropriate controls are limiting

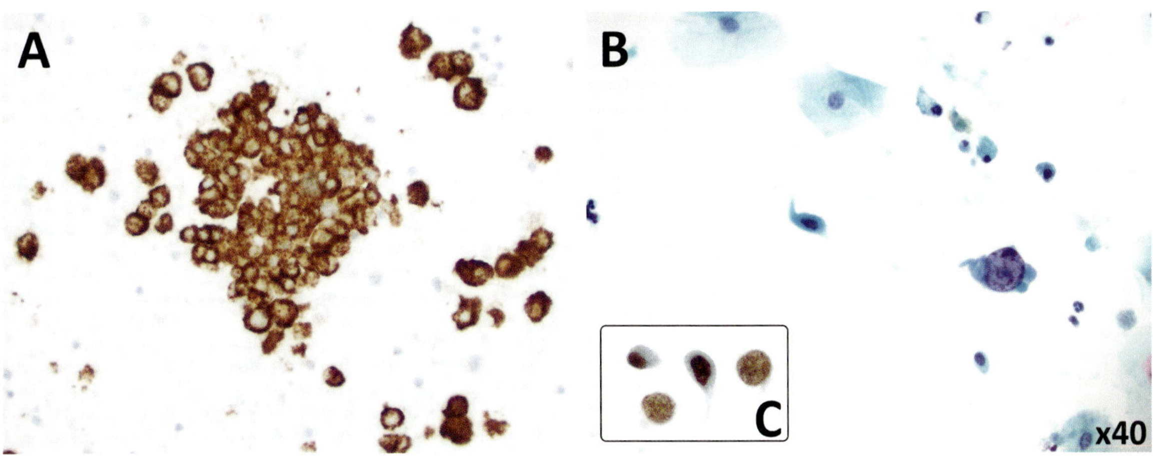

Figure 4.18 Immunohistochemistry on FNA lymph node for ALK D5F3 (A) and pap-stained urine (B) with corresponding SV40 IHC for polyomavirus (C)

factors with IHC on smears. Ongoing in-house verification of staining results in the laboratory may be accumulated over time.

Double Labelling with the BenchMark ULTRA

Staining two or more antibodies in the same tissue section is useful in cases where minimal tissue is available and when the markers complement each other, making it easier for the pathologist to piece together the clinical picture. The ability to visualize two or more antibodies in the same tissue section affords efficiency in reporting and interpretation, but these multiplex assays are technically more difficult with longer assay times and more costly to perform.

There are two strategies to employ double labelling. A simultaneous method occurs when a cocktail of different antibodies raised in different species (such as one antibody raised in mouse and another in rabbit) or antibodies raised in the same species with different isotypes are applied to the tissue section all at once followed by the detection systems. A sequential protocol is where the primary antibody is applied and detected (OptiView DAB), followed by the application of a second antibody developed with another chromogen such as alkaline phosphatase red. This method ensures one label staining technique is completed before the other.

Sequential Double Immunohistochemical Staining

Simultaneous (parallel) IHC staining protocol is not available on the Ventana ULTRA. Sequential double IHC staining, however, is available on this platform. The primary antibody is visualized with one detection kit followed by the second antibody being visualized by another detection kit. Commonly, the first primary antibody is developed with a DAB detection kit followed by the second primary antibody being developed with alkaline phosphatase red detection kit. Each antibody is optimized for each corresponding detection kit before performing double labelling. This form of sequential double IHC staining requires the antigen retrieval conditions of both antibodies being closely matched to each other. Ideally, the initial antigen retrieval is sufficient for both antibodies. Use of enzyme digestion on its own or in combination with HIER may reduce quality of tissue morphology. Use of control tissue is essential to monitor the method, reagents and instrument performance. Protocol selection includes choosing the antibody for the brown chromogen followed by the second antibody for the Fast Red chromogen. After the first chromogen is used, the slide is heated to 90°C to remove unbound primary antibody and ready the slide for the second antibody reaction and detection, seen in Appendix 5, step 18.

If the two or more antibodies require significantly different retrieval regimes, there is the option to add another retrieval step after the first chromogen is developed for more optimal staining of the second antibody. In this scenario, the simpler retrieval protocol is done first and developed with DAB before additional retrieval is carried out for the Fast Red chromogen. For instance, if antibody A requires CC1 for 10 minutes and antibody B needs CC1 for 20 minutes, the logical protocol would be to program the VSS for a 10-minute CC1 retrieval, apply and develop antibody A with DAB before subjecting the slides to a further 10-minute burst with CC1 so antibody B can be applied and subsequently developed. As no 'cocktails of antibodies' are involved, the antibodies are applied and developed independently and 'sequentially', one after another. Best practice is to use an initial antigen retrieval method that would suit both antibodies.

An example of a dual IHC stain performed regularly at the RMH is the SOX10 and Melan A combination. Demonstrated in Figure 4.19A, the transcription factor SOX10 is a nuclear marker developed with DAB to be brown in skin melanocytes and melanoma cells. This is followed by Melan A cytoplasmic staining with alkaline phosphatase red chromogen in melanocytes and melanosomes. A red stain for melanoma workup is useful due to the often observed brown melanin pigment present in these types of cases.

An example of a 'triple' stain is the PIN4 IHC assay for prostate investigations. In this context, the 'triple' stain does not refer to three colours. Instead three antibodies are developed into a two-colour system as shown in Figure 4.19B. The antibody cocktail includes a basal cell anti-p63 marker, high-molecular-weight, anti-34βE12 cytokeratin and anti-AMACR (P504S) prostate cancer marker. Both p63 and 34βE12 are developed with DAB via peroxidase to visualize the basal and myoepithelial cells seen in normal prostate glands. Although both markers are observed as brown entities, it is simple to distinguish between the two. Nuclear staining represents p63 whilst cytoplasmic

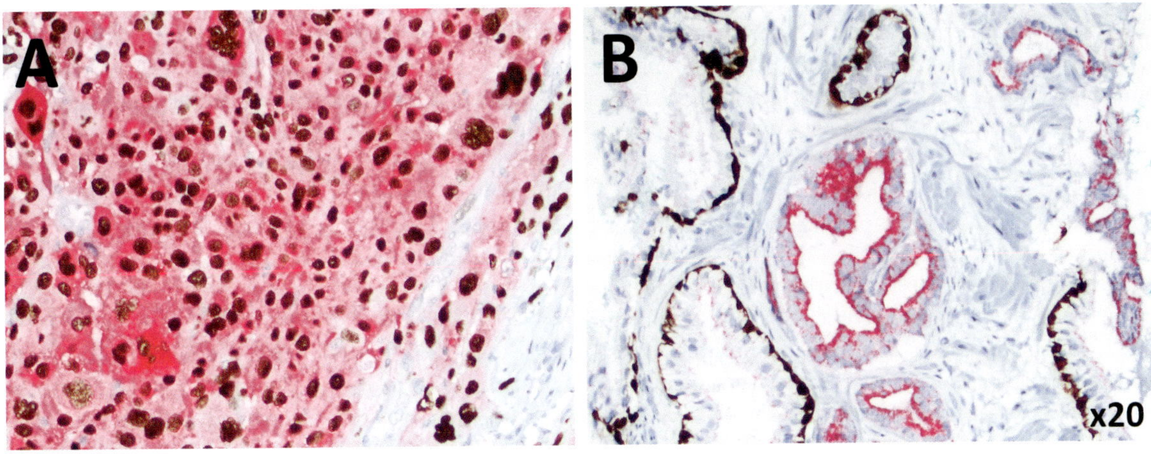

Figure 4.19 Double immunohistochemical staining using SOX10 brown and Melan A red (A). Cocktail of p63/34βE12 brown and AMACR red (B)

development is due to 34βE12. The AMACR is then established with Fast Red along the alkaline phosphatase pathway to highlight neoplastic prostate cells. Appendix 5 shows the PIN4 procedure using both OptiView DAB and UltraView Universal Alkaline Phosphatase Red detection kits in the dual colour IHC assay.

Ventana Quality Control

The Ventana system records all data, including case, stain, protocol and reagent lot number details, along with any errors or interruptions to the routine procedure, including RAPs. The information is backed up on an external data storage device. Generally there is easy, convenient access to slide, case and assay reports.

Quality control is defined by Cartun et al. (2019) as 'the aggregate of processes and techniques so derived to detect, reduce and correct deficiencies in an analytical process'. Ultimately, quality control starts with appropriate handling of fresh tissue and continues with every preparation step thereafter. The most common fixative is 10% NBF. It chemically stabilizes molecular structures by creating links in proteins. Fresh tissue needs to be fixed as soon as possible to reduce ischemic effect and the repercussions of lost antigenicity and tissue denaturation. The recommended fixation time is between 8 and 72 hours depending on the type and size of tissue. Subsequent steps of tissue processing, sectioning, microtomy, choice of slide type and baking times and temperatures all affect the IHC outcome.

Quality control activities such as daily monitoring of all staining results, regular maintenance of instrument and reagents as well as using same-slide external controls all help in the surveillance of poor staining results and reduce the number of IHC assays being repeated. The theory behind placing both positive and negative tissue controls on the same slide as the test section is that it allows exposure to the same conditions, reagents and protocol steps during the assay. This common practice also scrutinizes the instrument, antibodies and detection kits, ensuring all aspects of the IHC assay are performing as expected. The VSS provides options for recording information on control blocks and slides. Participation in external quality assurance programmes and laboratory accreditation systems ensures monitoring, conformance with continual improvement in the quality and safety of the IHC tests in the laboratory. Turnaround times and in particular trends in positive, equivocal and negative staining should be monitored especially for predictive markers.

Control tissue is best fixed and processed in the same way as the tissue sample being tested (Torlakovic et al. 2015). A weak staining positive control (low expressers) is more suitable as an indicator for optimal staining. Negative reagent control substituting the antibody with diluent buffer only tests for non-specific staining. Negative tissue controls are known to not contain the epitope. The BenchMark ULTRA monitors for errors and sounds an audible alarm when there are inadequate reagent volumes or expired reagents, or when there is uncertainty with barcode and lot number tracking within the reagent inventory management. Each slide report details all reagents and steps carried out to follow staining trends for troubleshooting. Regardless, human error cannot be entirely eliminated as the wrong sample may be submitted for staining or an incorrect external tissue control selected. These mistakes cannot be attributed to the instrument.

The overall laboratory workload, staff numbers, hours of operation and workflow considerations must be taken into account when organizing the logistics of staining slides on the BenchMark ULTRA to achieve maximum efficiency. At the RMH, the IHC facility operates Monday to Friday between 8:00 a.m. and 5:15 p.m. Upon staff members' arrival in the morning, slides stained overnight are removed from the instrument and appropriate post-staining procedures are applied. The biggest advantage of employing robotics in IHC is the ability to regularly set and perform assays overnight when all staff have left the laboratory. Slide drawers are checked for the presence of a blue LED light designating slides that need special attention. An urgent case or special post-staining protocols are highlighted. The VSS is checked for messages such as empty antibody dispensers or instrument errors. Stained slides are labelled, checked for quality assurance and, if successful, sent out to the reporting pathologists. Post-staining routines on the BenchMark ULTRA include slide drawer cleaning, priming ULTRA, bulk solution refills and waste management duties. Antibodies are removed from the instrument and stored at 4°C. New assay requests are sectioned and loaded onto the instrument continuously until 1:00 p.m. The scientist in charge of IHC is permanently rostered in the facility with one other staff member assisting on a daily rotation basis. Most scientists in the laboratory are adequately trained and capable of working independently in the IHC area. This allows other staff to 'drop in' to the IHC laboratory to help whenever the roster permits. Staff rostered in IHC also help in other laboratory sections, especially in the morning.

Maintaining a fresh stock of tissue controls, diluting antibodies from concentrates and regular instrument maintenance are performed whenever possible throughout the day. Urgent requests are loaded on demand. Although loaded reagents can be viewed via the VSS, it is convenient to fill in a form for each instrument listing the loaded antibodies and detection kits on board as a quick check sheet because user-fillable prep kits are only listed by their prep kit number without their designated antibody identification. There is no problem if vendor RTU antibodies are loaded. Another handy feature of the VSS is the pick list highlighting reagents no longer required when loading more slides on the instrument. The day's work is sent out as case runs are completed. The afternoon's requests and their reagents are sorted and loaded for the overnight run. The blue LED light is very useful for highlighting slide drawers that require the operator's attention as the stained slides are removed from the BenchMark ULTRA the following morning.

Maintenance on the BenchMark ULTRA

There are daily, monthly and quarterly maintenance schedules for the BenchMark ULTRA. Maintenance logs and reports are accessed using the maintenance 'gears' icon in the instrument view. Daily tasks include simple wiping down of the surface of the instrument and slide drawer cleaning to remove residual wax and reagents. The slide drawers should have a clean cycle run at least once a day. Although it can be difficult to find time in a busy facility, this task is important to keep the instrument optimal. The BenchMark ULTRA is placed into sleep mode and the 'clean' icon is initiated. The EZ prep and heat are employed to clean all 30 drawers at once and takes about 15 minutes to complete. During this 'down time' bulk fluid levels should be checked and waste containers emptied manually. Follow local regulations for DAB waste and oily chemical waste disposal. Remember the LCS technology Roche uses literally separates waste into two layers. The DAB waste resides in the aqueous layer and the LCS oil-based waste sits atop. The instrument is primed daily to clear the tubing of air bubbles and clean bulk reagent delivery nozzles.

On a monthly basis, the slide waste tub and drain are wiped down. The instrument is placed in 'ready mode' to allow fluid drainage before the slide thermo pads are cleaned with a brush dipped in soapy water. This task is followed by cleaning the slide drawers before the BenchMark ULTRA is used for staining. Take care not to pour water at any time into the trays as the electronics are very close to the surface. The waste tubs have been upgraded and retrofitted to all BenchMark ULTRAS by Roche in 2020 to improve safety. The bulk containers are rinsed with distilled water monthly before refill. This provides the operator with an option to decontaminate individual bulk containers on a monthly basis (not used at the RMH). Individually apply a sticker on each container recording the date it was last cleaned/decontaminated and when the opportunity arises (when the container is empty) near the monthly schedule, it is cleaned before refill.

Quarterly maintenance tasks include a major decontamination of the instrument, bulk fluid reservoirs and bulk fluid bottles. The recommendation is to decontaminate all bulks at once using the tubing manifold method even though decontaminating an individual bulk container is possible. This procedure takes about two to three hours with the instrument not available for staining during this time. The VSS issues an alert when this task is due (red maintenance icon) but has enabled the operator to decide a suitable time to initiate the process. Approximately 20 litres of disinfectant and 20 litres of distilled water are needed. Roche recommends 'Viraclean' or 'Lysol IC' for decontamination purposes. Adequate volumes of bulk reagents are needed to refill the bulk containers. The two waste containers must also be empty before starting. Heavy containers are being handled performing these tasks so safe manual handling methods should be employed. Use a mechanical lifter where possible to prevent injury. Once the decontamination cycle has initiated, there are manual intervention points requiring the operator to perform duties. Thus decontamination is not fully automatic.

The instrument starts with a purge of all the contents of the internal reservoirs into the waste containers. Unfortunately, there is an element of reagent wastage at this stage because the purged solutions cannot be recovered. A suggested workaround to minimize reagent loss is to deplete as much reagent as possible from the internal tanks prior to decontaminating. In order to do this successfully, disconnect all front bulk reagents from the instrument after an IHC or ISH run has commenced. The instrument will need all bulk containers connected at the start of the protocol run but will happily continue without the connected containers. The operator has effectively forced the instrument to deplete the internal tanks whilst purposefully preventing refill. Less reagent in the internal tanks means less wastage during the decontamination procedure.

The operator needs to remove all of the front bulk containers from the instrument. A tubing manifold method is used to introduce the disinfectant. The tubing is clicked into the bulk reagent points to access all the internal reservoirs. Note the one exception is the LCS reservoir, which does not require decontamination. The LCS cannot be contaminated with any water content. The machine pumps the disinfectant into each of the internal reservoirs and then pumps it out after the designated incubation time period. The same process occurs with the distilled water to rinse out any remaining disinfectant.

The front bulk reagent bottles do not need to be emptied and disinfected at this time if the monthly clean schedule described previously has been adhered to. Otherwise, the bulk fluid bottles are manually decontaminated, thoroughly rinsed in distilled water and refilled by the operator. All the external bulk fluid containers are reconnected, ensuring they are at least 75% full so the instrument can refill the internal reservoirs. Bulk reagents bottles may also be individually decontaminated. This is done if an individual bottle is contaminated or has been inadvertently filled with incorrect solution. This is especially relevant for the option carboy filled with UltraView silver wash solution, a troubleshooting action that may resolve silver dusting artefact on silver ISH-stained slides. The system is primed after the decontamination procedure, ready for use. Pre-planning for decontamination is required to reduce reagent wastage thereby reducing operational costs for the IHC facility. The VSS automatically records decontamination events within the maintenance log.

In addition, other maintenance tasks are performed as the need arises. The VSS is maintained via regular database backups. Data are automatically saved by the software program at the start of each run and as product data buttons are registered. A USB device is used to back up system data. It is important to properly exit the VSS before the computer is shut down in order to prevent data from being accidentally lost. Data archiving is performed at least annually by transferring old data from the VSS and storing it in an archive file. Unfortunately, this cannot be done when the connected instruments are running. The amount of time needed for archiving depends on the amount of data being archived. The instruments cannot be running when archived data are retrieved for viewing. Also, a disk clean-up can be performed to increase disk space on the computer.

Barcode readers are used for reading information on slides and reagents in the carousel. Occasionally, they may become dirty, resulting in failed reads. When it becomes difficult to register information from a barcode, the sensor on the reader must be cleaned. Laboratory staff should be able to follow the procedure outlined in the operator manual as the barcode readers are nestled inside the carousel.

Temperature verification tests are initiated to check for faulty heat pads inside slide drawers, particularly relevant if errors have been registered at particular slide positions during a staining run. Slide drawer temperature malfunction and broken posts are the main reasons for slide drawer replacement. Faulty slide drawer errors are reported to Roche technical support for replacement or repairs.

Preventative maintenance service reminders are built into the VSS. Instruments used for IHC only are serviced by Roche field service engineers every 12 months or after 12,000 slides have been stained. BenchMark ULTRAs which are used to run SISH or Dual ISH staining are serviced every 6 months or 6,000 slides. Maintenance service by Roche engineers takes at least a few hours. Preventative maintenance service keeps the instruments in optimal working order and should therefore be adhered to. Technical support in the form of application specialists is always available from Roche. Roche remote support systems are also available to aid in trouble shooting, updating and maintenance, which makes Roche a rather good company with customer support post instrument purchase.

Conclusion

The Roche Ventana BenchMark ULTRA efficiently automates the processes involved in IHC staining and ISH on FFPE sections on positively charged slides suitable for diagnostic histopathology. Fresh frozen sections and cytology cell block sections are also stained on this instrument. The ULTRA is a self-contained, free-standing, all-in-one platform that can execute slide baking, dewax, epitope retrieval with low- and high-pH cell conditioning solutions and heat, enzyme pretreatment, detection and counterstaining whilst monitoring accurate temperature and reagent volume. The workflow is flexible with batch and individual continuous slide loading, enabling the positive outcome of reproducible, accurate, high-quality results, reduced operator intervention and improved turnaround times. Flexible titration protocols ensure straightforward optimization of new antibodies. Roche Ventana offers a broad range of RTU antibodies and DNA and mRNA ISH probes including companion diagnostic predictive assays such as PD-L1, ROS1, ALK D5F3 and HER2 Dual ISH. The protocols for these assays are partially locked by the manufacturer, increasing standardization in the laboratory.

The unique technology behind the ULTRA lies in the ULTRA LCS, individual slide drawers, ability to perform manual primary antibody application, ultimate RAPs that allow for continuous, on-demand loading of slides (especially valuable for urgent cases), the range of detection systems available, multimer detection, proprietary reagents and the reagent delivery method.

The software is user friendly and the basic use of the platform is intuitive and quick to learn. There is visual management of slide activity and completion time. The reagent management screen shows dispensers on board the carousel and number of tests available. Protocol or antibody panel selection, generating slide labels and general routine operation are straightforward.

Quality control is covered by the VSS, which enables tracking of all slide and case runs with slide identification, staining protocols, error messages and reagent lot numbers. The ULTRA may be connected to the laboratory information system. These features enhance the laboratory quality assurance and control. Optimization of Roche Ventana RTU and antibody concentrates is made possible with the primary antibody titration function for determining antibody concentrate working dilution, and flexible protocol selection.

The ULTRA has some limitations. The rigorous decontamination maintenance procedure on the ULTRA and the preparation of 20-litre bulk reagents is time-consuming and poses a manual handling hazard. A safer mode of hazardous waste disposal is also required, as the existing waste management procedure is suboptimal. The best feature of this platform is the slide drawers, which are excellent for individual slide on-demand staining; however, they are notorious for heating pad temperature errors and other issues requiring attention and service. The dispensers also have their limitations, as their function declines randomly, dispensing more or less volume than they should.

The Ventana ULTRA is very efficient when every step of the process is carefully monitored – starting with optimal fixation of tissue in 10% NBF, processing, sectioning, use of recommended slides (correct storage, labelling and baking conditions), instrument maintenance, water quality, bulk reagent preparation and pH, dispenser checks, accurate post-staining procedures for coverslipping, staff training, quality assurance and strict monitoring of stain quality. Additionally, Roche Ventana provides excellent technical assistance from friendly and helpful application specialists and prompt service maintenance. Ultimately, the Roche Ventana ULTRA is an efficient and reliable system which improves workflow, generates faster turnaround times, reduces the risk of errors and produces accurate, high-quality results.

Appendix 1 Ventana General Buffers with Corresponding Histology Nomenclature

Common nomenclature	Ventana equivalent	Comments
Dewaxing solution	EZ Prep	Available as 2 L concentrate and must be diluted 1:10 with distilled or deionized water. Contains an aqueous-based detergent solution with 0.5% ProClin 300 as a preservative.
Technology to assist with reagent incubations	ULTRA Liquid coverslip (LCS)	Available as 2 L ready-to-use pre-dilute. Contains a low-density, paraffin hydrocarbon with mineral oil.
General wash buffer	Reaction buffer	Available as 2 L concentrate and must be diluted 1:10 with distilled water. A Tris-based buffer with preservative at pH7.4–7.8
Antigen retrieval high pH buffer	ULTRA Cell conditioning 1 (CC1)	Available as 2 L ready to use pre-dilute. Tris-based buffer and preservative at pH 8.0–8.5.
Antigen retrieval low-pH buffer	ULTRA Cell Conditioning 2 (CC2)	Available as 1 L ready-to-use pre-dilute. Citrate-based buffer pH 6.0 required for ISH and some IHC protocols. If not needed, fill bulk container with reaction buffer.
Antibody diluent	Antibody dilution buffer (green)	250 mL bottle. Contains phosphate-buffered saline containing stabilizing protein and 0.1% ProClin 300.

Appendix 2 Ventana Immunohistochemistry Reagents with Corresponding Histology Nomenclature

Common nomenclature	Ventana equivalent	Comments
Antigen retrieval low- and high-pH buffer	ULTRA Cell conditioning 1 (CC1) and ULTRA Cell conditioning 2 (CC2)	CC1 is 2 L ready-to-use Tris-based buffer with preservative at pH 8.0–8.5. CC2 is 1 L ready-to-use citrate-based buffer at pH 6.0 required for ISH and some IHC protocols.
Detection kit with multimer technology (enzymes conjugated to the secondary antibody via long-arm linkers)	UltraView Universal DAB OptiView DAB kit UltraView Red kit	UltraView and OptiView peroxidase based with DAB chromogen. UltraView Red Alkaline phosphatase based with Napthol Fast Red chromogen.
Signal enhancement	OptiView DAB Amplification kit	Used for low-expressing antigens/epitopes. For use with OptiView DAB IHC detection kit.
Enzyme retrieval (IHC)	IHC Protease 1/2/3	IHC Protease 1 is strongest: 0.38 mg/mL alkaline protease enzyme activity in an enzyme-stabilizing solution containing 0.01% sodium azide. Protease 2 and 3 (weaker) are also available.
Counterstain/Bluing reagent	Haematoxylin II/Bluing reagent	Both are acquired separately to the detection kit.
Open reagent container used for antibody concentrates	Prep kit user-fillable dispenser: 50 test/100 test/250 test	Antibody concentrate diluted in Ventana antibody diluent buffer or RTU antibody sourced from other vendors.

Appendix 3 Ventana *In Situ* Hybridization Reagents with Corresponding Histology Nomenclature

Common nomenclature	Ventana equivalent	Comments
Wash buffer for ISH applications only	Sodium Salt Citrate (SSC)	Available as 2 L concentrate and must be diluted 1:5 with distilled water. Contains sodium chloride, sodium citrate and a preservative at pH6.5–7.5.
Low-pH silver wash for silver ISH (SISH) only	Option bottle for SISH: UltraView Silver Wash II	Available as 2 L ready-to-use pre-dilute for stringency wash. Contains ~0.5 M citrate buffer and preservative at pH 4.0. If not needed, fill bulk container with reaction buffer.
Hybridization solution for ISH procedure	HybReady for ISH	Formamide based pre-hybridization buffer with < 55% formamide.
Detection kit for ISH	ISH iView Blue kit VENTANA Silver ISH DNP detection kit VENTANA Red ISH DIG detection kit	Chromogenic ISH for optical microscopy. Blue chromogen based on BCIP-NBT and alkaline phosphatase. Silver ion-based oxidation from peroxidase to black precipitate and red chromogen based on Napthol Fast Red chromogen and alkaline phosphatase.
Enzyme retrieval (ISH)	ISH Protease 1/2/3	ISH Protease 3: 0.24 casein U/mL is the weakest in a Tris-based enzyme-stabilizing solution containing sodium azide. ISH Protease 1 and 2 (stronger) are also available.
Red counterstain	Red Counterstain II	Purchased separately to the detection kit.

Appendix 4 SATB2 Immunohistochemistry Staining Protocol with OptiView Detection and Diaminobenzidine Chromogen

Step	Reagent	Temperature	Incubation time
1	On-board baking	65°C	8 min
2	Deparaffinize (EZ Prep)	72°C	~16 min
3	EZ Prep	Ambient	rinse
4	ULTRA CC1	100°C	48 min
5	Reaction buffer	Ambient	rinse
6	SATB2 RTU antibody	36°C	20 min
7	Reaction buffer	36°C	rinse
8	Peroxidase block	36°C	4 min
9	Reaction buffer	36°C	rinse
10	HQ linker	36°C	8 min
11	Reaction buffer	36°C	rinse
12	HRP multimer	36°C	8 min

(cont.)

Step	Reagent	Temperature	Incubation time
13	Reaction buffer	36°C	rinse
14	H_2O_2 and DAB chromogen	36°C	8 min
15	Reaction buffer	36°C	rinse
16	Copper enhancement	36°C	4 min
17	Reaction buffer	36°C	rinse
18	Haematoxylin II	36°C	12 min
19	Reaction buffer	36°C	rinse
20	Bluing Reagent	36°C	4 min
21	Reaction buffer	Ambient	rinse

Appendix 5 PIN4 Protocol Using OptiView Diaminobenzidine and UltraView Red Detection in a Sequential Dual-Colour Immunohistochemical Stain

Step	Reagent	Temperature	Incubation time
1	On-board baking	65°C	8 mins
2	Deparaffinize (EZ Prep)	72°C	~16 min
3	EZ Prep rinse	Ambient	rinse
4	ULTRA CC1	100°C	48 min
5	Reaction buffer	Ambient	rinse
6	34BE12+p63 (Primary antibody)	36°C	20 min
7	Reaction buffer	36°C	rinse
8	Peroxidase block	36°C	4 min
9	Reaction buffer	36°C	rinse
10	HQ linker	36°C	8 min
11	Reaction buffer	36°C	rinse
12	HRP multimer	36°C	8 min
13	Reaction buffer	36°C	rinse
14	DAB chromogen	36°C	8 min
15	Reaction buffer	36°C	rinse
16	Copper enhancement	36°C	4 min
17	Reaction buffer	Ambient	Rinse
18	Reaction buffer	90°C	4 min
19	Reaction buffer	36°C	4 min
20	AMACR (DS antibody)	36°C	40 min
21	Reaction buffer	36°C	rinse

(cont.)

Step	Reagent	Temperature	Incubation time
22	Red Universal Multimer	36°C	12 min
23	Reaction buffer	36°C	rinse
24	Red enhancer	36°C	4 min
25	Naphthol and Fast Red chromogen	36°C	8 min
26	Fast Red B	36°C	8 min
27	Reaction buffer	36°C	rinse
28	Haematoxylin II	36°C	4 min
29	Reaction buffer	36°C	rinse
30	Bluing reagent	36°C	4 min
31	Reaction buffer	Ambient	rinse

References

Cartun RW, Taylor CR, Dabbs DJ 2019. Techniques of immunohistochemistry: Principles, pitfalls and standardization. In Dabbs DJ, ed. *Diagnostic immunohistochemistry: Theranostic and genomic applications*. Saunders; 1–46.

Conde E, Hernandez S, Benito A, Caminoa A, Garrido P, Lopez-Rios F 2021. Screening for ROS1 fusions in patients with advanced non-small cell lung carcinomas using the VENTANA ROS1 (SP384) rabbit monoclonal primary antibody. *Expert Rev Mol Diagn* **21**:437–44.

Coons AH, Creech HJ, Jones RN 1941. Immunological properties of an antibody containing a fluorescent group. *Proceedings of the Society for Experimental Biology and Medicine* **47**(2):200–2.

FDA 2021. List of cleared or approved companion diagnostic devices (in vitro and imaging tools). US Food and Drug Administration (online). Available at www.fda.gov/MedicalDevices/ProductsandMedicalProcedures/InVitroDiagnostics/ucm301431.htm (Accessed 21 January 2021).

Lin F, Shi J 2015. Standardization of diagnostic immunohistochemistry. In Lin F, Prichard J, eds. *Handbook of practical immunohistochemistry: Frequently asked questions*. Springer; 17–30.

Myers J 2004. Automated slide stainers for special stains, immunohistochemistry, and in situ hybridization. *Medical Laboratory Observer* **36**(1):28–30.

Patel SP, Kurzrock R 2015. PD-L1 expression as a predictive biomarker in cancer immunotherapy. *Mol Cancer Ther* **14**(4):847–56.

Prichard J, Biting AK 2015. Automated immunohistochemistry overview. In Lin F, Prichard J, eds. *Handbook of practical immunohistochemistry: Frequently asked questions*. Springer; 31–8.

Shi RS, Key ME, Kalra KL 1991. Antigen retrieval in formalin-fixed, paraffin-embedded tissues: An enhancement method for immunohistochemical staining based on microwave oven heating of tissue sections. *J Histochem Cytochem* **39**(6):741–8.

Sternberger LA, Hardy PH, Cuculis JJ, Meyer HG 1970. An unlabeled antibody enzyme method of immunohistochemistry: Preparation and properties of soluble antigen-antibody complex (horseradish peroxidase–anti-horseradish peroxidase) and its use in identification of spirochetes. *J Histochem Cytochem* **18**(5):315–33.

Torlakovic EE, Emilia E, Soren N, Mogens V, Clive TR 2015. Getting controls under controls: The time is now for immunohistochemistry. *J Clin Pathol* **68**(11):879–82.

Ventana 2011a. Protease 1. Ventana Medical Systems Inc. (online). Available at https://pim-eservices.roche.com/eLD/api/downloads/69d63ce1-4133-ea11-fc90-005056a71a5d?countryIsoCode=au (Accessed 24 January 2021).

Ventana 2011b. Protease 2. Ventana Medical Systems Inc. (online). Available at https://pim-eservices.roche.com/eLD/api/downloads/b9e19050-4333-ea11-fc90-005056a71a5d?countryIsoCode=au (Accessed 24 January 2021).

Ventana 2012. BenchMark ULTRA Advanced Staining System Operator Guide. Ventana Medical Systems Inc. (online). Available at https://pim-eservices.roche.com/eLD/api/downloads/feb1a30c-5c0e-e411-1db5-00215a9b0ba8?countryIsoCode=au (Accessed 21 July 2021).

Ventana 2014a. VENTANA Ultra Cell Conditioning Solution (ULTRA CC1). Ventana Medical Systems Inc. (online). Available at https://pim-eservices.roche.com/eLD/api/downloads/87d39455-7733-ea11-fa90-005056a772fd?countryIsoCode=au (Accessed 21 July 2021).

Ventana 2014b. ULTRA Cell Conditioning Solution (ULTRA CC2). Ventana Medical Systems Inc. (online). Available at https://pim-eservices.roche.com/eLD/api/downloads/a96b5630-7733-ea11-fa90-005056a772fd?countryIsoCode=au (Accessed 24 January 2021).

Ventana 2014c. Anti-ALK (D5F3) Rabbit Monoclonal Primary Antibody. Ventana Medical Systems Inc. (online). Available at https://pim-eservices.roche.com/eLD/api/downloads/021ed24a-2436-ea11-fc90-005056a71a5d?countryIsoCode=au (Accessed 7 July 2021).

Ventana 2015a. Protease 3. Ventana Medical Systems Inc. (online). Available at https://pim-eservices.roche.com/eLD/api/downloads/e5ff24d9-4133-ea11-fc90-005056a71a5d?countryIsoCode=gb (Accessed 24 January 2021).

Ventana 2015b. ISH Protease 3. Ventana Medical Systems Inc. (online). Available at https://pim-eservices.roche.com/eLD/api/downloads/f6384c9d-6e33-ea11-fa90-005056a772fd?countryIsoCode=au (Accessed 24 January 2021).

Ventana 2017. Ventana PD-L1 SP263. Ventana Medical Systems Inc. (online). Available at https://pim-eservices.roche.com/eLD/api/downloads/176c3abe-2936-ea11-fc90-005056a71a5d?countryIsoCode=gb (Accessed 4 July 2021).

Ventana 2018. Ventana PD-L1 SP142. Ventana Medical Systems Inc. (online). Available at https://pim-eservices.roche.com/eLD/api/downloads/55b6cde7-2536-ea11-fc90-005056a71a5d?countryIsoCode=gb (Accessed 5 July 2021).

Ventana 2019. Ventana ROS1 (SP384). Rabbit monoclonal primary antibody. Ventana Medical Systems Inc. (online). Available at https://pim-eservices.roche.com/eLD/api/downloads/b1f4ca4d-3436-ea11-fc90-005056a71a5d?countryIsoCode=gb (Accessed 3 June 2021).

Ventana 2020. HER2 Dual ISH DNA Probe Cocktail. Ventana Medical Systems Inc. (online). Available at https://diagnostics.roche.com/content/dam/diagnostics/us/en/LandingPages/her2-dual-ish/VENTANA-HER2-Dual-ISH-Method-Sheet.pdf (Accessed 20 July 2021).

Ventana 2021a. ULTRA LCS (Predilute). Ventana Medical Systems Inc. (online). Available at https://pim-eservices.roche.com/eLD/api/downloads/bbd095de-7633-ea11-fa90-005056a772fd?countryIsoCode=au (Accessed 21 July 2021).

Ventana 2021b. UltraView Universal DAB Detection Kit. Ventana Medical Systems Inc. (online). Available at https://pim-eservices.roche.com/eLD/api/downloads/1a2df648-0b13-ea11-fa90-005056a772fd?countryIsoCode=au (Accessed 21 July 2021).

Ventana 2021c. OptiView DAB IHC Detection Kit. Ventana Medical Systems Inc. (online). Available at https://pim-eservices.roche.com/eLD/api/downloads/91aa0b07-1b36-ea11-fa90-005056a772fd?countryIsoCode=au (Accessed 21 July 2021).

Ventana 2021d. UltraView Universal Alkaline Phosphatase Red Detection Kit. Ventana Medical Systems Inc. (online). Available at https://pim-eservices.roche.com/eLD/api/downloads/e688db00-0b13-ea11-fa90-005056a772fd?countryIsoCode=au (Accessed 21 July 2021).

Ventana 2021e. ISH iVIEW$_{\text{Blue}}$ Detection Kit. Ventana Medical Systems Inc. (online). Available at https://pim-eservices.roche.com/eLD/api/downloads/e3d4d682-6e33-ea11-fa90-005056a772fd?countryIsoCode=au (Accessed 20 July 2021).

Ventana 2021f. Ventana Silver ISH DNP Detection Kit. Ventana Medical Systems Inc. (online). Available at https://pim-eservices.roche.com/eLD/api/downloads/091a97de-9662-ea11-fc90-005056a71a5d?countryIsoCode=au (Accessed 21 July 2021).

Ventana 2021g. Ventana Red ISH DIG Detection Kit. Ventana Medical Systems Inc. (online). Available at https://pim-eservices.roche.com/eLD/api/downloads/568df0ab-9662-ea11-fa90-005056a772fd?countryIsoCode=au (Accessed 21 July 21 2021).

Yaziji H, Barry T 2006. Diagnostic immunohistochemistry: What can go wrong? *Adv Anat Pathol* **13**(5):238–46.

Chapter 5

Automation and Robotics with the Agilent Dako Omnis

Andrew Dinan

Overview

Immunohistochemistry (IHC) automation is defined as a set of robotic processes performed by an instrument to alleviate the need for an operator to manually perform tasks required to achieve an IHC stain. The machines worth noting are ones that are fully automated, executing 'on board' dewax through to counterstain on formalin-fixed paraffin-embedded (FFPE) tissue. In addition to IHC, *in situ* hybridization (ISH) capabilities are also a necessity for most diagnostic histopathology facilities. The Alfred Hospital Melbourne has chosen two Dako Omnis instruments to fulfil these objectives and is the platform of which a closer examination is made from a user's perspective.

Formally released in 2013, the Omnis is Dako's answer to IHC and ISH automation. Subsequent to its official release, the company joined with Agilent, but the Dako name is still commonly used. The Autostainer Link 48 is Dako's previous generation IHC platform officially launched in 1996 and still in active duty in laboratories worldwide. Its longevity, owing to its 'open staining system', is still relevant, particularly in the research sector. In comparison, the Dako Omnis is a huge leap in technology, capability and design.

The instrument has a big footprint in the laboratory, standing at 1.77 metres tall, 1.5 metres wide and almost 0.8 metres deep (Agilent 2018). Figure 5.1 shows the distinctive design with a colour light strip

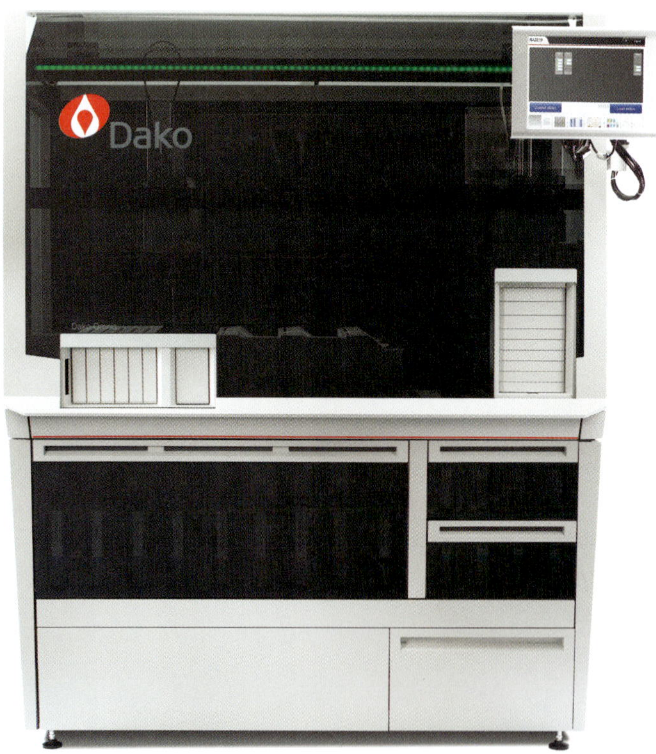

Figure 5.1 The Dako Omnis
Reproduced with permission Agilent Technologies, Inc.

across the front indicating machine status along with its dark, almost opaque front cover. All reagents necessary for IHC and ISH are concealed from view, only to be accessible when required and controlled via attached touchscreen tablet located in the top right corner.

The two machines are utilized every day, churning through thirty thousand slides a year with little interaction from the user. The technology employed to stain routine IHC assays on FFPE tissue, perform direct immunofluorescence on fresh frozen sections and ISH testing is explored in this chapter. The various components, epitope retrieval strategy and proprietary detection kits are analysed from a workflow perspective. Also included is a discussion on staining protocols, quality control measures and maintenance tasks. Dako markets the Omnis as a complete walk-away solution requiring minimal user interaction. This review tests that statement via experiences gathered from the two Omnis instruments employed at the Alfred Hospital Melbourne for IHC and ISH protocols.

Principle of the Omnis

The Omnis is based upon the Japanese 'poka-yoke' principle designed to minimize human error and enable processes to be as straightforward and streamlined as possible. Several design features are enlisted to achieve this objective. For instance, slides are clipped onto staining racks which can only be loaded into the drawers in a particular orientation via the location of holding pins. The same principle is extended to reagent vials, only fitting into the rack in a specified way. The racks themselves are also placed into the instrument in a particular fashion, guided by a 'lip' for a snug fit. This design enables the vial barcode to always face the reader.

Accidental loading of a reagent vial with the cap still fastened will cause the machine to go into alarm mode. This is due to an obstruction preventing the drawer from closing. The fine tolerances imposed on the instrument ensure no cap is accidently left on vials when loading reagents. The user is required to assign a reagent with its matched bottle number prompting a visual check for additional security. Retrieval solutions are differentiated by two distinct colours, minimizing errors attributed to reagent mishaps. The bulk containers also include plastic stoppers located at specific positions so as to alleviate mistakes made while loading reagents into the instrument. This endeavour makes it impossible to load a wash buffer in a position reserved for retrieval solution, for example. The poka-yoke standard is quite evident throughout the Omnis design.

Omnis Components

The engineering of the Dako Omnis layout is quite logical. As the operator is facing the instrument, the pathway from slide loading to slide exit is right to left. As highlighted in Figures 5.2 and 5.3, the main elements include:

a. the hood and touch screen	b. slide-loading drawers
c. pretreatment (PT) modules	d. staining modules
e. unloading station	f. reagent storage
g. mixing station	h. bulk reagent compartment
i. waste containers	j. PC and peripherals

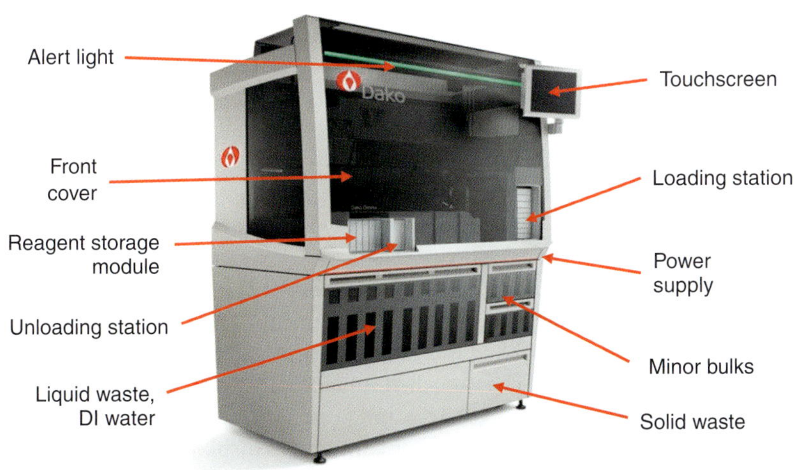

Figure 5.2 The Omnis layout
Reproduced with permission Agilent Technologies, Inc.

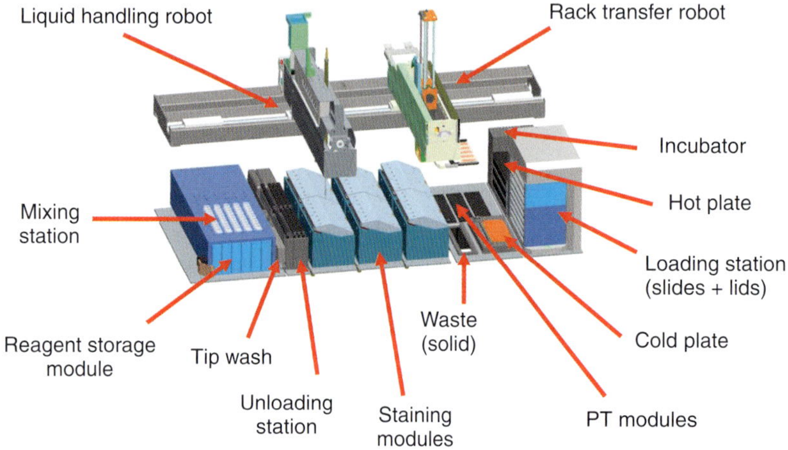

Figure 5.3 Schematic of the Dako Omnis
Reproduced with permission Agilent Technologies, Inc.

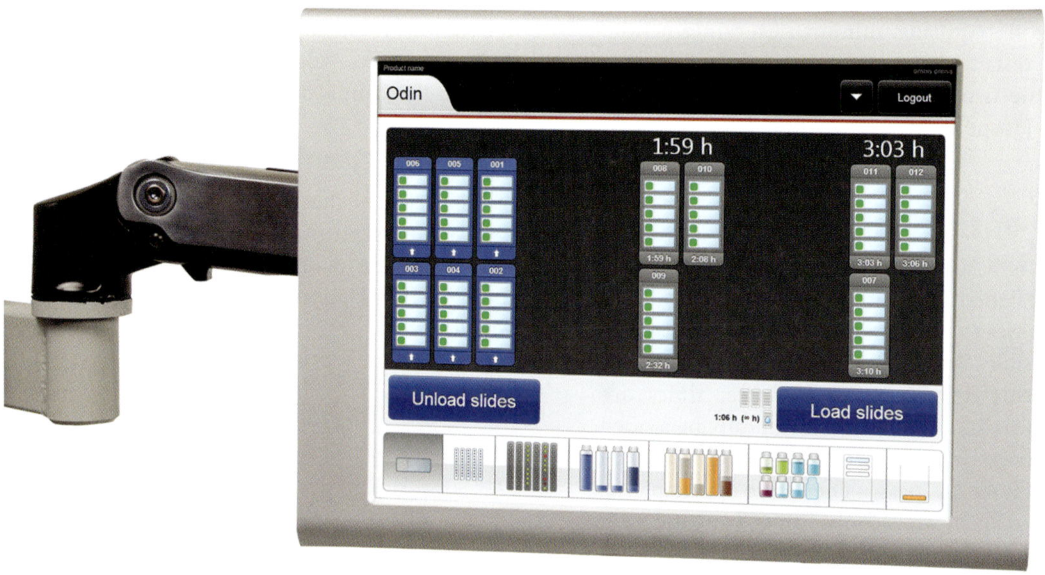

Figure 5.4 Attached touchscreen tablet
Reproduced with permission Agilent Technologies, Inc.

There are two robotic arms, one designated for liquid handling (LiHa) and the other to transfer slides.

Hood and Touchscreen Tablet

Across the top face of the Omnis is a light bar indicating various states the instrument is in. A green bar specifies the machine is working or is idle, ready for slides to be loaded. A yellow strip indicates user intervention is required before staining is initiated. For instance, slides may need to be unloaded in order to make room for newly finished slides or perhaps some reagents are missing and therefore need to be loaded to complete a staining protocol. A blue colour shows the instrument is in maintenance mode and blue flashing lights indicates user interaction is necessary. A red flashing light indicates the machine has encountered a problem. Complications can range from staining issues to mechanical glitches. The user is prompted to investigate by loading a list of all errors encountered since the last shutdown of the instrument. Error records are also displayed in a tab running along the top of the screen.

The attached touchscreen has several icons to select, giving a range of information and functions. Figure 5.4 shows the main display indicating slides

Table 5.1 Status bar

Icon	Tab	Function
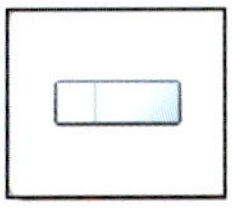	Slides	The slide tab will bring the user back to the main home screen.
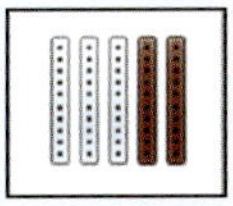	Mixing strips	This area is where diaminobenzidine (DAB) chromogen is prepared fresh as required. A used strip is indicated in brown, while unused strips and wells are indicated as white circles. Wells that are due to be used in the staining run are indicated in black.
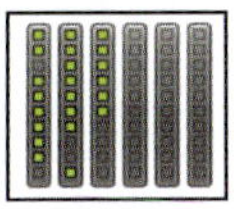	Vials	Allows access to vial loading drawers. Antibodies and detection kits are located here.
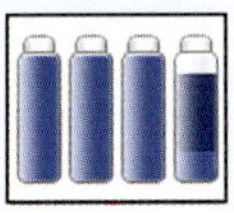	Water	Indicates deionized (DI) water levels on board and allows access to replenish these.
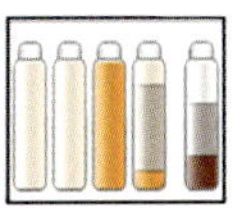	Waste	Shows the level of waste on the instrument. There are four normal waste containers and one hazardous waste container at the far right.
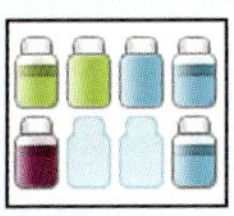	Bulks	Designates the levels of bulk reagent and identifies by colour all the reagents available. Darker shades forecast the amount that will be used during the run; these levels are shown in real time.
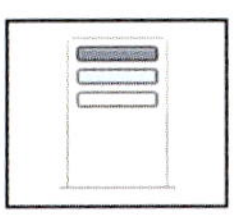	Lids	Permits access for loading ISH lids.
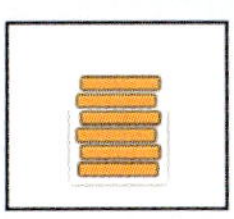	Used lids	Specifies the number of used lids which can be removed by pressing on this tab.

Icons reproduced with permission Agilent Technologies, Inc.

that have been loaded and are processing as well as slides ready to be unloaded. Slides progress from the right of the instrument to the left as the staining protocol advances. In the status-viewing area, the staining time to conclusion is shown over the racks so as to give the user an instant indication of what to expect. Further information can be displayed by selecting a rack to give information of the test and slide number.

Along the bottom of the screen is a status bar with icons that allow access to various functions. Summarized in Table 5.1, each icon has a specific function.

As highlighted in Figure 5.5, all tabs show real-time information and can be accessed at any time. Above these tabs are the load and unload slide buttons. Once pressed these take the user to the respective screens. Running at the top of the screen is the instrument name and on the right-hand corner is a triangle icon allowing access to the maintenance screen, scheduling and shutdown of the instrument. Next to this icon is the log-out/log-in function allowing multiple user accounts varying levels of access.

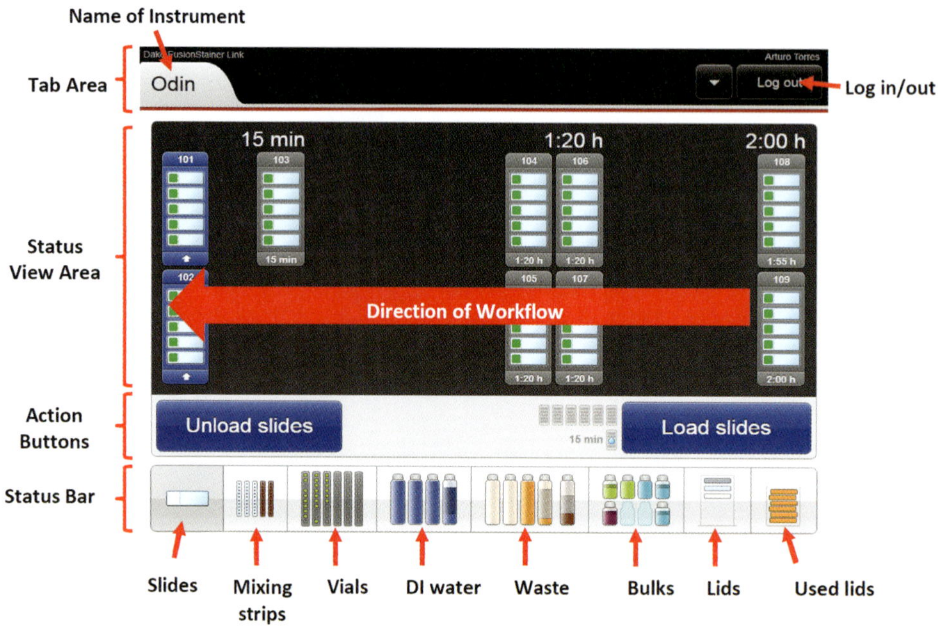

Figure 5.5 The main screen on the Omnis
Reproduced with permission Agilent Technologies, Inc.

Pressing each individual tab launches a separate window. Figure 5.6 shows the vial tab window after it has been opened. All vials currently on board the instrument are highlighted in lime green. Empty spots are dark grey. The capacity is six racks with 10 spots available per rack, giving a total of 60 places. The information is displayed visually, indicating the specific location of the vials, the names of the vials, the remaining volume and the expiration date of these reagents. The current temperatures of the vials are also displayed, usually around 18°C. Pressing the blue up arrow ejects the corresponding drawer to enable loading and unloading of reagents as needed.

To the right side of the display, the required reagents are listed as determined by the staining protocol of the loaded slides. The information contains the volume required along with the time by which the reagent is needed. If the required reagents are not loaded in time, the Omnis will abort the slide. This handy feature is utilized quite often to load the vials as required after slides have been loaded and committed to staining. The instrument examines every vial loaded by barcode scan to check for expiry dates and ensures there is an adequate volume required for the assay. If there is not enough reagent on board, that is indicated by a down arrow display on the right-hand side of the screen with an advisory 'not enough regent on board' message. Vials with past expiry dates are shown with an orange up arrow. Vials due to expire during the run are shown in orange with a clock symbol. This is a common scenario when running slides over night or slides that have been programmed for a delayed start.

When a rack with vials is loaded, a padlock symbol is displayed – a black padlock for reagents required by the slides that have been committed for staining and a white padlock for cases which have not yet been committed. In addition, a timer will then appear at the bottom of the rack icon. It remains blue until nine minutes before use and changes to yellow before turning red with less than five minutes before being required. The whole drawer is locked if a vial is currently being used, preventing access to the rack at that moment in time. Therefore, it is best practice to group and keep items of the detection kit together on a single rack, rather than spreading them out across several racks. For example, if multiple sulphuric acid vials were loaded across several racks, all racks would be locked when this item is in use. Antibodies are unloaded if they are no longer required during the day. Keeping to these simple procedures, the 60-place reagent drawers are adequate as we have not

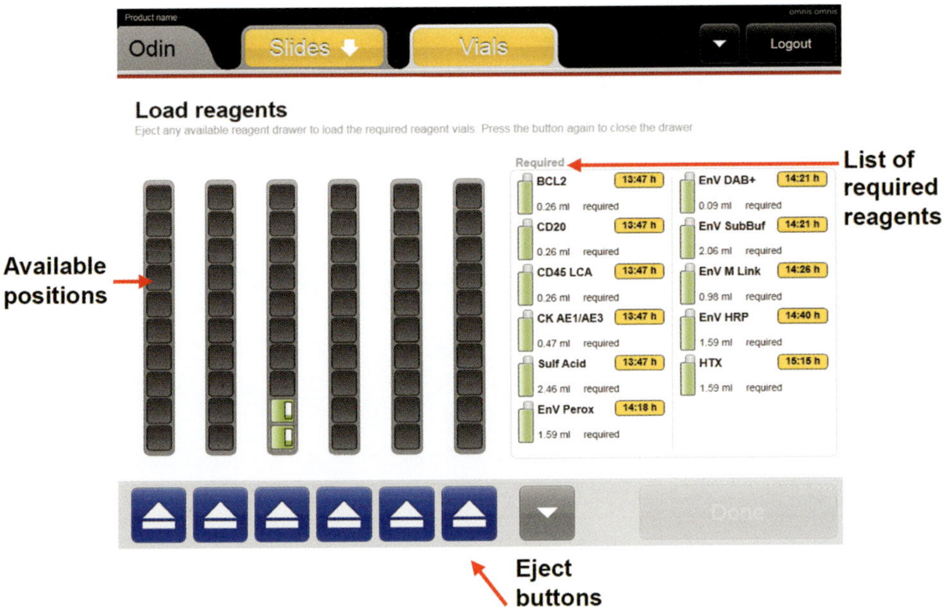

Figure 5.6 The vial tab window display

Reproduced with permission Agilent Technologies, Inc.

encountered capacity issues. Taking reagents off the instrument and back into 4°C storage helps with the shelf life and performance stability of the antibodies. The same system applies to ISH reagent vials as well since it is recommended to remove these after use and return the reagents to the freezer.

Slide-Loading Drawers

Routine FFPE IHC slides are classified as 'dry' and baked in an oven prior to loading. As shown in Figure 5.7, each drawer accommodates a rack which can hold 5 slides. A total of six racks can be loaded all at once offering a maximum of 30 slides. A further three racks can be loaded after the first three have moved immediately into the retrieval modules, resulting in 45 slides being loaded in one event. Figure 5.8 is the display of the corresponding loaded slides ready to be committed for staining. Icons with green colour mean all is well. A red colour indicates attention is needed. Table 5.2 highlights examples when errors have occurred.

The Omnis can also be configured to load 'wet' slides, which is useful for preparations of cytology alcohol-fixed slides, for example. The software notifies the user when the instrument can accommodate slides of this type by a visual countdown timer, and once loaded, a timer will show a maximum of two minutes for the slides to be committed to the run.

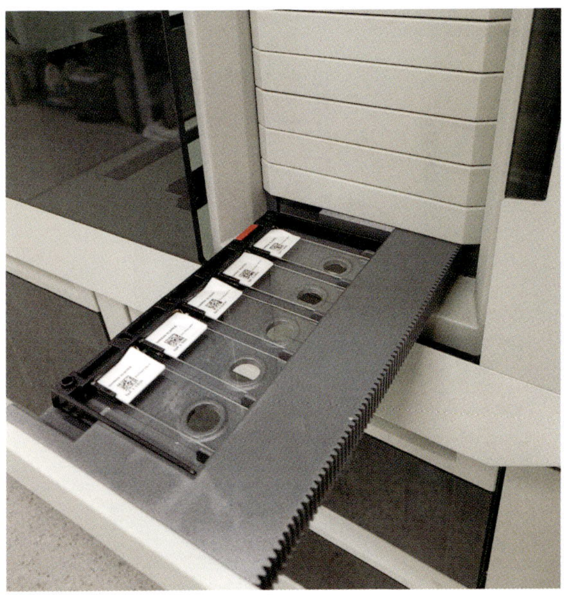

Figure 5.7 An opened Omnis slide drawer accommodating a rack of five slides

Table 5.2 Common errors that occur during slide loading

Icon	Error	Remedy
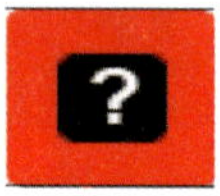	Bar code cannot be read	Ensure label is centred. Reprint label and apply again.
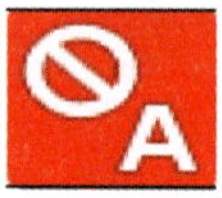	Incompatible protocol – immediate attention required	Incompatible slides must be removed and the rack reloaded to commit the slides to the run. Most commonly this is when high- and low-retrieval protocols are loaded onto the same rack.

Icons reproduced with permission Agilent Technologies, Inc.

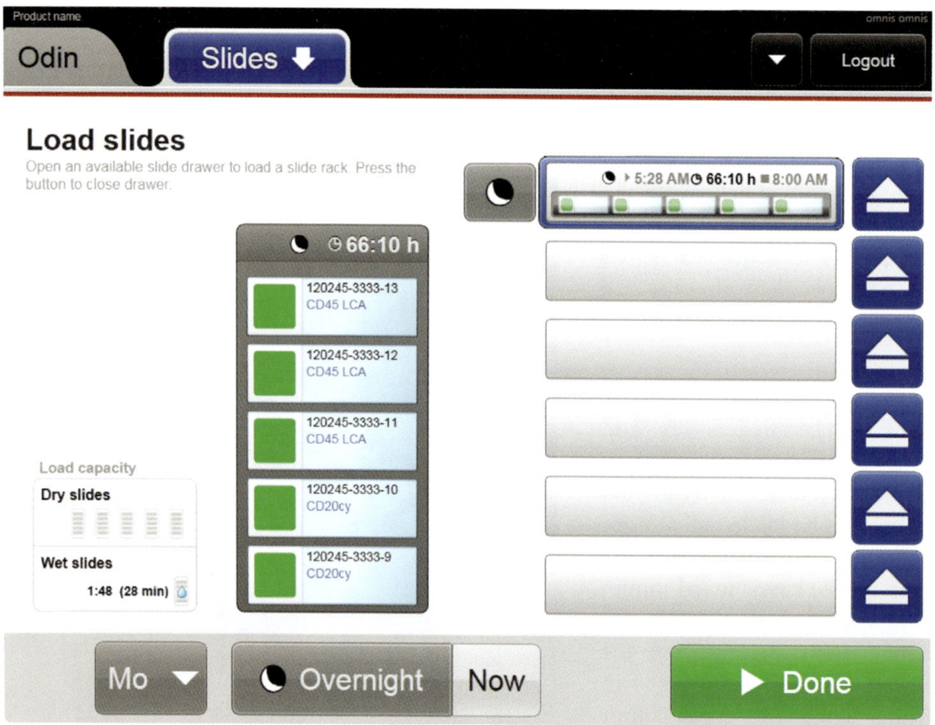

Figure 5.8 Loading screen showing a rack loaded and ready to be processed
Reproduced with permission Agilent Technologies, Inc.

Barcoded information contained within the slide label directs the Omnis to download the appropriate protocol stored on the server in the laboratory. These protocols are validated by the user on initial set-up of each antibody assay. The software gives visual information as to the slide details, the antibody assay and the total staining time of the loaded protocol. Knowing when slides will finish enables the Omnis to delay the start if the finish time is after laboratory operating hours. However, there is an 'override' function if the user wishes to proceed immediately. Delay starts can also be programmed for up to three days if required.

The instrument displays the required amount of reagent for the slides that are loaded; this is found on the first tab, labelled 'vials', which activates when slides are loaded. The Omnis records all reagent volumes used on the instrument and deducts the required volume after each use during staining. When the instrument does not have enough reagent to carry out the run, the display is changed to a 'down' arrow. If during staining, the machine encounters an empty or insufficient amount in a vial, then the instrument will cancel the slide and transfer it as 'completed'. The slide is marked with a red X, indicating that the test has been cancelled. The machine also flashes red and alarms to indicate to the user there has been an issue or insufficient reagent on board to complete staining. Unfortunately, unlike the Link 48, the Omnis does not give the user a chance to replace the reagent before it is required. Affected slides are cancelled and do not receive any more reagents. Other slides on the rack of differing protocols will carry on being stained.

In theory this situation should not occur as the instrument subtract reagents as it uses them, but for a small number of times, this has not always happened. A common reason can be bubbles in the vials, especially effecting the 2 mL vials. We find it best to check and minimize movement of vials. We have also found some vial racks not level, giving a slightly inaccurate reading of the vial volume quantity. Evaporation is also a possible reason for insufficient volumes, but in the vast majority of cases, the Omni is accurate in its estimation of reagent volume. Standard practice is to routinely check that antibody vials have a bit more than enough reagent to complete the run and, when starting an overnight run, that sufficient wash buffer and water are on board to complete the assays loaded.

Pretreatment Modules

The rack transfer robot moves the loaded rack and positions it into one of the three pretreatment (PT) modules. These tanks allow epitope retrieval on a maximum of five slides at one time. Some logistical manoeuvring is required to ensure all slides have the same PT regimens. For instance, loading slides requiring both low-pH and high-pH epitope retrieval onto the same rack is not possible. The user is notified of this error before loading as shown in Table 5.2. A useful method to separate slides by retrieval method is employing colour tabs on the rack as indicated in Figure 5.9. As there are only three modules, the Omnis can only retrieve three racks at a time. There are, however, six slide-loading drawers, so careful planning is required to get around this potential bottleneck. This theme is explored further when discussing workflow logistics.

The racks are lowered in vertically and if the slides are in 'dry' mode, Dako's Clearify dewax reagent is pumped in followed by wash buffer. As the Clearify is hydrophobic, the aqueous wash buffer raises the solution, starting from the bottom to the top of the slides in order to ensure complete dewax. Epitope retrieval then commences with reagent type and incubation conditions dictated by the IHC protocol of the slides. The Alfred Hospital keeps to a 'standard' retrieval parameter of 30 minutes at 97°C. Deionized water is used to wash and cool the slides before a wash buffer rinse in preparation for transfer to an available staining module.

Staining Modules

Temperature and humidity levels are controlled by the instrument in the staining modules, a feat made possible by its design and enclosed engineering as shown in Figure 5.10. The temperature is set to a 'standard' 32°C for IHC assays and each module utilizes cover plates to create the proprietary 'dynamic gap' technology for reagent incubation and staining. The LiHa robot is fitted with a probe to dispense all reagents from the vials. The probe actively detects liquid by using a sensitive coating and it is important to eliminate bubbles in the vials so as to ensure accurate detection. The software minimizes this error by inserting the probe up and down into the vial several times before drawing up reagent.

Unloading Station

Figure 5.11 shows the unloading station removed from the instrument accommodating the capacity for six wet racks divided into two main compartments. Filled with distilled water, the slides are held there until they are manually offloaded to undergo the laboratory's dehydrate, clear and coverslip protocol. If for any reason the unloading drawer is full with six racks awaiting unload, the Omnis can hold a further

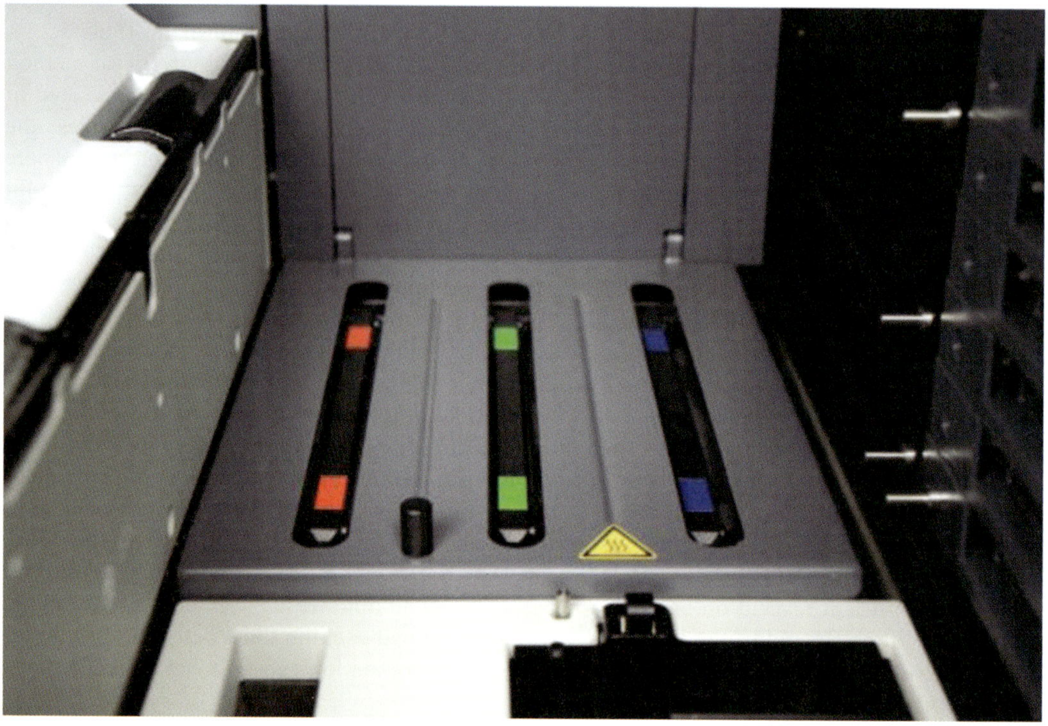

Figure 5.9 Pretreatment modules filled with slide racks
Reproduced with permission Agilent Technologies, Inc.

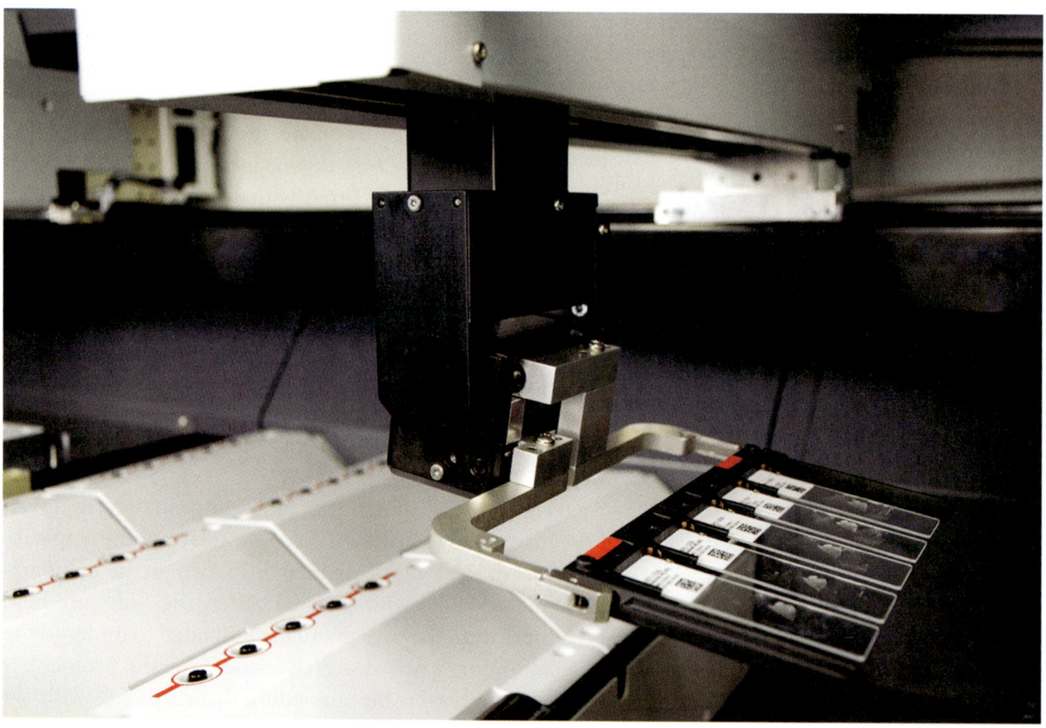

Figure 5.10 A staining module accepting slides
Reproduced with permission Agilent Technologies, Inc.

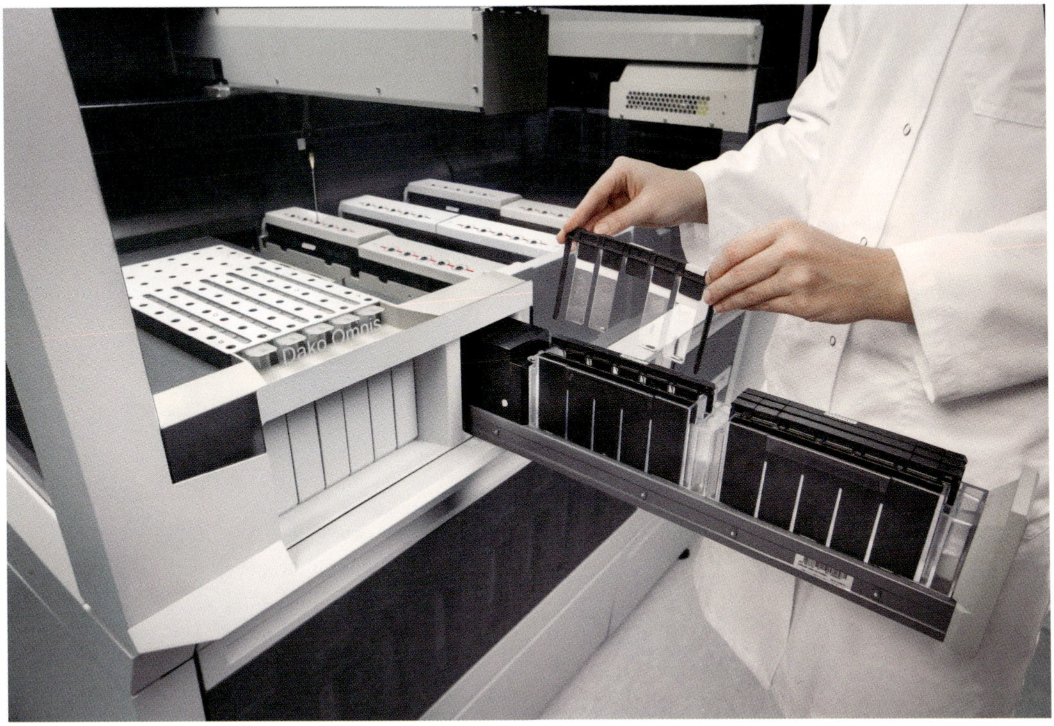

Figure 5.11 Unloading slides from the Omnis
Reproduced with permission Agilent Technologies, Inc.

six racks in the staining modules at the conclusion of staining. In this instance, the instrument cannot accept any more slides committed for staining until the completed racks are removed.

Reagent Storage

On-board storage of vials containing antibody and detection kit components is located on the left-hand side of the instrument. Six drawers are employed to accommodate racks manufactured for 10 vials each. A total of 60 spots is adequate for routine operations with the ability to add and remove vials as the Omnis is operating. The compartment has an ambient temperature of 18°C. Drawers are accessed from the touchscreen, moving in and out mechanically as highlighted in Figure 5.12. A small limitation to this design is that there are specific moments when the Omnis will not allow rack removal if the instrument requires a vial that is positioned in that rack. To minimize this predicament, the advice is to group reagents together – for example, reserving a rack to house all the detection kit reagents. Overall, access to the racks is not an issue if some thought is initially invested. A big advantage of having the reagent drawers accessible is that slides can be committed to staining without requiring all the necessary vials on board at the start. The Omnis can begin epitope retrieval protocols whilst the user is still loading the required vials into the drawers. However, a failure to load all reagents within the time limit will result in the machine aborting all of the slides.

Mixing Station

Standard practice for preparation of DAB chromogen is to formulate the reagent fresh just before use. The Omnis achieves this with a mixing station containing small single-use wells made from plastic. The software allocates colour to visually display the status of use. Figure 5.13 shows brown strips indicating the well has been used, black designates a well is reserved for use soon, and white denotes unused wells. The mixing station can accommodate five mixing strips with each strip containing 10 wells. Figure 5.14 demonstrates how the plastic strips are manually removed and replenished by the operator.

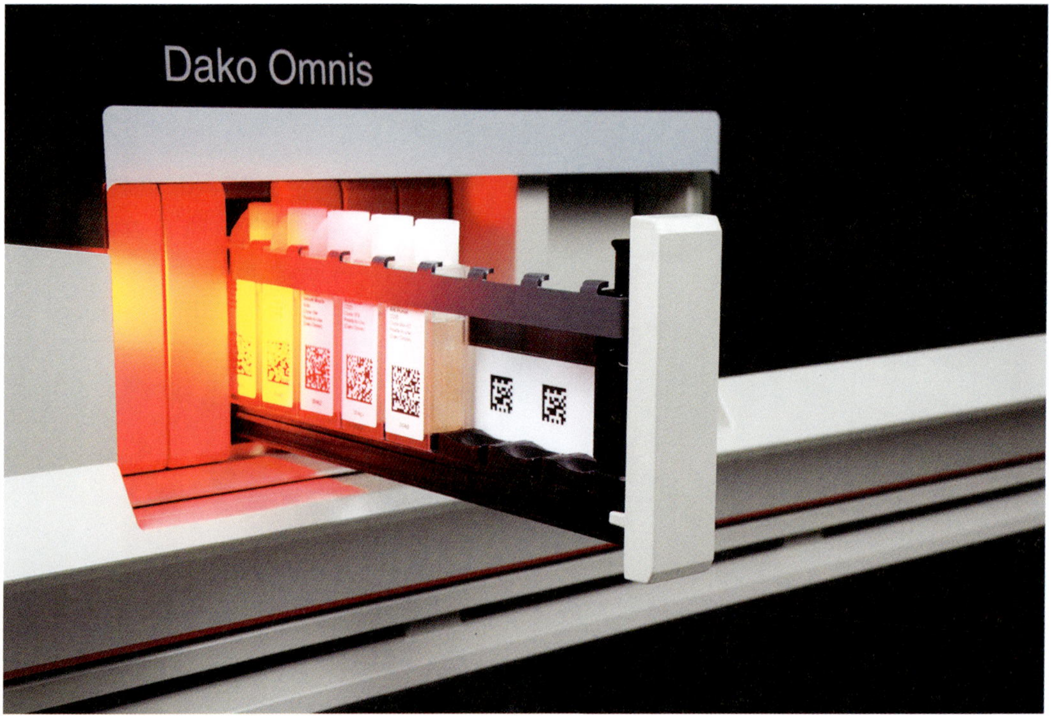

Figure 5.12 Reagent access showing vials being loaded and barcode read on the Omnis
Reproduced with permission Agilent Technologies, Inc.

Bulk Reagents

Similar to other IHC vendors supporting their own platforms, Dako supply all of the consumable bulk reagents for the Omnis. The instrument has capacity for seven bulk solutions in addition to a single Clearify dewax bulk reagent bottle. Shown in Figure 5.15, they are stored under the load drawers with each container able to hold three litres of reagent. Keeping to the poka-yoke theme, bulk reagents are added to each container filled with deionized water up to the fill line. Excluding Clearify, the reagents are supplied as a concentrate diluted to a working strength and correct pH with deionized water. Each container has a convenient specified line marking on the bottle indicating the water level before concentrate is added. All reagents are registered in the software by clicking the 'register new reagent' icon and scanning the barcode located on the bottle. The necessary barcode information contains the lot number and the expiry date of the reagent. The Omnis tracks reagent usage and nominates a working shelf life of two weeks, regardless of the expiry date displayed on the reagent concentrate. The ISH reagents are treated in the same way. Each bulk reagent has a weigh scale, allowing the machine to track the amount of reagent in the container and forecasting how much reagent will be used by the slides onboard. The software allows for viscosity differences between reagents.

A standard set-up is two wash buffers and two high-pH retrieval bottles with a Clearify bottle and a single low-pH retrieval bottle. Two spaces are reserved for ISH bulk reagents. When not in use, these are stored in the fridge in order to prolong the shelf life. Bulk reagents can be ejected on demand if currently not in use by the attached touchscreen tablet. Deionized water is also kept on board and held in four separate seven-litre containers. A lock symbol for all bulk reagents is shown when a particular bottle is in use.

Waste Containers

Waste is separated into hazardous and non-hazardous categories. Four containers each holding seven litres of non-hazardous waste are available in addition to one seven-litre container reserved for hazardous waste as highlighted in Figure 5.15. They are colour

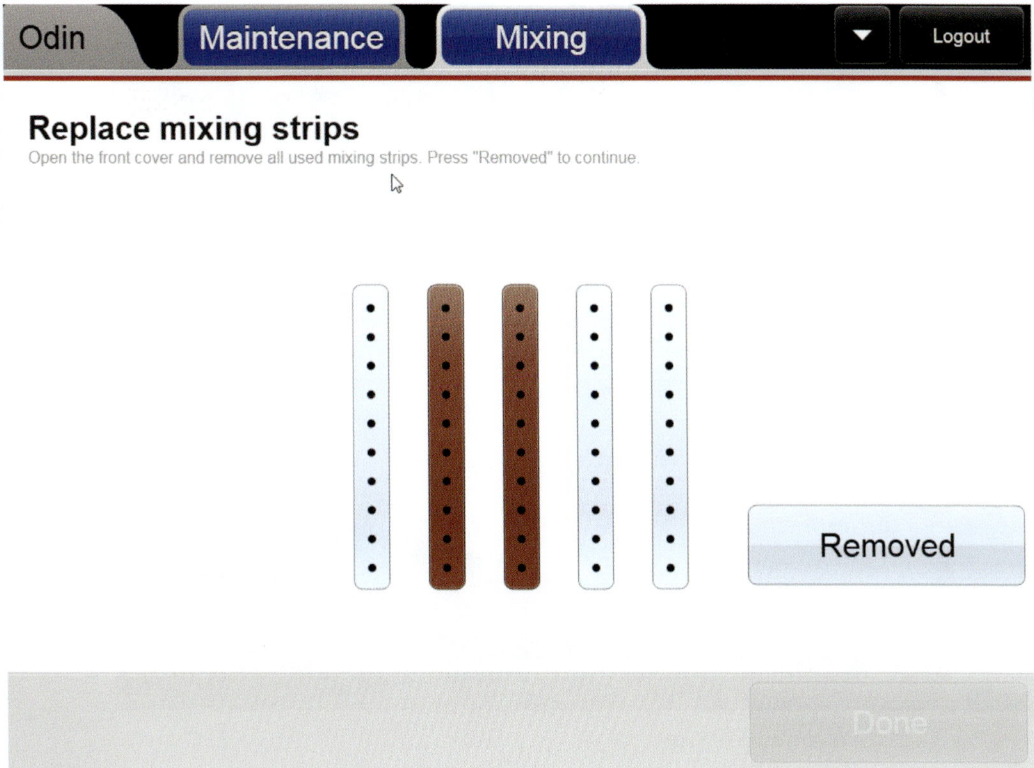

Figure 5.13 Colour designation of mixing wells
Reproduced with permission Agilent Technologies, Inc.

coded. Non-hazardous waste is housed in the four orange containers and is safe to be poured down the sink while the hazardous waste (brown bottle) containing used DAB and Clearify is disposed of via an external company. A non-hazardous waste container can be ejected at any time only if an alternative container is available. Hazardous waste, on the other hand, can be removed only once all slides on board have completed the chromogen step. Ensuring this hazardous waste container is empty at the start of each day will guarantee slides are not held up unnecessarily. Like the bulk reagents, each container sits on a weigh scale.

Personal Computer and Peripherals

Slides are requested through the Omnis workstation software on a personal computer (PC) by selecting the 'request slide' tab. The information that appears on the label can be customized depending on what information is required in the laboratory. Water- and xylene-resistant labels are printed out via the attached slide label printer. All of these items are supplied by Dako along with the Omnis instrument. At the Alfred Hospital Melbourne, batch loading is preferred. Loading slide racks when they are full ensures maximum throughput. The Omnis is capable of processing IHC and ISH slides simultaneously. The vendor claims the Omnis can process 165 slides in a typical day. A realistic benchmark in our laboratory is typically 150 slides in an eight-hour shift.

Setting up and registering new reagents along with entering slide labels are also dealt with from the Omnis workstation. Seen in Figure 5.16, the main screen of the workstation contains information regarding the instrument, slides waiting to be loaded, slides being stained and assays which have been completed. The workstation allows users to access individual screens where they can create new products and protocols, check inventory items and search for tests.

The software on the workstation tracks all antibodies and consumables. In the inventory tab, all reagents are shown and can be filtered to show those

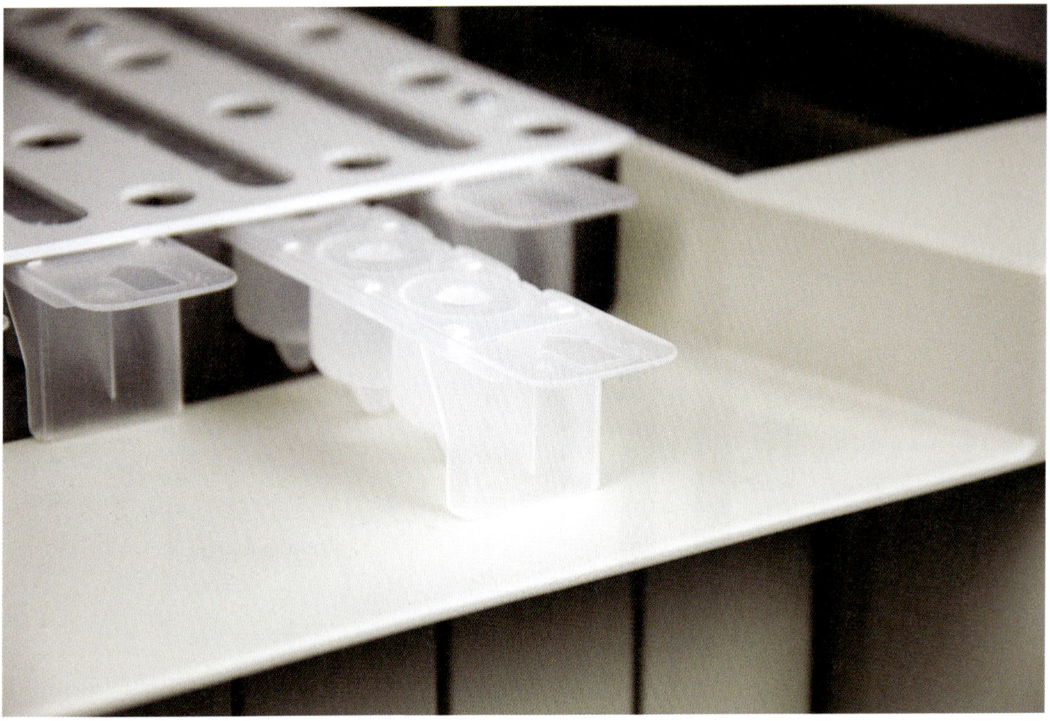

Figure 5.14 Mixing strip loading/unloading into the station
Reproduced with permission Agilent Technologies, Inc.

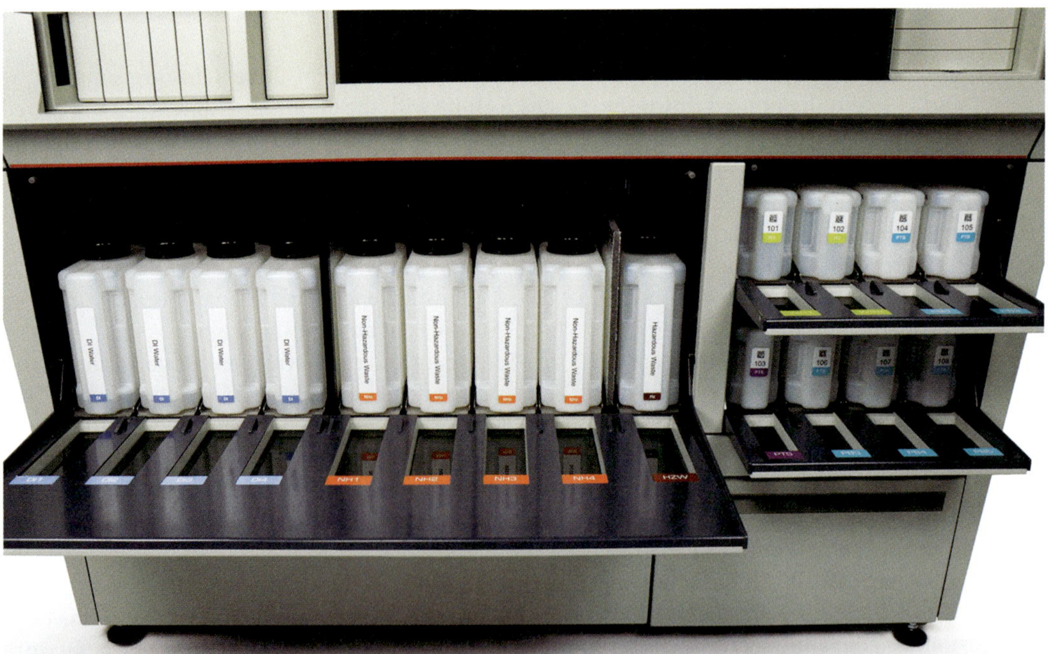

Figure 5.15 Bulk reagents, deionized water and waste bottles
Reproduced with permission Agilent Technologies, Inc.

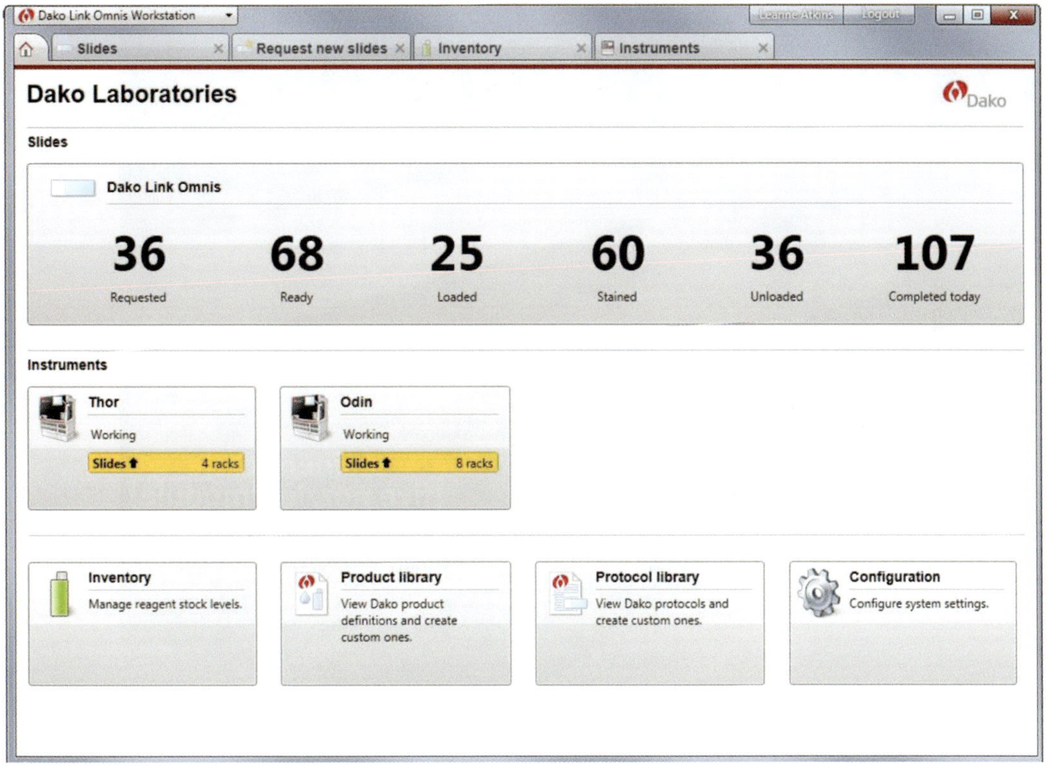

Figure 5.16 Main screen of the Omnis workstation
Reproduced with permission Agilent Technologies, Inc.

that are in use and their locations along with any suspicious or discarded items. Reagent levels with lot numbers and expiry details are also shown. Items can be looked up by typing the name of the reagent or barcode scanned to display the information. The Omnis will automatically discard reagents when they have expired as well as when they have less than one test remaining. There are times when this has not always been the case as some vials have 85 µl remaining and are yet to be discarded. The dead volume is 300 µl for a 2 mL vial. Fortunately, reagents can be discarded manually. This action allows users to identify reagents that are currently in use and it is convenient to know reagent volumes prior to loading as slides can be triaged prior to committing.

Dynamic Gap Technology

The dynamic gap technology sets the Omnis apart from its competitors. Dako have been able to achieve a staining area to cover the majority of the slide, with complete, even staining. The module opens to allow the rack, at a 25° angle, to slide inside the chamber as seen in Figure 5.17.

Figure 5.18 explains the dynamic gap lids in operation. When reagent is applied through the nozzle on the lid (A), the cover plate will move upwards to allow reagent to enter and close at the end (B and C). The cover plate is then lowered, allowing for a homogenous reaction during the incubation and washing steps (D). The capillary gap uses forces to draw down liquid and keep it between two surfaces. This ensures even reagent distribution (E). The plate then remains in position while deionized water is added, resulting in the whole slide being washed evenly (F). The technology will increase the gap in order to ensure thorough and complete washing. The plates minimize the amount of reagent required to cover a slide and also reduce evaporation. Removal of the slide is the reverse of loading, with the plate opening, allowing the robotic arm to access the rack.

After the retrieval protocol is completed, slides are cooled in a chamber with deionized water before transfer by a robotic arm to a vacant staining module.

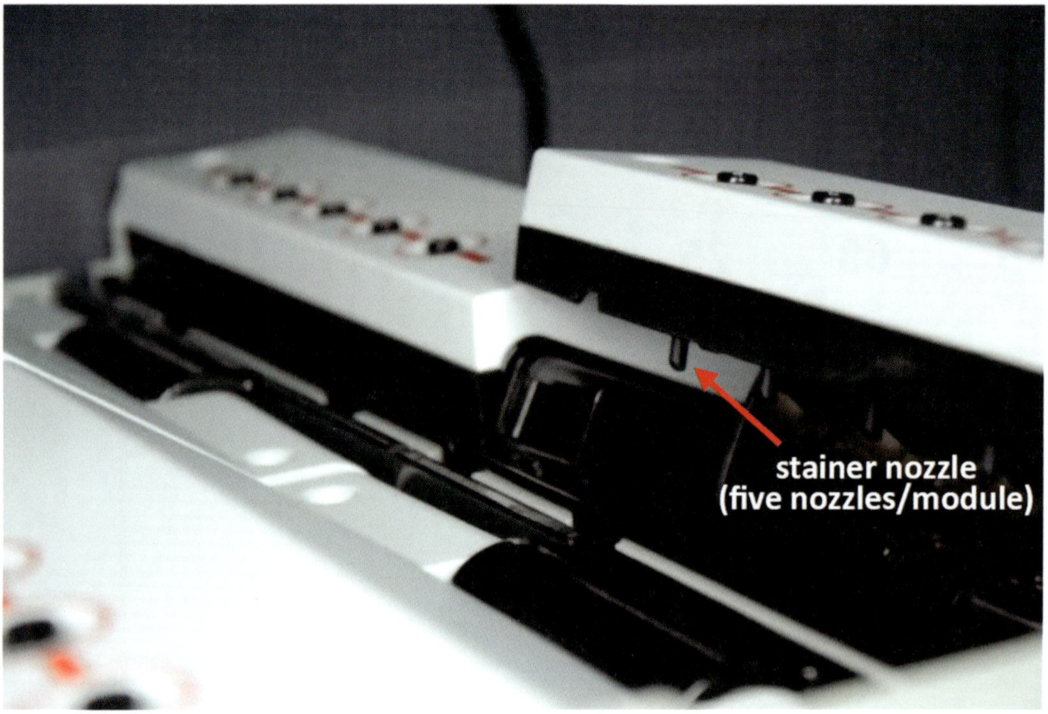

Figure 5.17 Opened staining module
Reproduced with permission Agilent Technologies, Inc.

The glass dynamic gap lids are then lowered on top of the slides. Dako believe dynamic gap technology is the answer to many problems associated with inconsistent staining, edge and air bubble artefacts. This strategy is based on capillary action which eliminates 'dead zones' through the even application and distribution of reagent over the entire slide. Due to the unique design and the dynamic action of the glass cover plates, reagent is pulled down over the slide equally after passing through the staining nozzle. Reagent is then continuously moved around on the slide.

Unlike similar capillary technology from other vendors, the lids are independent and free to move, and are set in motion via dynamic wings inside each of the six modules. This aids in the reagent mixing in 30-second intervals of movement during incubations and allows for a homogenous reaction across the entire slide (Rasmussen et al. 2014). There is none of the zonal depletion that can be sometimes seen with capillary action techniques, while the movement also ensures efficient washing steps and the constant high humidity within the chamber reduces the chance of reagent evaporation during staining. When the lid is in the open state, reagent overlay protects the tissue from drying out. The lid then closes and remains in that position until slides are removed by the arm, and if necessary, deionized water is applied so as to ensure slides do not dry out.

The continuous motion of the lids during incubation also aids in the elimination of air bubble formation in addition to air bubble traps within the supply lines from the bulk reagent containers. These are horseshoe-shaped tubes with a release valve at the top to allow gas to escape when opened. Periodic degassing takes place during staining and when the instrument is idle.

Areas at the top and bottom of the slide receive equal staining. Although Dako testify that the staining area covers 17.5 mm x 45.0 mm, users must be mindful of the slide edges. The cover plate can under certain circumstance scratch off tissue that is close to the edge during staining, resulting in edge artefact as shown in Figure 5.19.

Localization Antibodies

Dako is a reputable vendor of antibodies and offers an extensive catalogue with an increasing amount provided in ready-to-use (RTU) form. They are identified

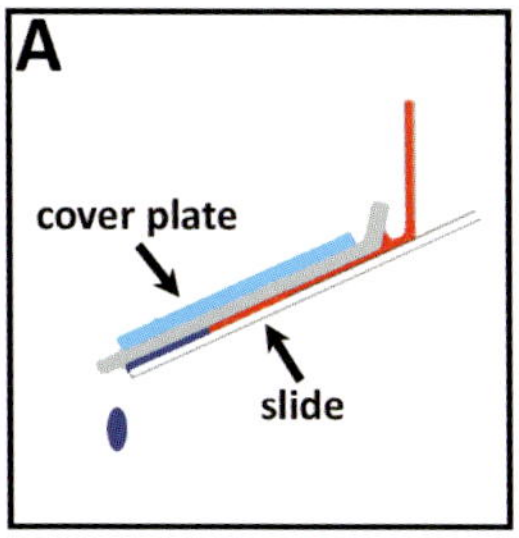

Figure 5.18 Movement of dynamic gap lids with reagent
Reproduced with permission Agilent Technologies, Inc.
Figure 5.18a When reagent is applied through the nozzle and the lid, it expels the previous solution from the slide.

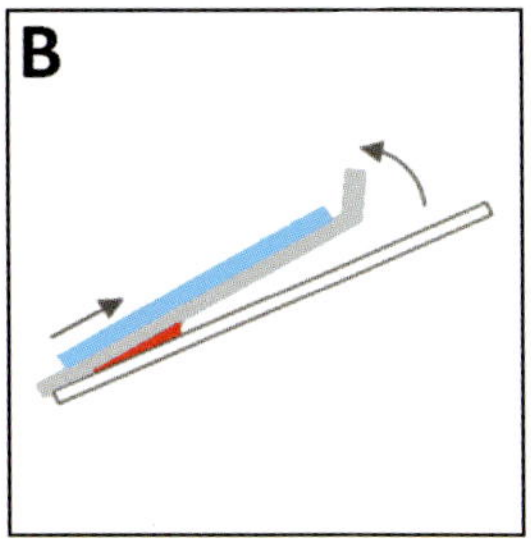

Figure 5.18b To prepare for incoming new reagent, the cover plate begins to lift upwards only at one end.

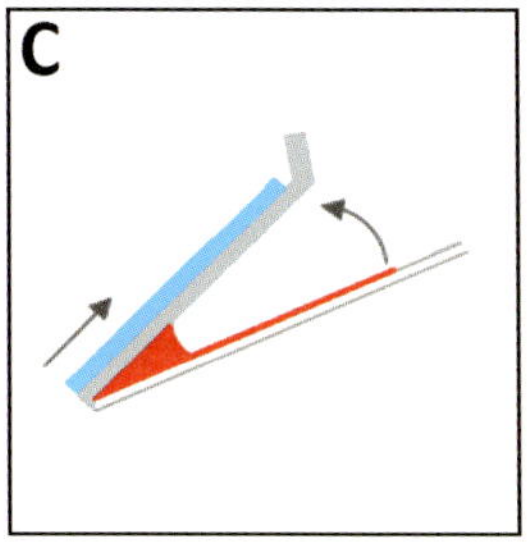

Figure 5.18c As the cover plate opens, there is no loss of reagent because the angle is closed at the other end of the slide.

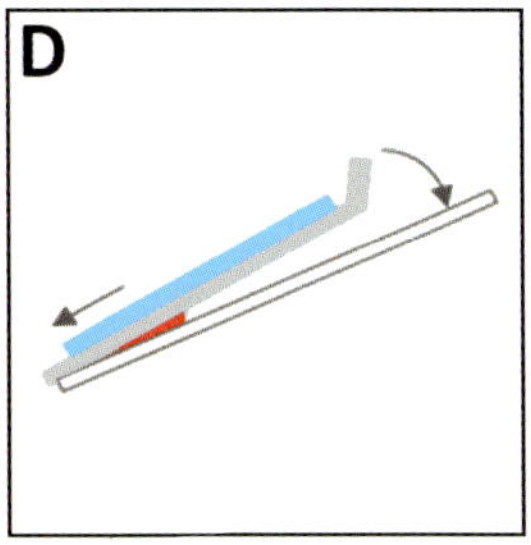

Figure 5.18d The cover plate is then lowered to allow for homogenous reaction incubation and washing steps.

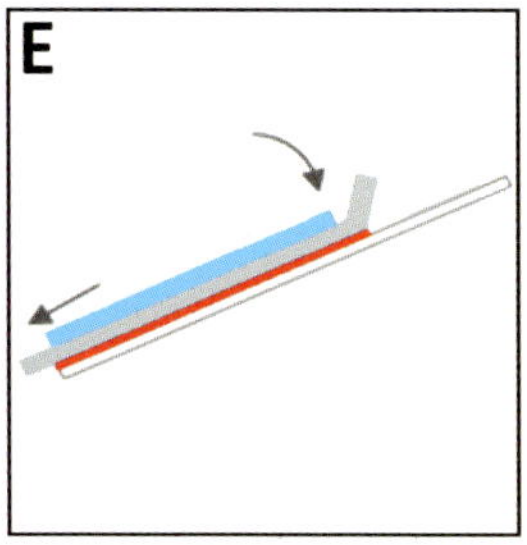

Figure 5.18e The capillary gap keeps reagent level between two surfaces. This ensures even reagent distribution.

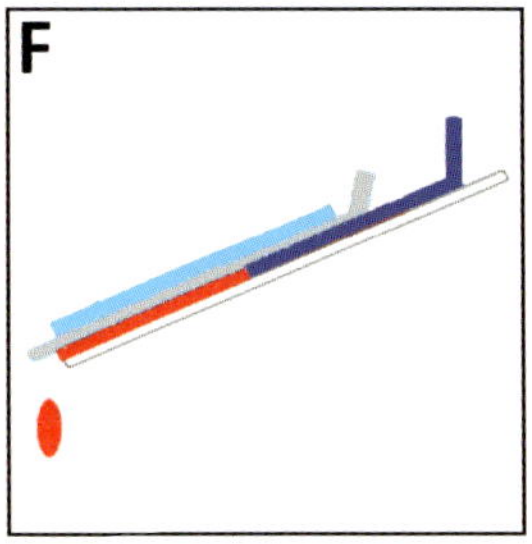

Figure 5.18f The cover plate remains in position while deionized water is flushed through to wash the whole slide evenly.

in two groups: GA vials and IR vials. The latter is designed for use with the Dako Link48, but after pouring the contents into a user-fillable vial, it is compatible for use on the Omnis and the software has been designed to accommodate IR vials. An example of a GA vial is shown in Figure 5.20 (A) and can be loaded directly with no prior scanning. The 'ears' (B) on the lids allow for the caps to be bent back and clipped to the side of the vials. The vials can be loaded in this position and when in storage, lids can be placed back on top. This can prevent spillage and evaporation. This is a neat design, but we have found the lids unnecessary and often snap them off in order to enable quick loading on the racks.

The vials have a distinctive rectangular shape and come in two sizes – 30 mL and 2 mL – chosen according to specific needs. Each vial has unique barcode information printed on it. The RTU vials have the name of the reagent, along with lot number and expiry information. Each vial has a screw top containing a

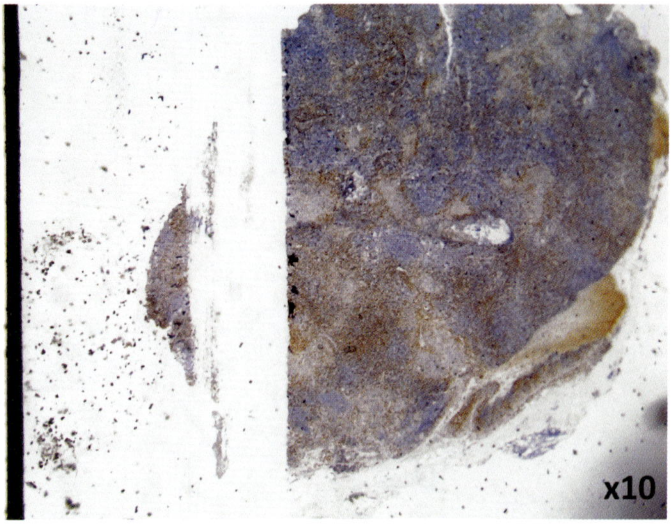

Figure 5.19 Lymph node demonstrating edge artefact caused by the cover plate

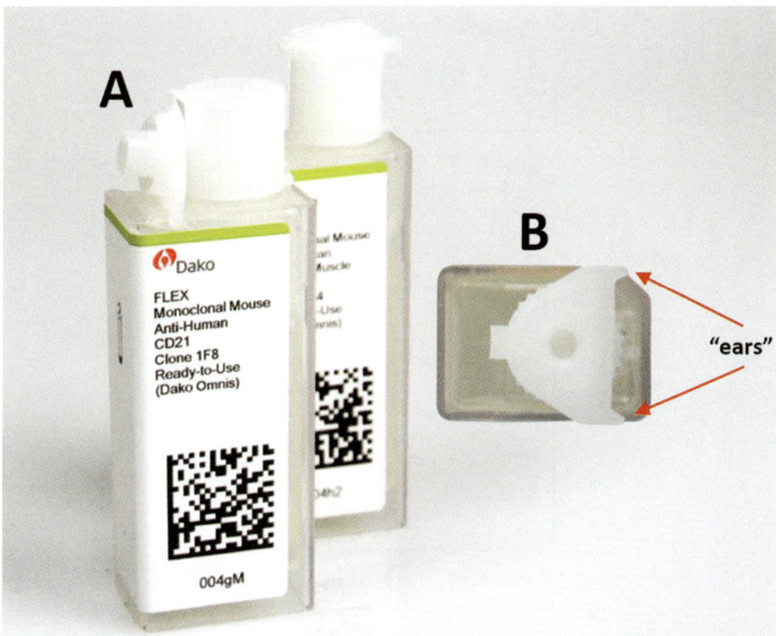

Figure 5.20 An Omnis GA vial containing ready-to-use CD21 (A), and a top-down view (B)

Reproduced with permission Agilent Technologies, Inc.

perforated inner lid, allowing the probe to enter, but when not in use it minimizes evaporation and spillage.

Antibody concentrates offered by Dako are still available with product code 'M'. For instance, catalogue #M0750 is Dako's PSA concentrate. These concentrates are used in accordance with the manufacture recommendations found on the product sheets and diluted out into Dako Omnis vials. Careful validation is required when using concentrates.

Omnis Detection Kits

Detection reagents for the Omnis consist of multiple products, all supplied by Dako but not necessarily all inclusive as one complete kit. A 'main kit' is sold under the catalogue# GV800 and marketed as 'EnVision FLEX High pH'. The kit contains the following five reagents:

(1) Hydrogen peroxide to block endogenous peroxidase activity.

(2) Horseradish peroxidase enzyme coupled to a dextran backbone with antibodies derived from goat.
(3) 3,3' diaminobenzidine tetrahydrochloride (DAB) chromogen.
(4) Substrate buffer containing hydrogen peroxide to facilitate DAB development.
(5) Tris/EDTA antigen retrieval buffer at pH9 in a 50x concentrate.

The exclusion of haematoxylin counterstain and the inclusion of a high-pH retrieval solution in this kit are interesting decisions from Dako. This means that the corresponding low-pH retrieval solution along with secondary linker antibodies and wash buffer reagents all need to be purchased separately. The detection kit is manufactured for 600 slides. Therefore the equivalent amount of other consumable reagents is needed. Experience has shown that when racks are stained at full capacity, an excessive amount of high-pH retrieval solution, DAB chromogen and substrate buffer reagents is left over when the kit has been 'exhausted'. Unfortunately, Dako do not offer hydrogen peroxide block or peroxidase dextran polymer reagent as stand-alone items. It is these limiting items that dictate the kit's end of life. In reality, a great deal of surplus reagents has to be discarded. Rabbit and mouse linker antibodies are also separated from this kit. They are available as two distinct reagents and utilized according to the primary antibody species. A rabbit linker is used for rabbit primary antibody, for instance. These secondary linkers are employed in the majority of IHC assays and are therefore considered necessary.

In addition to the traditional DAB chromogen, Dako offers an EnVision FLEX HRP Magenta stain similar to the red chromogen other vendors sell. Figure 5.21 shows the components of the kit packaged similarly to the DAB detection. The only difference is the magenta chromogen is substituted in place of the DAB; otherwise the magenta chromogen can be purchased separately (GV925), with other consumables being used from the standard EnVision FLEX kit (GV800). As the name suggests, it is a peroxidase system whereas some other vendors utilize alkaline phosphatase for the red chromogen. Applications for magenta chromogen include differentiation from endogenous melanin pigment as well as for double IHC staining because of the good contrast it offers to brown.

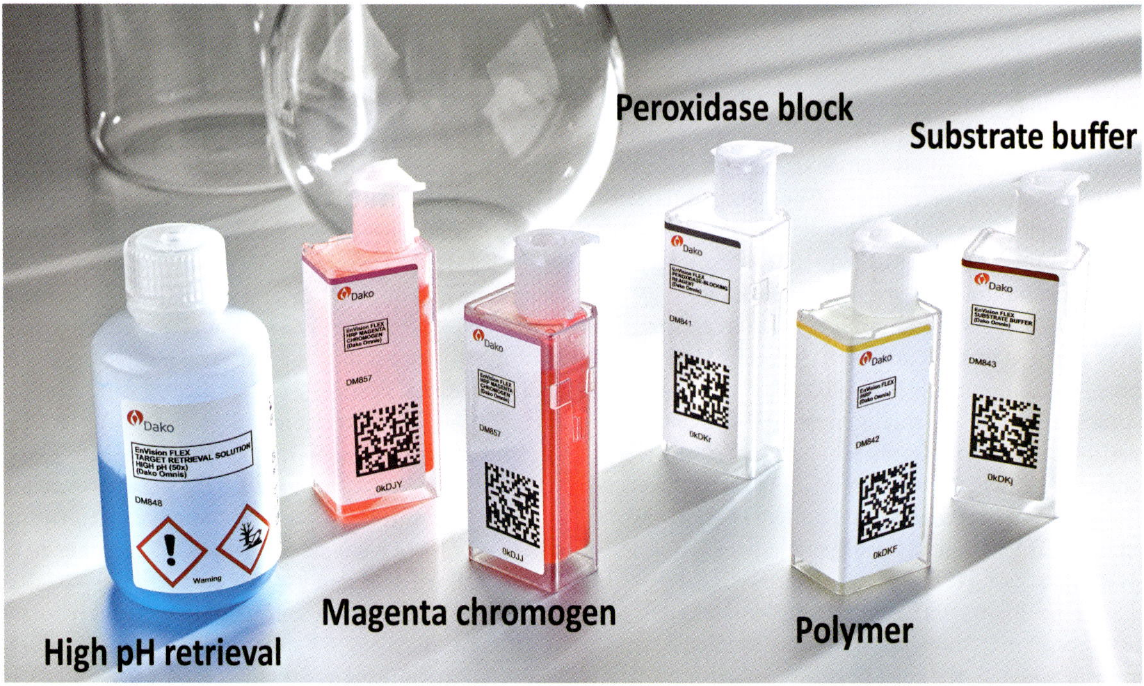

Figure 5.21 Magenta peroxidase detection kit (GV900)
Reproduced with permission Agilent Technologies, Inc.

Staining Protocols

The Alfred Hospital Melbourne currently employs two Omnis instruments for routine chromogenic IHC on FFPE tissue, fresh frozen sections and cytology preparations. Diagnostic IHC assays on FFPE tissue and cytology cell block material make up the majority of situations. Immunohistochemical assays on fresh frozen sections are also performed on muscle biopsies due to the co-location of the Victorian Neuromuscular Laboratory Service on campus. Direct immunofluorescence is implemented on fresh frozen skin biopsies and, lastly, ISH assays are accomplished on a limited number of probes.

Routine Immunohistochemistry

Figure 5.22 represents the standard protocol for chromogenic IHC at the facility. The Omnis is entrusted to automate the entire IHC assay from dewax to counterstain. Similar to other automated platforms, epitope retrieval is executed first with either heated low- or high-pH buffers or via protease enzymatic digestion. Wash buffer is applied after each reagent step for 2 minutes with 10 cycles. The primary antibody is then employed with the incubation conditions determined at antibody validation. The empirical standard of 20 minutes at 32°C incubation is nominally followed. Endogenous peroxidase block is implemented next for 3 minutes before a secondary linker antibody (if required) is applied for 10 minutes. Detection with peroxidase-dextran-goat antibodies is initiated for 20 minutes before the freshly prepared DAB chromogen is utilized. Counterstain is with haematoxylin and once completed, the racks are moved to the unloading drawer awaiting subsequent dehydrate, mount and coverslip protocols.

To ensure zero contamination of reagents, the LiHa probe is washed after each step and decontaminated with sulphuric acid as required. The Omnis has a practical solution to mixing fresh DAB on board the instrument. The plastic disposable mixing strips are employed in which one part of DAB chromogen is mixed to five parts of substrate buffer. There is always sufficient DAB reagent freshly made per mixing well for each rack of five slides.

The haematoxylin counterstain is acceptable for most occasions. Problems are observed after a weekend run when slides have been immersed for a prolonged time in distilled water at the unloading drawer after an immediate start on a Friday. A workaround is to counterstain these slides on the laboratory's automated H&E stainer. There is no impact on the IHC stain because a special programme is used only to apply haematoxylin. Another issue with the counterstain is seen with IHC on renal biopsies. Routine section thickness is a very thin 1 μm, which results in the Dako haematoxylin imparting a very weak counterstain. A resolution was achieved by introducing the laboratory's haematoxylin on board the Omnis as an alternative counterstain in the renal IHC protocol.

Cytology cell blocks are created using thrombin and occasionally agar. They are then processed routinely in the same manner as tissue samples through to paraffin wax and IHC stained on the Omnis using normal IHC protocols. Consistent high-quality staining is regularly achieved. However, no attempts have been made to do the same on cytology smears. Doing so would open many quality assurance issues pertaining to controls, consistency and reproducibility. Although the Omnis would be able to perform IHC protocols on cytology smears, the results cannot be properly verified, and this must be made clear to the individual evaluating the slide.

Dako has been at the forefront of companion diagnostic testing for a while. The HercepTest for breast cancer was launched in the late 1990s when Herceptin (Trastuzumab) humanized monoclonal antibody was approved for treating patients with Her2 overexpression (Brenner and Adams 1999). This is an example of identifying a patient population who would benefit from a specific targeted therapy. Currently the DAKO HercepTest CE-IVD kit is not available for use on the Omnis. Therefore our laboratory uses monoclonal Anti-ErbB2 SP3 clone for Her2 screening of breast cancers with equivocal 2+ and 3+ IHC scores reflexed to Her2 FISH testing. We have had a preference and historical association to this clone, favouring it over the polyclonal Dako c-erbb-2 oncoprotein.

Another common companion diagnostic is PD-L1 status for lung adenocarcinoma. The 22c3 clone (Figure 5.23) has recently been CE-IVD approved for use on the Omnis. There is a choice of performing this assay from a concentrate or as a RTU pharmDx kit. A full workup and assessment of the Dako 22c3 concentrate clone was comparable to the kit form. Although there is a 60-slide limit to the kit and an increase in running costs, the ease of use and IVD certification from the manufacturer proved advantageous.

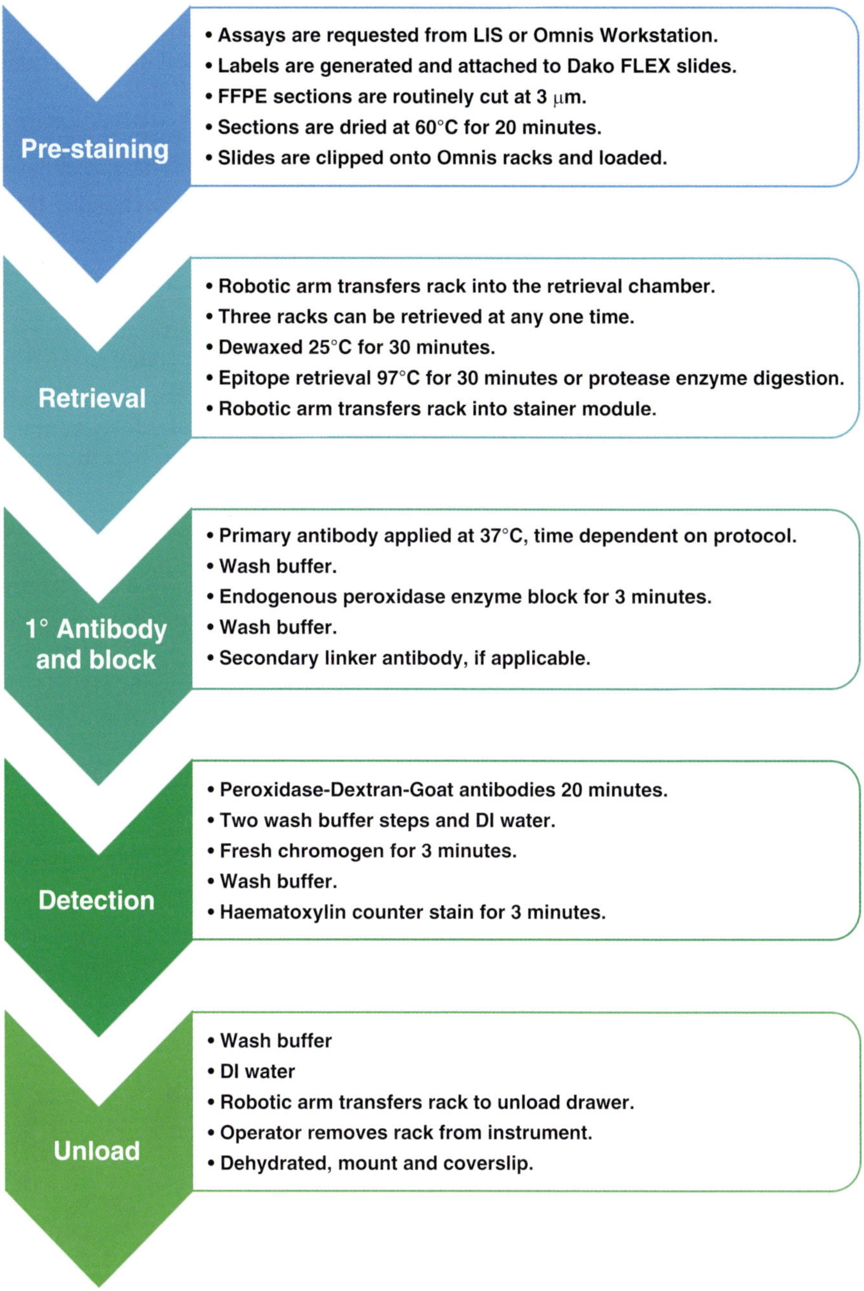

Figure 5.22 Routine immunohistochemical protocol for formalin-fixed paraffin-embedded tissue on the Omnis

Dako have been slow to convert existing RTU antibodies on the Link48 platform over to the Omnis instrument. This is surprising since the Omnis is the flagship model. Granted, the Link48 RTU antibodies can be easily adopted for Omnis duties, but the extra work to transfer reagent from one vial to another and the additional effort needed to programme the software makes it more complicated than it should be.

One other point to raise, and it is dependent on individual preference, is the lack of DAB enhancement with reagent containing copper or nickel. As highlighted in Figure 5.24, staining is clear and crisp and there is good intensity between weakly positive and strong staining. Take for example CD10 IHC (A); an opinion can be made that there is no need for chromogen enhancement. Traditionally a low-expressing (weak positive) antibody, the Omnis has managed to label CD10 in tonsil a rather strong reaction. Dako have tuned the detection system to be precise enough to differentiate between different levels of expression. The pan-cytokeratin marker AE1/3 (B) shows the staining gradient between proximal and distal tubules in the kidney. Overall, there is a noticeable difference in the shade of brown when compared to other manufacturers that offer DAB enhancement. Excluding their PD-L1 kit, Dako do not include an enhancement step within the IHC protocol. If a darker shade of DAB brown is wanted, it must be performed manually off-board the instrument.

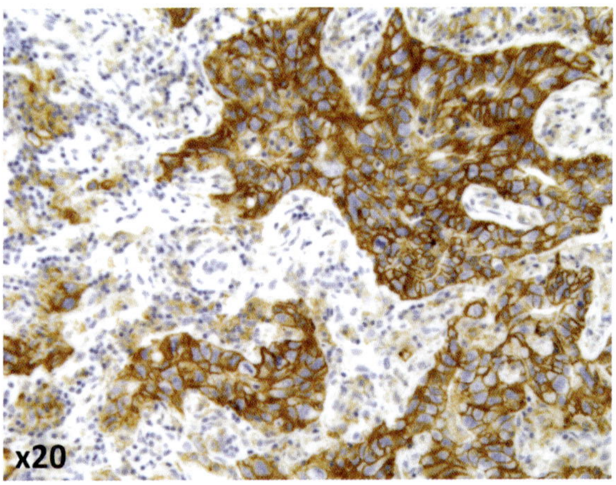

Figure 5.23 PD-L1 (clone 22c3) immunohistochemical staining of lung adenocarcinoma on the Omnis

Immunofluorescence Protocol

Investigations of autoimmune skin bullous-type lesions are best performed with direct immunofluorescence (IF) assays on fresh frozen sections (Diercks et al. 2017). This rather quick and straightforward protocol does not require epitope retrieval steps. The routine panel consists of FITC conjugated to the following antibodies: IgG, IgA, IgM, C1q, C3 c, albumin and fibrinogen. The staining protocol is forty minutes at 32°C in duration and it is advised to circle the tissue section with a permanent marker prior to loading. The permanent marker stays on during the staining and helps the technician to find the section at microscopy. After the slides are removed from the instrument, they are coverslipped using an aqueous liquid mountant.

The laboratory uses the Leica DM7 microscope to view IF staining. The light source is metal halide 120 W and supplied by Leica, EL6000. We have customized our microscope to have the capacity for six filter cubes as outlined in Table 5.3 and a scanning stage. All filters are supplied by Chroma. This set-up is also used for FISH purposes, hence the additional filters. For direct IF, a FITC filter is all that is needed. The emission spectrum is between 495 nm and 519 nm, which gives the green characteristic colour of IF-stained slides evidenced in Figure 5.25. The

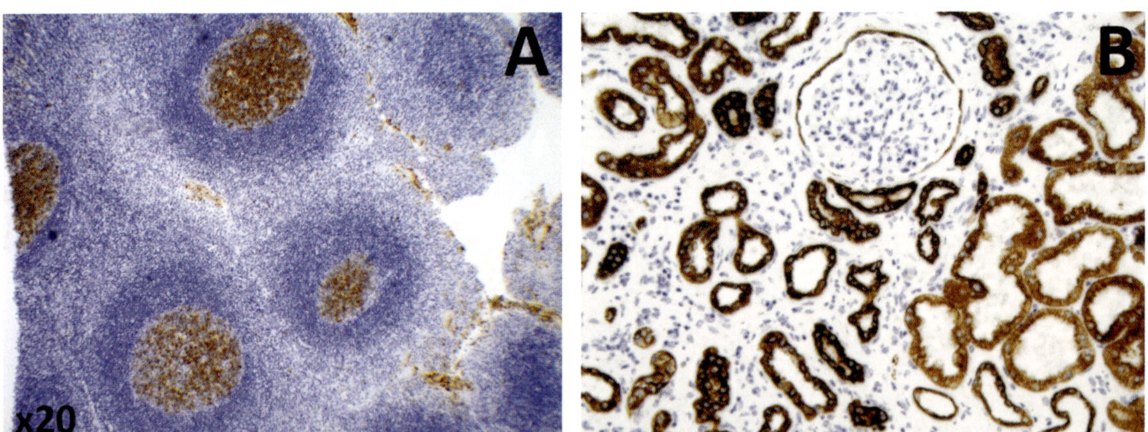

Figure 5.24 CD10 immunohistochemistry in tonsil (A) and CK AE1/3 in kidney (B)

image shows IgG (A) and C3c (B) linear deposits seen in bullous skin disorders.

Recently IF has commenced on FFPE sections with the Omnis. The protocol firstly dewaxes the slides and then applies proteinase K. The slides are then stained with FITC-labelled antibodies. We have used this staining method for renal native biopsies when no fresh tissue was available and have achieved excellent results. Validation of this protocol involved parallel staining of samples on both fixed and fresh tissue.

There has been no detrimental loss of staining or any unwanted background staining with the FFPE sections. Formaldehyde-induced fluorescence has not been encountered, possibly due to the nature of the tissue and rapid fixation. Another theory may be related to the clearing agent, Clearify. This product is based on naphtha isoparaffinic hydrocarbon, which may remove aldehyde groups, but this theory has not been substantiated.

An example of the IF technique on FFPE tissue is shown in Figure 5.26. In this case study, IHC was performed on an FFPE renal transplant core biopsy. The IHC panel consisted of IgA, IgG and C4d antibodies. Initial staining showed focal granular deposits for IgA at the glomerular basement membrane (A) indicated by black arrows. Subsequent complement protein IHC was ordered but showed no reactivity. With no unfixed tissue to use for IF staining, FFPE was used. The results showed a similar focal granular staining pattern designated with white arrows (B). The IF image is easier to see because IF is a more sensitive assay. The sample was sent for electron microscopy studies which confirmed deposits within the mesangial matrix, suggesting early IgA nephropathy. Our experience with IF staining on FFPE tissues shows a high degree of confidence confirmed by correlation with electron microscopy.

Table 5.3 Filter sets for immunofluorescence

Cube name	Colour range	Excitation wavelength (nm)
GFP ET	blue	470/40
TX2 ET	red/green	560/40
Y3 ET	green	545/25
LMD GFP/CY3	green; red	470/40; 550/20
G/R	blue; green	470/40; 570/35
Dapi	blue	350/50

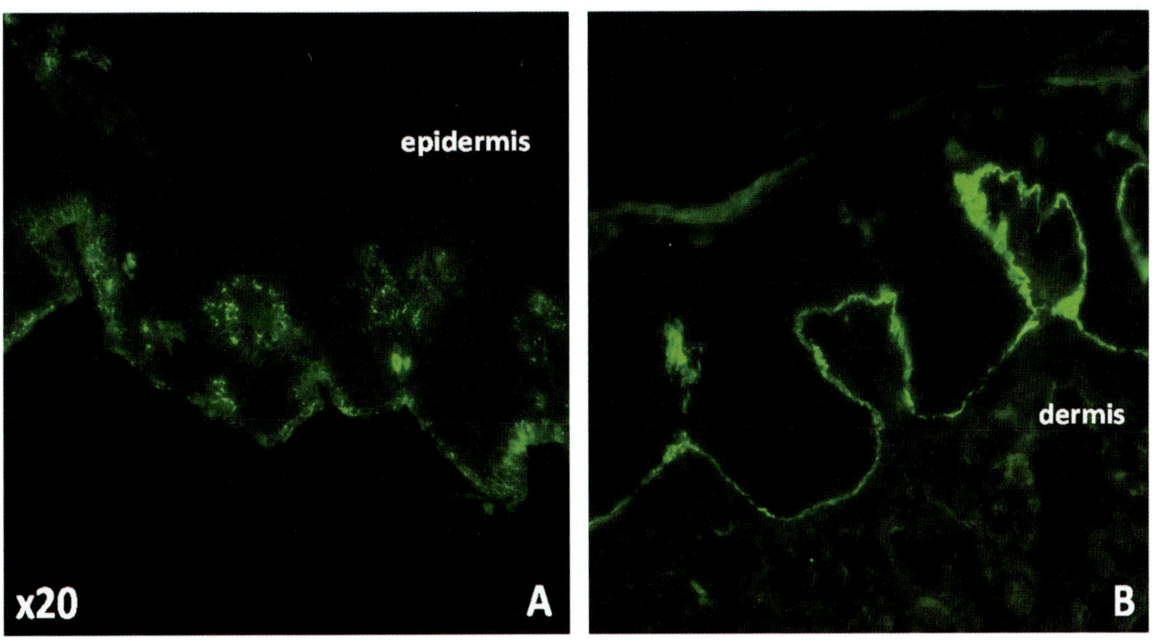

Figure 5.25 IgG-FITC (A) and C3c-FITC (B) on a skin biopsy

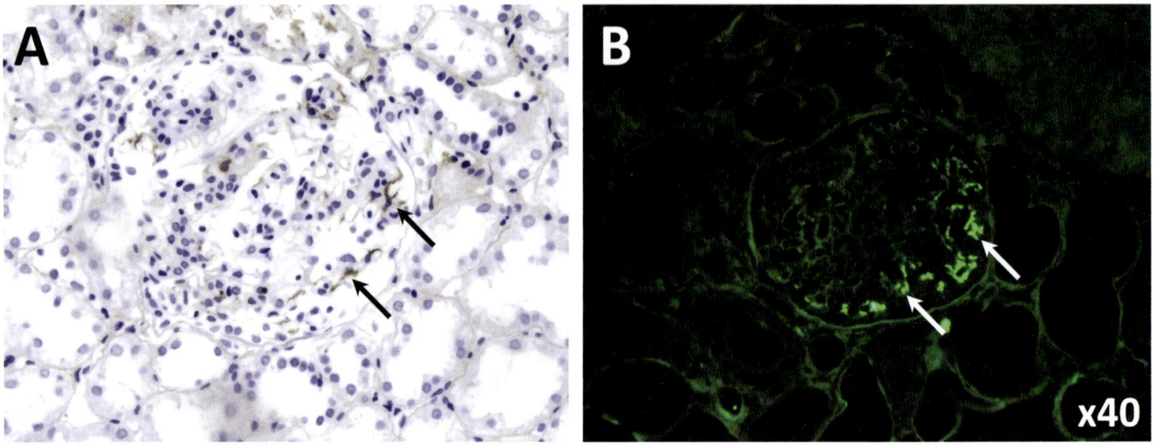

Figure 5.26 Immunoglobulin A immunohistochemistry (A) and Immunoglobulin IF with FITC (B) on formalin-fixed paraffin-embedded renal tissue demonstrating IgA deposits

In Situ Hybridization

Meeting the molecular frontier as it blends into traditional histopathology methods, the Omnis is capable of performing *in situ* hybridization (ISH) assays simultaneously with IHC staining. Omnis has joined with Agilent, a company renowned for molecular technologies, and an extensive catalogue of FISH probes is available. Three routine diagnostic ISH tests are currently offered at the Alfred Hospital Melbourne – the HER2 FISH, 1p19q FISH and EBER ISH assays.

Dako's Her2 IQFISH IVD kit is produced and approved for use on the Omnis. Similar to current trends in companion diagnostic testing, this kit is presented as a 'plug and play' assay offering three preprogrammed protocols which require minimal set-up from the user. The protocol has a number of parameters which are locked by the vendor. Therefore it is not possible to change options such as time and temperature conditions associated with hybridization or denaturation steps. A slight 'tweak' to the pepsin treatment time was needed in order to achieve optimal hybridization. Apart from this there were no other parameters that required changes to make the assay interpretable. The Her2 FISH protocol takes three and a half hours to complete, enabling it to be performed alongside IHC slides during the day. There is a hesitancy to run the protocol overnight because the probe needs to be mixed just prior to use. There was a robust validation process to certify the kit fit for purpose. Slides were initially compared to normal tissue in order to establish a baseline for pepsin digestion. After an optimal digestion time was achieved, the protocol was further examined using known amplified cases in a variety of tissue size and amplification status. Finally, select cases were performed in parallel using an external reference laboratory to evaluate concordance.

The Omnis requires two bulk reagents, pretreatment solution and hybridization buffer to be loaded prior to the ISH assays. These are supplied by Dako as pre-filled concentrates to be diluted with deionized water before use and registered in the same manner as other bulk reagents. These solutions will have an expiry of seven days if stored on board and one month if stored at 2–8°C. Reagents must be brought to 18°C before use. Other required solutions include pepsin, ethanol and ISH clean reagent. Pepsin is stored in the freezer and thawed prior to use. We keep our bulk reagents on board the instrument because of the time it takes to warm to the correct temperature. The probe is kept in the freezer and usually thawed an hour before use.

Figure 5.27 shows a cover plate containing glass lids utilized to spread the probe over the section evenly during hybridization. The slide heating apparatus can also be seen towards the top of the image. When the lid drawer icon is pressed on the touchscreen, the lids are loaded and ready for the transfer robotic arm to lower them onto the slides after probe application.

Both the rack and the lids are picked up together to be firstly dried and then transferred to the on-board heater for hybridization. After hybridization has

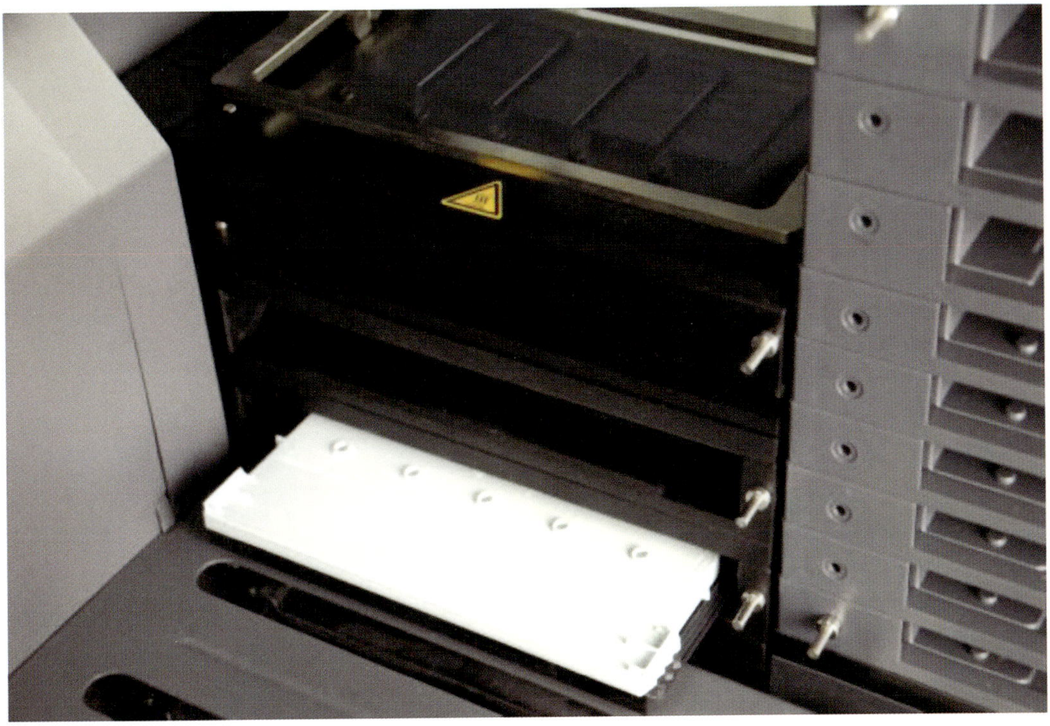

Figure 5.27 Cover plate lid entering hybridization
Reproduced with permission Agilent Technologies, Inc.

finished, the rack and lids, still intact, are transferred to the cold plate once again. It is here that the lids are separated and disposed down a chute to be removed from the instrument. The rack containing slides is then transferred to the PT module for a stringent wash buffer step carried out at 57°C. Slides, unless a further FISH protocol is needed, are dried on the hot plate at 45°C before transfer to the dry unload drawer. There is little chance FISH signals are weakened by photo reactivity due to the opaque drawer. Mounting is achieved with Dako liquid mountant containing DAPI and left to develop for approximately 15 minutes before being viewed under the fluorescence microscope. Figure 5.28 summarizes the FISH protocol on board the Omnis.

A major issue with the FISH assay is achieving adequate staining intensity. For example, the HER2 IQFISH assay for breast cancer offers a good intensity of red signal, but it is a struggle to achieve the same for the green signal. Several different techniques and protocols have been tried without success. A suitable workaround is to employ image processing with Leica's LAS X software coupled with the Leica DM7 microscopy system. The FISH probes can be viewed with reasonable results from the microscope but with a greater sensitivity when using the LAS X software demonstrated in Figure 5.29. Although not strictly ISH related, it is essential to consider the fluorescence microscope capabilities when viewing and considering the suitability of FISH assays.

Our laboratory technique is to take individual images of an area of interest indicated on the slide by the pathologist. A programmed Z-stack is employed whilst ensuring the correct aperture is used for each probe. The images are then combined displaying all the probes of interest on a single plane. Post-capture enhancements of the final image include removal of background shading and boosting the red and green points of the image for scoring Her2 status.

Other problems have been encountered with the Dako sureFISH probes and are centred around the limitation of the Omnis and protocol programmes. Traditional ISH protocols require careful time and temperature controls with hybridization usually overnight. The Omnis with its sureFISH probes method has a hybridization step limited to two hours. In

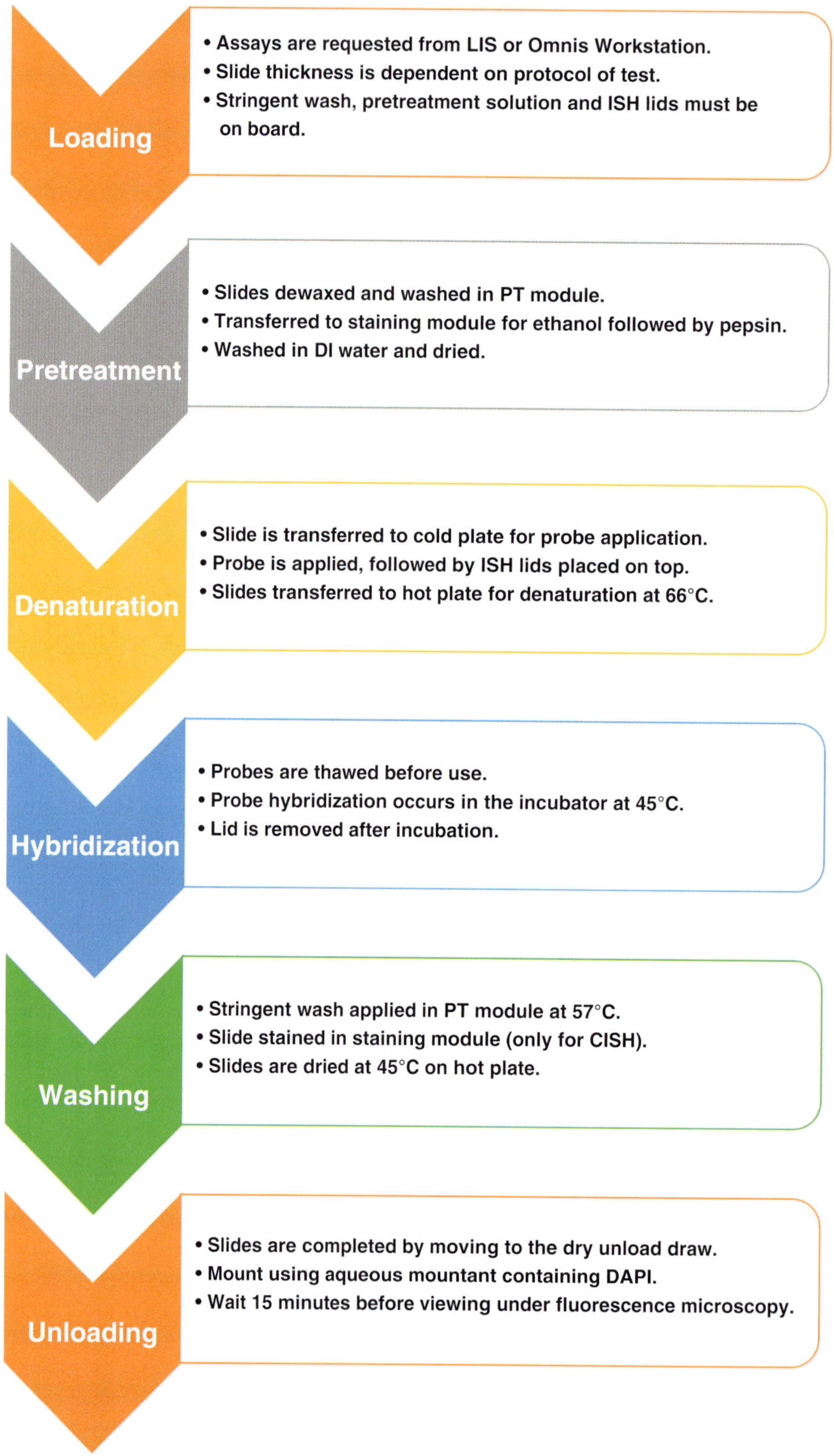

Figure 5.28 FISH protocol on board the Omnis

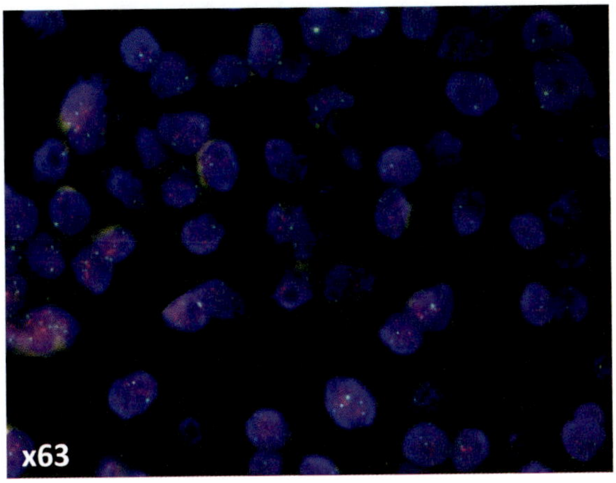

Figure 5.29 HER2 FISH assay. Combined image of the HER2 probe (red) and chromosome 17 (green)

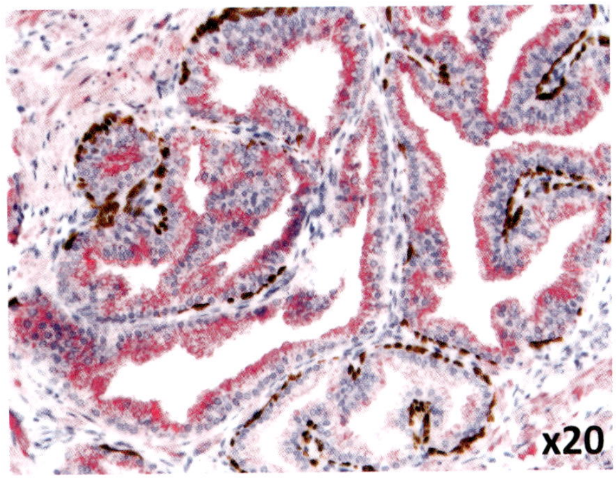

Figure 5.30 Double immunohistochemical stain with AMACR (red) and P63/34βE12 (brown) in prostate

addition, the stringent wash also has a limit on time and temperature parameters. The temperature might be too low to achieve optimal assay conditions and may be a factor of weak signals for some probes.

Chromogenic ISH is utilized for the Epstein Barr–encoded RNA (EBER) ISH assay. Switching the traditional label for ISH assays from fluorescence to a chromogen, adequate results have been obtained for this probe. The EBER ISH kit was initially designed for the Link48 instrument but has recently been offered for the Omnis with comparable results. All ISH products and reagents are supplied directly from Dako. There have been no attempts to try third-party reagents or probes. The biggest advantage the Omnis has over other platforms for ISH assays is the rapid protocol time. Currently, the Omnis remains the only integrated IHC/ISH platform to process ISH assays within four hours, bringing huge benefit to clinicians and patients.

Research Protocols

The Omnis has been employed for research purposes and is more than capable of performing in this role with certain caveats. Protocols are relatively open for modification just as long as the generic template is followed and within this template, primary antibodies of any nature can be used. The antibodies must be able to bind to the goat antibodies used in the detection system if using the peroxidase-DAB chromogen method. Research work can be stained alongside routine diagnostic slides without any glitches. Most research applications involve working up an unknown antibody in much the same way as that of a new diagnostic antibody in the laboratory. Sometimes researchers prefer to design their own protocol and run their own slides. Dako detection reagents must be used on the Omnis platform regardless.

Double Labelling with the Omnis

Double staining has a huge advantage when dealing with minimal tissue, as it can demonstrate multiple antibodies on the one section. Although double IHC assays are technically more complicated, the rewards are worthwhile if performed correctly. Multiplexing with fluorophores has not been tried on the Omnis at the Alfred Hospital Melbourne. All double-staining efforts have been performed with peroxidase-based DAB and magenta chromogens using a 'sequential' methodology. This approach involves application and development of the first antibody before submitting and elucidating the second antibody. There are preset protocols on the Omnis for this type of sequential staining and the routine pair is DAB with the magenta chromogen.

A useful assay is combining AMACR and p63 for transrectal ultrasound resection of prostate (TURP) biopsy investigations. Demonstrated in Figure 5.30, the Omnis double-stain protocol allows the user to select the first primary antibody and detection with DAB chromogen before applying a blocking step. The second primary antibody is then directed onto the same slide to be developed with the magenta chromogen. This sequential method requires both primary antibodies selected to have the same retrieval method. In this instance, both AMACR and p63 epitope retrieval involves the high-pH Tris/EDTA buffer. The protocol only allows the second antibody to have the option of a linker antibody applied, but the order of chromogen development is independent and can be switched depending on preference. As both chromogens in this example are peroxidase based, only one endogenous peroxidase-blocking step is required.

A further enhancement to the prostate double IHC assay is to add another basal marker to the mix. The addition of 34βE12 high-molecular-weight cytokeratin to p63 gives both a nuclear and a cytoplasmic signal of the basal cells in the prostate glands. In effect, this cocktail takes the total number of antibodies to three, albeit resulting in a two-colour IHC stain. Other examples of double IHC assays to be diagnostically useful include CD31 and CK AE1/3 along with CD3 and CD31 combinations.

These double-staining protocols take one hour longer to perform due to the extra blocking and further incubation of the secondary antibody. The Omnis is not capable of sequential staining beyond two protocols. It would be theoretically possible to apply a third chromogen, but this would involve taking slides off the instrument after the double stain and reloading them 'wet' onto the Omnis for an additional protocol. Currently, there are no set template protocols for multiplexing with more than two labels.

Similarly, simultaneous (parallel) double IHC assays have not been performed on the Omnis. This strategy involves a cocktail of different antibodies applied to the tissue section at one time and then developing the reaction with two different enzyme systems for dual colour chromogen development. A classic example is using peroxidase for DAB and alkaline phosphatase for Fast Red.

Antibody cocktails are routinely employed at this facility, but they are only for single-colour IHC. For example, CK AE1/3 is mixed with CK Cam 5.2 for an IHC assay that is sure to highlight almost all tumours epithelial in nature. The same strategy is employed for melanoma investigations whereby HMB45, Melan A and tyrosine antibodies are combined in a cocktail for a single-chromogen IHC assay.

Managing Workflow Logistics

An additional investment in a second Omnis instrument has changed the workflow dynamics compared to when only a single machine was available. The anatomical pathology department at the Alfred Hospital Melbourne does not operate a 24-hour service, which meant processes had to be streamlined in order to get the maximum capacity out of each instrument within the routine 8:00 a.m. to 5:00 p.m. operating hours. Efficient workflow not only involves the user operating the instrument; there is also a dependence on the instrument to be reliable without unplanned downtimes.

The IHC laboratory is separated from the main histology facility and is self-contained; all reagents and consumables are available for paraffin sectioning, frozen sections and staining. Managing stock and inventory for efficient workflow is easier to achieve within this set-up. Staffing includes a senior scientist in charge of inventory management, quality control measures and validating new antibody assays for the facility. One other staff member rotates through who is responsible for sectioning and managing the daily staining requirements.

Each day starts with the removal of the stained slides from the overnight run and preparations for the day's workload. It is essential to empty the solitary hazardous waste container and used mixing strips first thing in the morning. Failure to do so means the machine will not be able to operate at full capacity during the day. Bulk reagents and water bottles are then filled before any maintenance tasks are dealt with and new slides are loaded for staining. Staffing the facility with two members allows for a smooth workflow as one can unload and check the quality of staining while the other loads slides and prepares the antibodies and reagents. A target of about 30 racks per day is achievable when full racks containing 5 slides each are loaded in groups of three. This will give a total of 150 stained slides in a day. The Omnis can accommodate 9 racks loaded within a short time frame – 3 racks in the PT modules and 6 racks in the load drawers. That is 45 slides committed for staining in about 10–15 minutes. A big advantage is the ability to commit the slides without all the necessary reagents on board. On-board dewaxing and epitope retrieval are completed within 60 minutes, ample time to prepare and load primary antibodies and detection reagents. Bulk reagents such as Clearify, high-pH retrieval and wash buffer must be loaded prior to committing the slides. We ideally keep cases together and aim for groups of 3 racks to be loaded. We find that this is the most effective way of processing cases;

as it has been found that an average case number is 4.5 slides, we find that working in this way allows us to hand out cases faster and achieve more from the instrument.

The Omnis is a stable machine. The software is reliable and is relatively fast when loading large number of slides. To maintain this, however, the instrument requires a shutdown procedure every three weeks. A busy laboratory running the instrument at full capacity will struggle with this task, but if it is not performed regularly, that will be detrimental. One key sign is the instrument starts to run slow. This is noticeable when the slides are flagged as suspicious due to the difficulty the processor has in dealing with the data requirements. As such, the protocols get delayed by a few seconds, causing a suspicious flag to be placed on the slide. On occasion, slides have been aborted due to the instrument freezing and becoming unresponsive with the only solution being a hard shutdown and manually retrieving the slides from the instrument. It is therefore imperative that the machine is restarted regularly in order to avoid these issues. The other shortcoming is that at some point after slides have finished, the instrument must remain idle while the hazardous waste is removed. At this time, it is also best to remove used mixing strips as well because they can only be changed when the instrument is idle. Although these tasks are quick to perform, they disrupt the flow of work and delay slides being loaded on the instrument. As a matter of principle, it is best to perform these tasks in the morning after the overnight run is unloaded. The machine should then be ready for all the slides loaded that day and the forthcoming overnight run.

The Omnis software will alert the user if there is an insufficient amount of reagent before the run has commenced. Accessing the 'vials' tab, a list of necessary items is displayed and shown in order of requirement antibodies and reagents, including those from the detection kit that will be needed during the staining process. A time icon is displayed next to these items to indicate when they will be utilized. If an item is missed or insufficient reagent levels are detected, the Omnis cancels the slide. It is best not to leave loading of reagents to the last minute and to load them in advance, especially when making dilutions from antibody concentrates. Long-term storage of concentrates is in a −30°C freezer. Repeated freeze-thaw cycles are avoided by freezing small aliquots of the concentrated antibody and thawing each aliquot only when required. Ready-to-use antibodies and vials of diluted antibody are stored at 4°C except for ISH probes and certain antibodies which must remain frozen between uses. Storage policies are made in accordance with the manufacturer's guidelines.

Registering antibodies made from concentrates via the workstation software is 'clunky' and not as streamlined as it could be. In-house-prepared diluted antibodies that are required will be shown in the 'register new items' tab on the workstation. This tab is accessed from the 'inventory' tab. Reagents that are needed during the run will appear in the 'required' drop-down field. Every other product will appear in the 'all' drop-down field. Products that are RTU will not appear in these lists as they do not need manual registration.

To register an item, select the product from either list to display the product, diluent option and container information. The user will then need to add the new product lot number and expiry date to which the same process is done for the diluent or any other secondary reagent. The container is then scanned into the system to allocate the vial to the reagent. After this is done, three green ticks will let the user know that the process is complete and that the product has been successfully registered. Figure 5.31

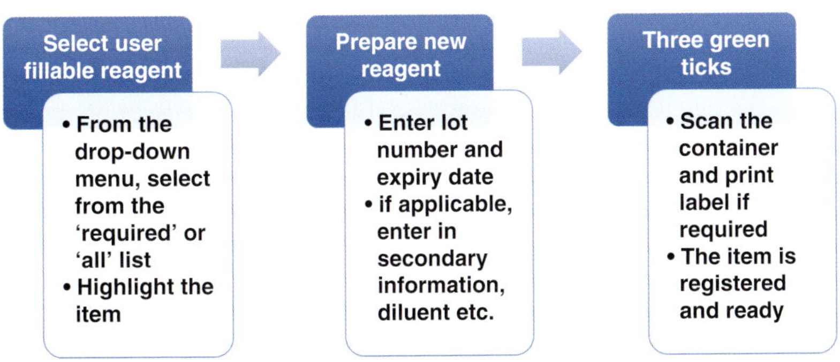

Figure 5.31 Registering an in-house manufactured antibody

summarizes the steps involved. There is also an option to generate a label. From experience, we have learned it is best to prepare the dilution first and then register the product to ensure only one product is registered at a time. After a vial is scanned into the system it cannot be altered, so care is needed to ensure the right product is highlighted. Vial operating volumes can be adjusted, but the vial type, either 2 mL or 30 mL cannot be. Optimal dilutions should be known from validation studies and are set at the time of creating a new product.

The IHC facility with its dedicated microtome brings workflow advantages as sections can be cut on demand quickly. Block alignment, however, is a real issue for histology laboratories with multiple microtomes. It is imperative to consciously keep the IHC microtome aligned with all the others in the facility. This is a feat that is easier said than done and requires a high degree of acumen to avoid wastage of precious tissue. The act of trimming into the block unnecessarily to achieve a full face because it is out of alignment is a common problem faced by histology professionals all over the world. This dilemma is magnified by several degrees in the case of small and thin tissue cores. Regular surveillance by technically proficient staff should ensure minimal tissue wastage.

To improve efficiency all tissue control sections are pre-cut, meaning a stock of control slides is always available for each antibody assay. The test tissue is freshly cut and mounted onto the same slide containing the control. There are arguments for and against this practice. The biggest criticism against pre-cut controls is the notion that both test and control tissue must be treated equally and that this is not the case if one section is freshly cut and the other has been cut already. Considering all control tissues are optimally fixed and processed to paraffin, tissue degradation of the block should not be a concern. To alleviate any concerns once a section is generated onto a slide, the pre-cut controls are stored in the freezer until required. They are cut in batches, testing the last slide of each batch in order to ensure the expected staining is present throughout the batch. The details of this quality control endeavour are all recorded and include tissue type, date of preparation and storage conditions.

Experience has shown acceptable IHC staining in pre-cut control tissues stored for greater than three months at −30°C. For consistency, pre-cut controls are nominated to be used within three months at the Alfred Hospital Melbourne. When adhering to these measures, there have not been any issues with the staining quality. In the initial workup, validation studies were performed so as to ensure pre-cut slides retained their antigenicity when stored for this length of time. Less commonly used control slides are cut in smaller batches in order to minimize wastage. The advantages of pre-cut controls far outweigh the negatives, especially when it comes to efficiency gains in workflow.

The majority of requests for IHC are made from 11:00 a.m. onwards, so there is pressure to get these sections cut, dried and loaded onto the Omnis. The cut-off time is 1:00 p.m. for same-day turnaround IHC. Ideally, to achieve maximum capacity, full racks containing five slides in groups of three are loaded, even if there is a brief period of time waiting for the necessary numbers to eventuate. Often, by the end of the day, partially full racks are loaded for an overnight run in order to achieve turnaround targets. The cut-off time to make the overnight run is 4:30 p.m. so as to ensure adequate time for the slides to dry before being loaded.

The addition of the second Omnis has made it easier to load slides based on cases, which in turn has resulted in faster turnaround times. When there was only a single instrument available, more planning around logistics had to be implemented before slides were loaded. Priority cases had to be committed first and various protocols were scrutinized before loading so as not to create bottlenecks within the system. The second Omnis brought more capacity whereby any protocol could be loaded without the need to worry if the slides will hold up more urgent cases. This is especially true for FISH and direct IF assays as they are now performed alongside routine IHC slides.

Although the aim is to load full racks for the machine to be at full capacity, this does not always eventuate smoothly. The main issue occurs with assays that require enzyme retrieval. Currently, 2% of protocols need proteinase K pretreatment and these slides seem to cause temperature fluctuations in the PT module if loaded just before or alongside another rack undergoing heat-induced epitope retrieval (HIER) in another PT module. The slides are aborted because the instrument's sensors would often detect higher than specified temperatures, resulting in an error event due to a thermal regulation failure. Note that the routine HIER is at 97°C and enzyme digestion is at 65°C. The difference in temperature of the two epitope unmasking procedures seem to account for the temperature error. A breakdown service visit from the Dako engineer normally follows in order to check the sensors and valves, resulting in downtime of the machine.

A workaround to this problem is to load slides requiring enzyme retrieval first thing in the morning or on a delayed overnight run. Waiting until proteinase K digestion has finished and vacated a PT module before loading other assays has stopped this error from happening. The wait is up to one hour, but the time is not lost as sections can be cut and preparations made for the next batch of IHC assays.

The PT module design is the biggest limitation of the Omnis platform for two reasons. The first is that there are only three modules servicing six staining drawers and each module can only accommodate one rack at a time, meaning that only 15 slides can be started at one time. The user can actually commit six racks at once, but only three racks are advanced to the PT modules for epitope retrieval, leaving three racks waiting. Secondly, all slides loaded onto a rack must undergo the same retrieval method. There cannot be two slides loaded for high-pH buffer and three slides for low-pH retrieval on the same rack, for example. The reality of this predicament is that there will be single slides taking the space of a whole rack because it is required to complete a panel.

The Omnis can notify the user of protocol conflicts as displayed on the screen. Incompatible assays are marked with a red square containing a letter. For example, protocols with mismatched retrieval will display as A and B, as highlighted in Table 5.2. The operator is required to take these slides back and redistribute them on another rack. Slides flagged with a red square without a letter mean there is a set-up error when programming the assay into the workstation – for example, a buffer wash step being omitted at the initial set-up. A red square with a question mark indicates a barcode which has not been read correctly or has been used before.

The two instruments allow performing IHC assays by patient case and not dictated by the antibody already loaded onto the instrument. Agilent's transparent cost per slide model means that all the necessary reagents, including localization antibodies, are packaged in the one price. Therefore multiple vials of each antibody are available, one for each instrument to be utilized at the same time if required without incurring any additional operational costs. Cost per slide transparency enables managers to easily monitor the budget forecasts. The inherent flexibility of swapping reagents and antibodies between instruments as required makes it simpler for the user to load patient cases rather by antibody type. Take for example the following scenario involving multiple patient cases all requiring CD20. If only one Omnis instrument was available, cases were more likely to be loaded as dictated by the antibody availability, meaning panels were often split up in order to utilize the CD20 antibody preloaded on the instrument. Completion of patient cases was then delayed, waiting for the full panel requested because finish times were not closely synchronized. The addition of a second Omnis enables CD20 IHC assays to run concurrently on both machines because two CD20 vials are available. Complete patient cases can now be loaded and finished at the same time, improving workflow. There has not been a noticeable rise in overall reagent usage. As a specific number of assays is performed each year, a certain volume of reagent is required to meet this demand. The volume is the same amount whether there is one Omnis or two. The difference is that the reagents are now being split between two machines, therefore the operational costs should not be adversely affected.

A downside of two working instruments is the fact that maintenance tasks are doubled and managing stock inventory has become more involved. The laboratory has staggered the schedule for maintenance duties so that the more involved jobs are completed on separate weeks, ensuring a machine is always available when maintenance tasks are required. Managing stock consumables can be laborious but is necessary for smooth IHC operations. Delays on reagent delivery can have serious implications for the availability of tests. To appreciate the consumable demands for an IHC facility with an output of three thousand slides, Table 5.4 lists the monthly requirements.

Reliability has been acceptable with the majority of issues resolved either over the phone, or a workaround solution can be found until the technician can come in. For instance, the Omnis has a feature that enables the user to disable a troublesome PT module or a malfunctioning staining module, allowing normal staining to continue, bypassing the affected module. At other times, a workaround solution cannot be found. One of the major issues with the Omnis is reagent leakages. The instrument is designed to detect

Table 5.4 Monthly reagent consumables excluding primary localization antibodies

Reagent	Quantity per month
Mixing Strip, 25 strips	2
Reagent Vial, small (24 x 2 mL) pack	3
Reagent Vial, large (24 x 30 mL) pack	2
Sulphuric Acid 0.3 M (10 x 22.5 mL) pack	6
Wash Buffer (20 x 175 mL) 1,700 tests	3
Hematoxylin (8 x 22.5 mL) 600 tests	5
Clearify, 3.8 L	1
EnVision FLEX high pH, 600 tests	5
Target Retrieval Solution low pH, (3 x 68 mL) 225 tests	1
EnVision FLEX Rabbit LINKER, 75 tests	6
EnVision FLEX Mouse LINKER, 75 tests	10
FLEX IHC Microscope Slides, 5 x 100 slides	5
Antibody diluent with background-reducing components 125 mL	3

any leaks inside and is equipped with an overflow pipe. There have been several instances where clips have become loose from the tubing at the back of the instrument, resulting in the machine entering safe mode. This means assays already loaded are finished, but the instrument will not accept any new slides. Usually, from the overflow pipe, the user can determine from which bulk reagent the leak has occurred and remove the affected bottle if it is valve related. When the technician is on site, the fix is relatively simple and the instrument is back up and running. The Omnis is designed in such a way that if a leak occurs, the vital and sensitive electronic equipment is always protected.

Another issue that obstructs efficient workflow involves the clips that control the flow of solutions into the PT tanks. This has been especially problematic with non-retrieval protocols or protease K assays as these require large amounts of wash buffer at short intervals flowing into the chamber. The clips become 'sticky' over time and do not open fast enough, leading to the sensors detecting a blockage. As this is not a true blockage, there is no deleterious effect on dewaxing and washing slides, but the error does cause the slides to be cancelled. The only solution to this problem is for the technician to replace the tubing and valves. Since there is some regularity to this error and it is a job that involves several hours to complete, the decision has been taken to incorporate this task into the yearly service of the instrument. Overall, more downtime is encountered as the annual service is now managed over a number of days. The ability to split the service into several visits maintains workflow as slides can be stained overnight before the technician continues the following day. Replacing valves yearly has improved the reliability of the Omnis.

Another separate valve problem centres around the release mechanism of the waste bottles. They expand as a result of the warm liquid passing through, causing the valves to 'stick'. Ejecting waste bottles via the touchscreen does not translate to the bottles 'popping out'. The release mechanism can be heard working, but because of the sticking valve, it is unable to eject out. Counter-intuitively, manually pushing the bottle further into the instrument releases the waste bottles. The vendor has promised a redesign of the valve and connector to make it more durable, and this will be installed when available. Another redesign was made to existing PT tanks as the older modules suffered from corrosion due to solutions overfilling in the tanks. Minor issues such as these were expected as the new Omnis platform matures.

Omnis Quality Control

As highlighted in Chapter 2, quality assurance measures for IHC must be robust to guarantee assays are legitimate stand-alone medical devices as prescribed by the Therapeutic Goods Administration in Australia. Introducing automation to IHC assays brings a different set of quality considerations. The main one is assessing whether the machine is fit for purpose and whether the level of instrumentation can produce consistent and reliable IHC and ISH assays. Another important parameter is an appraisal of the instrument in fulfilling all the needs of the facility, such as optimizing new localization antibodies when there is a demand for new biomarkers.

Initial Validation of the Instrument

With any new equipment or technique, robust validation methods are essential to give confidence to the assays performed on the platform. The manufacturer dictates the appropriate initial validation protocol after installation and in the case of the Omnis, a Dako applications specialist is enlisted. Five slides are loaded to assess all areas of the instrument. To evaluate ISH performance, only two slides are required. After all slides have 'passed quality control', showing that all areas of the machine are working without any error, the laboratory validation of all IHC assays can begin.

After appropriate user training, validation of all the IHC, IF and ISH assays must be done before any real diagnostic cases are loaded. Each assay underwent an initial workup based on the current tried and tested method. The slides were then reviewed and adjustments made to the protocol accordingly. Personal preference and other external conditions dictate whether a facility employs localization antibodies in an RTU format or as a concentrate. A mixture of Dako RTU antibodies and concentrates sourced from manufactures such as Leica and Cell Marque is employed at this facility.

Dako RTU protocols are preloaded on the Omnis, making the use of RTU antibodies relatively hassle free. Most of the preparation and associated protocol optimization has been completed by Dako. The laboratory needs to apply the RTU on their own control tissue to assess performance. The high degree of standardization achieved at present, especially in pre-analytic parameters, means that often RTU antibodies are suitable without the need to 'tweak' any settings. The main advantage in this situation is that the assay is registered IVD from the vendor. Any changes made to the published protocol provided by the manufacturer change the IVD status to an in-house IVD test, which is the same if a concentrate was used.

Optimizing Immunohistochemical Assays

Antibody concentrates can be likened to the 'Wild West' of IHC. Any vendor, however big or small, can offer a concentrate for IHC claiming it is the best clone for certain applications. How does one tell if a concentrate will be useful? Reputable vendors and quality clones do get mentioned at conferences, meetings, quality assurance programmes, in journal publications and via word of mouth. Regardless, the choice often comes down to availability, price and performance. The Omnis caters for complete flexibility in the type of antibody and protocol used. The initial workup involves testing the concentrate on a range of dilutions and pretreatment strategies. The Omnis does not allow for any changes in naming of antibodies or protocols once saved, so blank templates are archived to be used as required in order to allow as much flexibility as the instrument will allow. For example, to test a new concentrate on a range of dilutions, there will need to be three or more protocols all using common reagents apart from the antibody. At this work-up stage, the antibody will be known as the titration value it is made at. This is taken as the 'protocol name'. The information is printed on the slide label so that in the future antibody and concentration can be traced back. This practice allows for multiple titrations to be compared at once, reducing the time required to optimize a new antibody.

Working antibody concentrations (titres) are based on initial workups and assessments. Quality assurance programmes and vendor recommendations are used as references, but working titres are ultimately based on the facility's processes and tissue types. No issues have been encountered when employing third-party concentrates on the Omnis. Generally the concentrate can be diluted further than what is recommended from the manufacturer by incorporating Dako's secondary linker antibodies within the protocol. A conscious effort has been made to keep primary antibody incubation times ranging from 8 to 30 minutes with the majority of assays utilizing 20 minutes.

The retrieval regimen can be a limiting factor. Although Dako offers both high- and low-pH buffers in addition to proteinase K, consideration needs to be paid to the time and temperature parameters. Due to the PT modules engineered to accommodate one rack at a time, all of the slides loaded on one rack must have compatible protocols. A concerted effort to keep incubation time and temperature consistent between all assays will enable a smooth workflow. For example, an assay requiring 20 minutes in high-pH buffer cannot be loaded on the same rack with a slide that requires 50 minutes in high-pH buffer, even though both use the same retrieval solution. To enlist a degree of standardization across all assays, the Omnis protocol does not give flexibility in the HRP detection and peroxidase block times. Staining is clean and crisp, but the DAB chromogen is not dark-black brown as seen on other platforms using copper enhancement. Preference is given to golden-brown DAB with no background staining. Most assays use a secondary linker antibody and there have no negative issues surrounding their use.

Setting up a new IHC protocol is managed by the desktop PC because the Omnis workstation is where all slide and reagent information is stored. The database keeps track of every reagent used along with every slide stained. Progress of slides on board the instrument in real time can also be found on the Omnis. Logs of any issues in the staining process will also be recorded in the slide history.

Getting used to the software can be challenging. It is not as intuitive as one would like. To introduce a new protocol involves many steps. Summarized in Figure 5.32, a new antibody must firstly be created. If this is a concentrate, then it is a two-step process. A concentrate must be first registered as a 'new product' before a name can be assigned, but this name should be different to the one used for the final antibody assay. A recommendation is to use the antibody name followed by 'conc' to designate the concentrated antibody. This is defined as a new product and preparation method is 'none' as it is only a product name. After the item is saved, the new reagent tab is opened once again and the antibody name is entered in, only this time with the final concentration as well. This information will be displayed on the required antibody screen. New reagent is selected again but for the preparation method, 'user fillable dilution' is selected from the drop-down menu. This displays an additional window. From the drop-down list, the concentrated antibody (recently named) is selected and in the second drop-down list, the antibody diluent is chosen. Care should be taken to select the right dilution at this stage as this will be displayed when making up new dilutions. In addition, the vial size can be nominated as either 2 mL or 30 mL vials. One important note is that once these products are created and saved, no amendments are possible. A new product must be created every time, even for a small change, with the exception of the vial size. The products also cannot be deleted once created, only put into a 'not for use' state.

For Omnis RTU antibodies, these steps are not needed as all required information is contained within the barcodes. Some Dako RTU antibodies are only available in Dako Link 48 vials. To utilize these RTUs on the Omnis, a 'new product' needs to be selected and the 'none' option chosen as the preparation method. The reagent must be transferred manually into an Omnis vial and processed via the 'register new items' tab.

After the antibody is registered, it can be linked to a protocol via the 'protocol' tab. A new one can be created from a blank protocol or duplicated from an existing template. Protocol names must be unique and cannot be changed once saved. Most of the

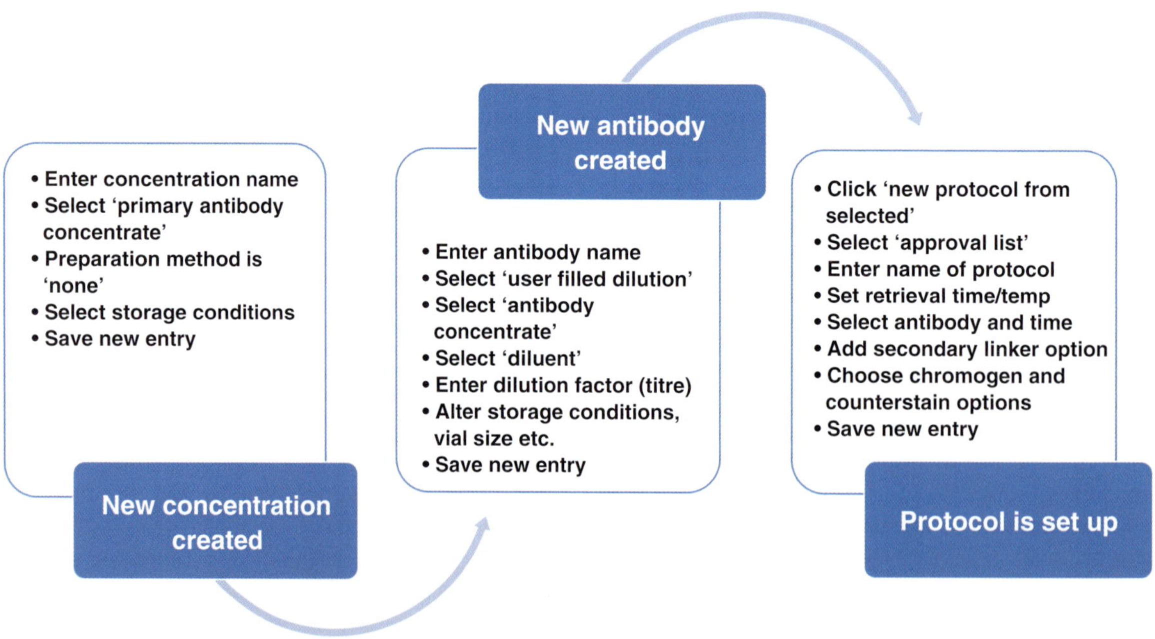

Figure 5.32 Flow chart of optimizing a new immunohistochemical assay on the Omnis

parameters of the protocol can be changed such as retrieval time and temperature, inclusion of enzyme digestion, antibody incubation time and addition of linkers. Peroxidase blocking and HRP detection steps are set and cannot be altered, as are the number of buffer wash steps. Chromogen development time can be modified along with the haematoxylin counterstain time. It is possible to use a different chromogen – for example, magenta – and a different counterstain if needed. Protocols are grouped as 'diagnostic' or 'non-diagnostic'. This feature is particularly useful when working up new assays to designate them in the non-diagnostic test category. Slides loaded for validating the new assay can be ordered in the 'non-diagnostic' tab. Protocols deemed 'diagnostic' have to be named in the configuration screen and then added to the test repertoire. The name chosen at this stage will be the test name used when being ordered. There is also the ability to print and track date changes to the protocol, although detailed information on changes made is not available. The final step is to map the protocol to the test and the instrument. The assay can now be ordered via the diagnostic tab or the LIS. Figure 5.32 outlines the steps covered.

Reagent volumes are set when new products are made but can be changed at any time. A single IHC assay consumes 300 μL of primary antibody to cover the whole slide and the dead volume for a 2 mL vial is 150 μL. In theory, the minimum volume required for a single assay should be 450 μL, but experience has shown the real value is 500 μL. A difference of 50 μL is not a huge concern, so this margin of error is acceptable. The laboratory prepares a 'standard' 5 mL working dilution from concentrates for commonly used antibodies. For less common assays, 1 mL dilutions are prepared from the concentrate form. Expiry is nominated at three months although the expected stability of antibodies is greater than this; there have not been in-house validation studies concerning longer shelf life. It is interesting to note that Dako RTU antibodies have an expiry usually of 18 months. Regardless, all reagents have an on-board lifetime that is measured in hours by the instrument. This is set at time of creation for user-prepared reagents while Dako reagents are factory set by the manufacturer and contained in the barcode. The user can access this information via the workstation anytime.

The LiHa probe on board the Omnis will accurately take a volume measurement of each reagent every time a new one is loaded. The initial amount is recorded and a deduction is taken on every occasion the reagent is used. The remaining volume is then used to assess whether the onboard quantity is sufficient to fulfil the required assays committed for staining. There have been very few occasions where the instrument has estimated an incorrect volume resulting in a cancelled assay. A possible explanation is perhaps a small amount of evaporation has occurred or a slight calibration error. The LiHa probe is extremely sensitive and overall, reagent volume management has been accurate. The only detrimental causation is the generation of bubbles inside the vials, a reason for inaccurate volume reading whereby vials can be discarded as empty by the instrument. It is essential when loading and preparing new concentrates that any bubbles are removed by inverting the vial several times prior to loading.

Monitoring for Quality

Most failed IHC assays are due to human error. Repeat tests are performed because the incorrect control tissue is selected or the wrong patient block was used. Both positive and negative tissue controls accompany every diagnostic slide. To minimize this error, multi-block controls are utilized and contain a variety of tissue types including normal and disease states. Assays which require staining intensity assessments need different specific controls to allow for an evaluation of various staining patterns. About 80% of IHC assays are covered by only three separate multi-block controls at the Alfred Hospital Melbourne, which has resulted in a decrease in repeat assays due to incorrect controls selected. Anecdotally the IHC facility sectioning all the test cases with a dedicated microtome has also contributed to this trend. Figure 5.33 shows the majority of issues are due to human error. Interestingly, the total number of errors due to instrument failure is less than 1%. Proprietary reagents supplied by Dako have consistently performed as expected between batches and lot numbers. All reagents are used before expiry and stored within recommended guidelines.

Slides can be tracked in real time on the instrument via the touchscreen or followed on the PC workstation. The tablet on the Omnis instrument shows the assays currently in process and relevant information is detailed by selecting individual slides. The information is displayed as the laboratory accession number and all the tests associated with it. The workstation provides

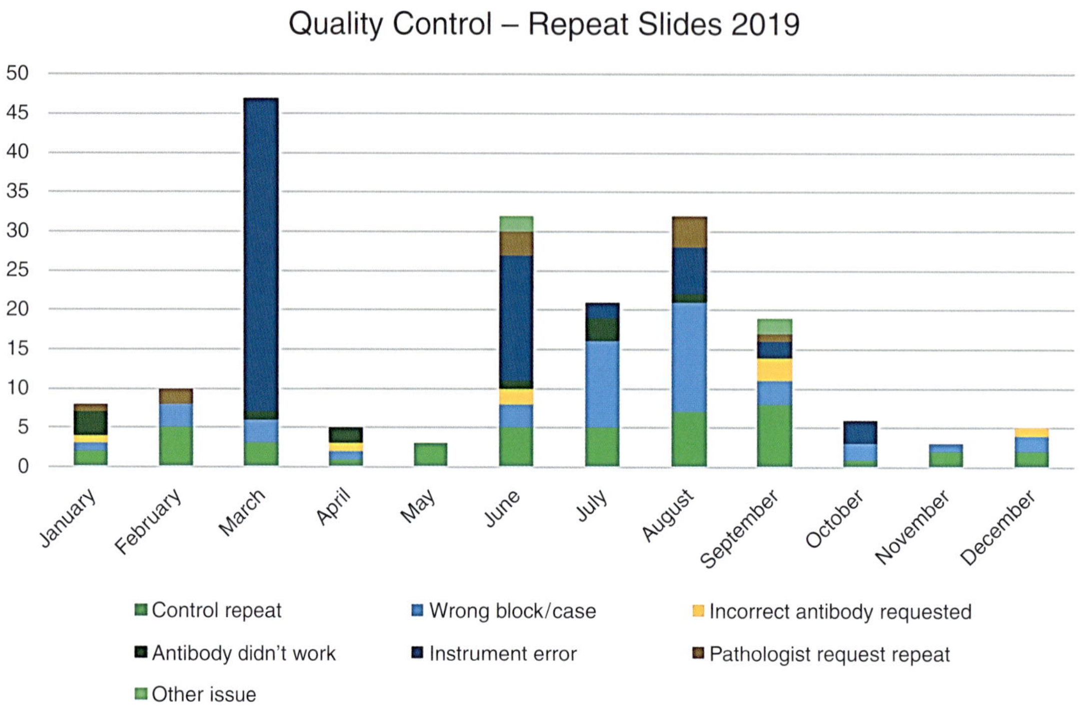

Figure 5.33 A record of errors in immunohistochemical assays for one year

faster and more detailed information via the 'slide' tab and selecting 'all' to input an accession number to conduct a search. The resulting data cover all assays attached to the case and include slides due to be completed in time scale form and if the slides are completed, the date and time this has occurred. This is a useful tool if slides are missing from the archives as the information will indicate when the assay was completed by the instrument. The Omnis has been successfully integrated into the laboratory's Cerner Millennium LIS enabling requests made by the pathologists to automatically queue in a 'requested' state waiting for loading. The software then progresses to 'staining', and when completed but not yet unloaded, they remain in a 'stained' state. After unloading, the slides are recorded as 'complete'.

The same principle applies to reagent monitoring with the information accessed via the 'inventory' tab. Experience has shown that it is easy to search for a reagent by typing in the first few letters of the reagent name in the search bar. The more information entered and the narrower the search becomes, it appears the less accurate the search is. It is better to have the information displayed with all reagents containing the letters searched for and then narrow down the search history as further filters can be applied. These include the type of reagent, the location being on board or in storage, as well as the state of the reagent, which can be normal, suspicious or discarded. Further information can be found on the reagent by clicking on the appropriate entry. This will display a range of information from date of registration, expiry and the volume remaining. A 'history' tab can be opened to access logs of all slides that have been stained using that specified reagent. Other information that is recorded includes each time a reagent is loaded and unloaded from the instrument under the specific username.

Assays can be flagged before being loaded as urgent and this will prioritize the rack that contains them. This only effects slides that are yet to be loaded, not slides currently on the machine. The user can assign slides tagged as a repeat assay or another customizable label, but this will have no impact on staining protocol. The instrument can flag assays as suspicious or cancelled. Suspicious slides can occur for several reasons – the slides may be stained with an expired reagent, the instrument may have encountered an issue while staining, or maintenance is overdue at the time of staining. These issues are recorded in the software and can be accessed when searching the run history of a particular slide. Slides that are cancelled by the instrument must be re-entered and a new barcode printed. Assays flagged as suspicious but not stained due to incomplete maintenance status can be changed from suspicious to normal in order to be reaccepted for staining.

Reagents are flagged in a similar way. The instrument can label an item as discarded or suspicious if there has been an issue with the item while on board. This is recorded in the software and can be filtered to display the suspicious or discarded items. It is possible to change a suspicious item back to a 'normal' status. This is particularly important if it is necessary to carry out a hard reset of the instrument and reagents cannot be removed before doing this. The regents on board will be flagged as suspicious and the instrument will not accept them for staining of slides. After an item is discarded, there is no way of reintroducing it for use. The software records the item as empty or expired and these details cannot be changed.

Record Logs

The instrument generates a large volume of data, recording each measurement of the process for each slide. This information is all stored on the server and can be accessed by searching or scanning a barcode of the slide. Time, temperature, measurements and any suspicious activity are recorded. This can be particularly useful when identifying staining issues. If needed, these log files can be uploaded and accessed by a service engineer. Depending on the issue, it might be necessary to call the Dako service engineer as they can give support over the phone to possibly resolve a problem quickly. All problems should be formally logged with the Agilent service desk. To retrieve the log files for any issues with the instrument, the user downloads them by selecting the drop-down menu accessed from the arrow on the top of the screen. Select the 'about' icon menu and pick 'create diagnostic archive'. This will back up all information and run logs from the machine since the last shutdown of the instrument.

To upload a log file for remote access by the Dako service engineer, first click on 'download log files' from the top left-hand corner of the Omnis workstation. This will prompt the user to select the instrument and the date range they wish to download. It is best to download dates that are only concerned with the incident as this will make the upload of the log files faster and easier for the engineer. The log file is then downloaded to the desktop of the workstation and saved in a zipped folder. The user then clicks on the icon on the desktop to upload the log files. The user is then taken to a Dako website and asked to fill in various information ranging from the instrument number and user contact details and a brief description of the issue. Then a prompt is made to attach the zipped folder of the log file. The form and log files are then automatically sent to Dako and the service engineer. From the data stored, the engineer can recreate an issue, detect if a particular valve did not work as expected or identify a sensor that has recorded a temperature out of a defined parameter. Users then can be given advice and determine the most appropriate course of action.

Quality Assurance Programmes

The laboratory is enrolled in the RCPA QAP for proficiency testing, which is essential to ensure the laboratory's output is acceptable according to set standards in the industry. This has been particularly important when assessing the quality of the Omnis as it is a new platform compared to other established instruments. Compared to proven benchmarks set by Leica and Roche Ventana, the Omnis has performed particularly well, achieving top scores in a range of antibodies. One point to mention when comparing RCPA QAP scores is the fact that although an expert panel of assessors is employed to evaluate the quality of IHC staining, this programme does not assess slides based on the same platform as the laboratory in question. Before assigning scores for each respective laboratory, a benchmark standard must be set for the type of automation of that facility. Each staining platform, be it Leica, Ventana or Dako, has different qualities that the assessor should consider. For instance, the Omnis has been criticized for the staining tone of the DAB chromogen and the haematoxylin intensity. NordiQC is a recommended resource because they have done an extensive comparison work on a wide range of platforms in addition to using a panel of expert assessors (Mogens and Nielsen 2016). This results in a huge resource for protocol comparisons and suitable antibody clone recommendations for which the Omnis has achieved a high degree of compliance.

Maintenance on the Omnis

There are two main categories of maintenance tasks – a liquid system clean and a dynamic gap lid clean. All other duties are considered minimal in user intervention. Notification of maintenance is always provided in advance via an orange bar appearing at the top of the touchscreen. This bar will turn red if the maintenance tasks are overdue. A tab will also be opened at the top of the screen and remains open while maintenance is due. The tasks can be accessed from the tab or by the drop-down menu at the top of the touchscreen.

Liquid System Clean

The liquid system clean is the most time-consuming of all of the tasks, requiring one hour and 20 minutes every month. The operator needs to be present during the clean and will be prompted at a number of stages to load and unload bulk containers. The aim is to clean and decontaminate the internal tubing of the instrument. It involves removal of all bottles from the Omnis, including all bulk reagents, water and waste. This step will reset the scales to zero and allow for accurate measurements of the bulk reagents. The next step is to load all empty waste bottles. The bubble traps are emptied, then one 7.5 L bulk bottle is loaded containing 4 M sodium hydroxide (NaOH), although five litres is sufficient for the task. The single bulk bottle is loaded where the water would normally be and a further two, smaller bulk reagent bottles are loaded where the wash buffer would normally be found and the other at the retrieval solution station. The system is then filled with 4 M NaOH and the process is repeated for each of the bulk reagent positions. The instrument will prompt the operator to move the bottles to the next location when required. The machine then primes the internal tubing and allows the NaOH to soak. The next step is to replace all bulk reagents with distilled water. The machine then pumps water throughout the machine and rinses all NaOH from the instrument. This task lasts for 46 minutes and at the end the machine will require two full wash buffer bulk reagents to prime the buffer lines. One final duty is to perform a liquid system leak test. It is best to conduct this at the end because it requires all the bulk reagents to be present and takes 6 minutes to complete.

Dynamic Gap Lid Clean

A dynamic gap lid clean is dependent on the number of racks processed, not necessarily the number of slides, but the total racks. At intervals of one hundred racks, the dynamic gap lid clean maintenance task should be performed. This maintenance task is designed to clean the glass lids inside the instrument to reduce and clear away build-up of DAB chromogen. The LiHa probe tip also undergoes a decontamination. The time required is 48 minutes in total. After initiating the task, the first step is to load six racks of blank slides into the Omnis. This is then followed by 25 mL of bleach into a 30 mL vial loaded onto the instrument. The bleach must be undiluted with no additives. The best kind is found to be the cheapest and most basic product from a local supermarket. The vial containing bleach is registered as a 'new reagent' and then loaded onto the Omnis in one of the vial racks. The tasks are then carried out automatically, first by decontaminating the tip, and then the arm will transfer each rack to the staining modules and pipette a small volume of bleach onto each lid, cleaning and removing the DAB residue. Once finished the machine automatically flushes each chamber sufficiently. Removing DAB residue via this method is more effective than manual cleaning of the lids with a brush. There have not been any ill effects on the staining intensity after this lid-cleaning process.

Other Minor Tasks

Highlighted in Table 5.5 are other minor maintenance tasks such as an accessory clean, which requires users to remove all items from the machine for cleaning. This duty is not routinely performed as contaminated reagent bottles are taken out of use if any issues arise. Other accessories are kept clean as an included task of routine laboratory cleaning regimen. Checking that the probe tip is intact and correctly centred above its positioning pin is included in the daily assessment of the machine, but the user is prompted to do this on a 30-day cycle. Another maintenance task is to check for lost slides in the machine, primarily in the PT chambers, monthly. This is something the user would only be concerned with if there was a known loss of slides. Flushing and pressurizing the system along with checking the robotic arm are carried out automatically at the end of each staining run while the machine is idle. All bulk reagents are primed before use by the machine, and in an idle state, the machine will also prime periodically.

Grouping the monthly maintenance tasks together minimizes instrument downtime. The longer tasks should be staggered to occur on separate days. There

Table 5.5 Omnis maintenance schedule at the Alfred Hospital Melbourne

Maintenance procedure	Default interval
Initialize robotic arm	After 24 hours of activity (automatic)
Flush system	48 hours (automatic)
Clean dynamic gap lids and decontaminate tip	Weekly
Clean ISH modules	100 ISH cycles
Liquid system leakage test	14 days
Clean liquid system	30 days
Clean stainer modules	30 days
Clean pretreatment modules	30 days
Clean accessories	30 days
Check liquid handling robot reference position	30 days
Check liquid handling robot	30 days

may appear to be an excessive maintenance schedule for the Omnis, but in practical terms, the maintenance tasks are all quite manageable and do not infringe on workflow if planned efficiently.

Green Credentials

Dako's packaging of their products produces a large volume of waste, mainly cardboard but also polystyrene and plastic. Each vial has a life in terms of expiry and life on board. At the end of this the vials must be thrown out. Bulk reagents are made up individually, therefore each time a bulk solution is prepared, an empty plastic container is thrown away. The Omnis uses plastic mixing strips that when full have to be disposed of, and as they contain DAB they cannot be reused. This can add up to a huge amount of waste that is not easily recycled.

Agilent as a wider company is committed to reducing waste and has a list of environmental policies it adheres to, and locally Dako have consolidated deliveries and packaging to reduce waste. As a laboratory we aim to reduce our waste by recycling locally as much of the reagent bottles and packaging as we can, but given that some of the containers are contaminated and cannot be reused, we find we are disposing of large quantities of this waste, especially hard plastics. Every 12 months included in the maintenance schedule is the replacement of all reagent bottles. This is a huge amount of plastic that has to be disposed of. We rely on reagents being disposable and one-time, one-use products, but without proper thought into reusing and recycling such items. In our laboratory we use approximately one hundred vials per year, along with more than 40 wash buffer bottles. All are plastic and we currently don't have the resources to reuse or recycle these items.

We think it would be highly desirable for manufactures to consider the environmental impacts of their products. Manufactures should place a higher emphasis on the waste produced by laboratories and specifically in IHC departments with respect to packaging and used containers. It would be beneficial to the whole industry if manufacturers worked towards gaining B Corp certification.

Omnis Version 2.0

The following paragraphs contain a few suggestions for Dako to consider if they were thinking of upgrading the Omnis to version 2.0. A major improvement would be a larger number of PT modules. The current three that are available are a major bottleneck for batch loading and throughput of assays. A further three PT chambers would improve turnaround times. Perhaps Dako could offer the Omnis in two 'flavours', one with ISH capabilities and one without, so that an extra three PT modules can be accommodated on the instrument that only offers IHC. There may be a market for an 'IHC only' Omnis as not all diagnostic anatomical pathology facilities offer an ISH service. Following along with this proposal is the need for an increase in bulk reagent capacity, especially for wash buffers.

Optional on-board slide baking or a drying cycle would be handy. The user should be able to switch this function on/off for individual racks as necessary. There should be a true urgent priority protocol where the Omnis has the ability to genuinely prioritize a slide or batch of slides over others currently staining. At the moment, there is a tag that is applied, but it doesn't make a huge difference in terms of time and priority.

The desktop workstation software could be redesigned to be more intuitive and more customizable and to give meaningful information. Currently the search function is difficult in terms of obtaining the information users want to see. On occasion, assays that have been stained do not display in the completed tab, but when the user exits the screen and a second attempt is made, the slides appear. There should be a separate tab for information about antibody levels for easy retrieval of data. It would be preferable for a symbol to appear when antibodies are loaded on the Omnis to indicate when the reagent has capacity for only one more test. Currently, users have to check individual vials, but this would be better highlighted by the Omnis so that the operator can plan to replenish antibody reagent for the next assay. Managing stock inventory would be helpful if there is a suggested list generated for reagents needed to be ordered that could be printed or emailed to allow streamlined ordering through Dako. This list could be generated from reagents that are due to expire or those that have low volume levels.

It would be beneficial to reorganize the creation of new protocols and products. Currently, too many steps are involved to produce a new protocol and for it to be available as a diagnostic test. If this could be managed in one application, it would reduce errors in protocol set-up and the duplication of steps. Note that these observations have been made from real experiences using the Omnis daily. Considering the numerous tasks the instrument does well, these comments can be taken as minor quibbles.

Five things which prevent the Omnis from being a better platform:

(1) Only three PT chambers servicing six staining modules.
(2) Rather lengthy and user involved maintenance schedules.
(3) Small volume of bulk reagents.
(4) Mixing strips and hazardous waste can only be changed when the instrument is idle.
(5) Convoluted way of generating new products for new IHC assays.

Five things that make the Omnis exceptional:

(1) Nine racks (45 slides) with antibodies and reagents can all be loaded in 15 minutes.
(2) Six staining modules independent of each other.
(3) Integration and full compatibility with laboratory's Cerner Millennium LIS software.
(4) Capacity to run IHC and ISH slides concurrently with ISH protocols shorter than 5 hours in duration.
(5) Access to bulk reagents and vial draws when instrument is operational.

Conclusion

The Omnis is a solid investment choice for automating IHC and ISH assays. Although a large instrument, its modern design aesthetic with attached touchscreen and status light bar is a highlight. The two imposing instruments certainly creates a talking point in the facility with visitors.

The software package manages reagent lot numbers, expiry dates and user profiles. It is clearly laid out and registering consumables via the workstation is straightforward. Slide registration is clear and accessible, along with slide details and progression of tests. The initial new product and protocol procedure is convoluted, but fortunately once created do not need to be accessed again. A redesign of the workstation to offer users a more intuitive experience is needed, but the touchscreen on the Omnis is user friendly and clear with the information that is displayed.

In today's IHC world, it is important to consider the flexibility of any platform for third-party products. Immunohistochemistry instrumentation should not be tightly 'closed' in terms of antibody assays the user wishes to employ. The Omnis is designed to utilize not only Dako antibodies, but also those sourced from other vendors. No one manufacturer can offer all the localization antibody a facility needs. The Omnis has produced excellent results using both Dako and non-Dako antibodies with the available protocols and detection.

The facility's external QAP and proficiency testing results have been to a high standard when compared to rival instruments. The instrument has increased efficiencies with a streamlined workflow of cut, load and unload slides. A reduced turnaround time means a larger number of assays achieving same-day completion. A contributing factor is the availability of RTU antibodies, which in turn means a greater level of matching pre-analytic standardization efforts between vendor and testing laboratory. With this workflow the machine has little idle time and allows the user to carry out maintenance tasks in the morning. The ability to process ISH on board with minimal user interaction and the short protocol time have also been a huge benefit. Especially beneficial at the end of the working day is the ability to load 60 slides or 12 racks in a relatively short time for an overnight run.

There have been minor issues with the instrument, but the laboratory has not encountered a problem causing the instrument to be down for more than a day. Most issues have a workaround so assays can continue staining. As the Omni is a relatively new platform, these issues are considered 'teething' problems and there is always adequate, rapid and professional service from Dako. Always reassuring is the constant stream of updates to hardware and software affirming the strong after sales support from the vendor. The requisite maintenance tasks can be inconvenient and always seem to arrive on a particularly demanding day. But in retrospect these tasks are manageable if planned properly and are relatively low maintenance considering the number of assays the Omnis performs. Employing dynamic gap technology to differentiate from other automation platforms, the Omnis is an ideal instrument in terms of capacity and ease of use for a busy IHC and ISH facility.

References

Agilent 2018. Dako Omnis: A comprehensive IHC and ISH solution designed for true patient case management. Agilent Technologies (online). Available at www.agilent.com/cs/library/datasheets/public/29067_dako-omnis-data-sheet.pdf (Accessed 1 March 2020).

Brenner TL, Adams VR 1999. First MAb approved for treatment of metastatic breast cancer. *J Am Pharm Assoc (Wash)* **39**(2):236–8.

Diercks GF, Pas HH, Jonkman MF 2017. Immunofluorescence of autoimmune bullous diseases. *Surg Pathol Clin* **10**(2):505–12.

Mogens V, Nielsen S 2016. Proficiency testing in immunohistochemistry: Experiences from Nordic Immunohistochemical Quality Control (NordiQC). *Virchows Arch* **468**:19–29.

Rasmussen OF, Binzer T, Rudbeck L 2014. Dynamic gap staining: A new IHC staining technology. Agilent Technologies (online). Available at www.agilent.com/cs/library/whitepaper/public/29079_dynamic_gap_staining.pdf (Accessed 1 March 2020).

Chapter 6

Immunohistochemistry for Research Applications

Trung Nguyen

Overview

Antibodies do not read textbooks and not all antibodies are created equal. This sentiment is often shared when unusual or unexpected results are obtained, which is unfortunately a real occurrence. The technique of immunohistochemistry (IHC) can be both simple and complicated. It all depends on the situation, the available reagents and the objectives of the researcher. It is not the intention of this chapter to provide protocols for every situation that can be encountered in the research sphere. Whether the investigator is diving into IHC for the first time or is a seasoned operator, the intention of this chapter is to highlight and explain specific areas of importance. These matters require careful consideration because they dictate the success or failure of an IHC assay.

Researchers' aim is to achieve a highly sensitive and specific IHC signal. They want a crisp, clean and reproducible stain for their projects. Most investigators will not have a grounding in traditional histological techniques, a necessity to understand the nuances in order to optimize IHC assays. Support is offered here via provisions of both theoretical and practical IHC principles so this knowledge can be applied to any IHC scenario. At the very least, it is hoped researchers can take an existing IHC protocol which has undoubtedly been handed down through the years from researcher to researcher and be able to refine them in order to gain efficiencies.

This chapter covers important parameters researchers need to know by first explaining the difference between IHC for diagnostic work in human pathology as compared to a broad research device for many settings. The importance of standardization is highlighted with reference to the concepts of pre-analytical, analytical and post-analytical stages. The format chosen is a discussion based on a template request form and explanations are conveyed as to why they are significant. Each segment of the template form is examined via a question-and-answer format because it is these responses that dictate the overall parameters of the IHC protocol.

After variables such as fixation, tissue type and visualization methods are decided, the IHC protocol is examined in detail with references as to how it can be optimized and adapted to any given research setting. The chapter concludes with practical tips shared for antibody titre preparations and handy hints to achieve efficient and reliable IHC assays.

Diagnostic Immunohistochemistry versus Research Immunohistochemistry

Immunohistochemistry in the clinical diagnostic histopathology setting is straightforward. The test tissue is always of human origin and routinely processed as formalin-fixed paraffin-embedded (FFPE) tissue blocks. The primary antibody is of either mouse or rabbit origin. Secondary antibodies and linkers comprising the detection kit are specified to work on either mouse or rabbit primary antibodies. The enzyme label of choice is peroxidase obtained from the horseradish plant and therefore blocking is tuned for endogenous peroxidase activity. The 3,3' diaminobenzidine (DAB) chromogen is the conventional choice with haematoxylin as the counterstain. Standard practice ensures buffer washes, incubation time and temperature parameters for detection are kept consistent. If this can be achieved, then the only variables left to be concerned with are the antigen retrieval and working antibody concentration. From so many variables, now there are just two. This can be decreased to just one if ready-to-use (RTU) antibodies are employed.

Immunohistochemistry for research purposes, on the other hand, can be complicated because of the many variables attributed to the IHC assay. An explanation of why this is so can be found when addressing the many reasons IHC is employed for research applications. Some projects require one colour (label) IHC while other endeavours may need multiplexing to highlight different proteins of interest. An investigation may employ antibodies derived from the same species as the test tissue – the so-called mouse-on-mouse studies are an example. A concerted effort is needed to shape the IHC assay to be fit for purpose and tailored to the researcher's specific requirements. Unfortunately, there is no one IHC solution that fits for all purposes. The investigator must understand that if an antibody has been successfully verified in a Western blot, this does not necessarily mean IHC success for tissue sections.

To achieve a methodical approach, the IHC assay is split into three main areas known as the pre-analytical, analytical and post-analytical segments. Using this classification allows the investigator to impart a degree of standardization to the IHC assay. In this chapter the three stages are taken from the context of the IHC assay only. It is important to state this unambiguously because confusion results when a clear definition is not provided as to which perspective is used. For example, when IHC is discussed as an analytical technique belonging to an arsenal of other histological methods such as H&E and special stains, the events within the pre-analytical domain are considered somewhat out of the control of the laboratory. Tissue sampling by the surgeon, cold ischaemic time and specimen transit time from operating theatre to laboratory are examples.

Parameters such as fixation, tissue macroscopic dissection, processing and microtomy are considered analytical in this context because they are variables that the laboratory can standardize and control. Remember that IHC in this setting is just one technique amongst others in the anatomical pathology laboratory. When the perspective changes and discussion is centred only around the IHC assay itself, the parameters of fixation, tissue dissection, processing and microtomy are now considered pre-analytical, albeit still under the direct control of the investigator if the project is planned in advance. Epitope retrieval, antibody concentrations and detection system considerations are examples of analytical factors within the IHC assay. To clarify further, take the situation where the laboratory has received an unstained section on a slide and has been asked to perform a CD20 IHC assay by another facility. Tissue fixation, section thickness and the type of microscope slide are all important pre-analytical variables because the facility receiving the unstained sections does not have any influence on these parameters. A similar set of circumstances arises when a researcher with a novel antibody asks the IHC facility to 'make it work' on tissue sections.

When a diagnostic IHC facility is approached for assistance from researchers, a good starting point is to make available a specific request form for the researcher to fill in. Figure 6.1 is an example of documentation researchers can apply in order to optimize IHC assays or request IHC services from an external laboratory. This form is also reproduced and made available as an appendix at the end of the chapter for practical use, designed as two pages to be printed front and back. To complement this questionnaire, the basic IHC protocol is outlined in Figure 6.7 as a flow chart. The combination of these two illustrations and the discussions associated with them should provide a sound basis for deep understanding of the IHC assay. The researcher should then be able to assess, adapt and tweak the IHC method for their individual needs.

Essentially, IHC optimization is an experimental process of trial and elimination. If the antibody assay doesn't provide satisfactory results, tweaking different retrieval regimens or attempting different working titres are standard practices until all avenues are exhausted. What the investigator really wants to measure and ascertain is how 'good' the antibody is. Is it a dud? If so, it must be proven so. It is incumbent on the researcher to measure the antibody's specificity and sensitivity by performing assays in conjunction with appropriate controls.

Pre-analytical Stage

As illustrated in Figure 6.1, the request form is divided into five sections. Figure 6.2 shows a cropped version of the form highlighting the section containing pre-analytical factors. This portion enables the laboratory assisting the researcher access to relevant information about the project. If careful thought has been placed into the design of the research project from the beginning, creating a suitable IHC assay should be straightforward because pre-analytical factors have been

Immunohistochemistry request form for research applications

Answer the following questions accurately. Refer to guidelines overleaf. If answer is unknown, please leave blank.

Researcher details

Name	Phone
Email	Institution
Background information	

Pre-analytical

Tissue origin	Tissue source	Section thickness
Nature	Fixation	

Analytical

Antibody name	Antibody source	
Host species	Aliquot contents	
Protein concentration	Lot/serial number	Manufacture date
Expiry date	Storage	Clonality & Ig class
Enrichment/purification process	Visualization	

Post-analytical

Localization	Staining pattern
Morphology requirements	

Quality control

Control tissue	Tissue source
Nature	Fixation
Have you successfully optimized a Western blot? Yes/No	Do you intend to apply stereological analysis? Yes/No

Figure 6.1 Request form for immunohistochemistry services

optimized for IHC purposes. Unfortunately, time and time again, IHC is an afterthought, and it can be challenging to achieve a suitable IHC stain from less than ideal pre-analytical conditions. The questions posed in this section are mainly centred around the material for testing and analysis.

Background information

Pre-analytical

Tissue origin	Tissue source	Section thickness
Nature	Fixation	

Figure 6.2 Pre-analytical information required

Background Information

What are you trying to achieve?

Have other research groups worked with this antibody before?

Are methods available with this antibody within the literature?

Just like trying to solve a crime, every little piece of information gained from the researcher helps when trying to work with a novel research antibody. A good place to start is ascertaining if other research groups have worked with this particular antibody clone and if journal papers are available. When external parties have already optimized the antibody, it is a waste of resources to essentially repeat the process. A better outcome is to use an established protocol to determine if it works and then decide if any tweaks or modifications are required to make the IHC assay better.

Tissue Origin

Is the tissue to be tested of human origin or from some other animal such as a rodent or a primate?

The reagents to be used for the IHC assay depend on the tissue of origin. Establishing whether the test material is of human origin or from some other animal species is important because of the need for immunological cross-reactivity. This is the hallmark of any IHC assay.

Tissue Source

Who is providing the test tissue?

Where did it come from?

Was it obtained from a tissue or tumour bank?

Was it taken from diagnostic pathology archives?

Is the test tissue derived from tissue culture, specific cell lines or FFPE?

Learning the exact source of the test material and how it was created offers insights to how fresh or old the material is. Tissue storage conditions and the way the tissue has been prepared are important considerations. Access to departmental records can be useful for the overall analytical process.

Section Thickness

How thick should the sections be?

Routine 2–3µm or thicker?

Immunohistochemical staining is a physical process and if there are thin or thick sections, parameters such as incubation times and temperature control may need to be matched for optimal results.

Nature

Is the test tissue fresh frozen?

Has the test tissue been through FFPE histological processing?

The IHC protocol for fresh tissue is different to that of FFPE tissue. Morphological information is better retained in FFPE sections, but antigen retrieval steps may be necessary. Fresh tissue in the form of cryostat sections may not require epitope retrieval, but certain enzymes may still be active. For instance, endogenous alkaline phosphatase is neutralized in FFPE sections but functional in frozen sections. Hence a block with levamisole is required if choosing an IHC assay based on alkaline phosphatase. Ponder and Wilkinson (1981) found levamisole unsuccessful in blocking intestinal-type alkaline phosphatase; in this case another label such as peroxidase of a fluorochrome should be chosen.

Fixation

Has the test tissue been treated with a fixative?

What type of fixative and for how long?

Is the test tissue fresh frozen?

Has the test tissue been through FFPE histological processing?

The standard fixative for tissue sections is 10% neutral buffered formalin. It is somewhat of a default choice because formaldehyde was used for its preservation of tissue morphology decades before the arrival of IHC technology (Fox et al. 1985). Certain fixatives are incompatible with good-quality IHC staining. Ingredients such as chromium, picric acid, mercury and other heavy metals can impede certain antibodies (Jackson and Blythe 2008). Another aspect for contemplation is that basic principles of fixation also apply here. It is a physical process requiring time and under the influence of temperature. 'Under' as well as 'over' fixation is known to lead to suboptimal IHC results.

Analytical Stage

The analytical stage is the nitty-gritty portion of testing the antibody to the tissue. Figure 6.3 contains questions relating to the antibody nominated for investigation. The answers obtained will assess the suitability of the clone for the planned IHC assay. Keep in mind that all of the pre-analytical factors discussed earlier impact the overall protocol design along with the antibody.

Antibody Name

Include other names by which the antibody is also commonly known in the literature.

There is no set convention when naming antibody clones. Even when there is a concerted effort, antibodies can often be referred to by their clone names. Using the clusters of differentiation (CD) nomenclature as an example, CD117 is commonly known as c-kit, CD15 is described as LeuM1 and CD274 is called PD-L1 (Fabrizio et al. 2018). As such, there are numerous examples of the same antibody being referred to by several different names. Her2, c-erbB2, neu and ERBB2 are all the same antibody (Busse et al. 2000).

Antibody Source

Commercial vendor or in-house preparation?

List the specific catalogue numbers from the manufacturer.

Knowledge of the antibody origin is useful because it offers an insight into how and when it was manufactured. Commercial antibodies sourced from biotechnology companies should have a specification sheet outlining useful information. Once again, there is no set convention to these data sheets, but at the very least, information pertaining to the host species, lot and serial numbers, protein concentration, additives and preservatives present, expiry dates, clonality and immunoglobulin class should be provided. Other information such as storage recommendations, verification or validation studies and perhaps a recommended protocol is considered a bonus. If the antibody was prepared in house, more effort is required to optimize the antibody because of the lack

Analytical

Antibody name		Antibody source
Host species		Aliquot contents
Protein concentration	Lot/serial number	Manufacture date
Expiry date	Storage	Clonality & Ig class
Enrichment/purification process		Visualization

Figure 6.3 Analytical questions

of a validation process provided by a vendor. Whichever situation plays out, it is best to gain as much information as possible from the researcher or the party responsible for manufacturing the antibody before commencing optimization.

Host Species

The animal from which the antibody was derived.

Knowledge of the species from which the test tissue was derived is equally important as the species from which the antibody was developed. The establishment of a reaction based on immunological principles is in question, especially the ability to detect and react to something that is foreign to oneself. There are instances when the test tissue and the primary antibody come from the same species. This situation should be avoided because of unwanted binding of the secondary antibodies with endogenous antibodies as well as the primary antibody. If this cannot be helped, special kits and protocols are available for this type of IHC analysis. Goodpaster and Randolph-Habecker (2014) describe a protocol for 'mouse-on-mouse' IHC – that is, using a mouse primary antibody on mouse test tissue. A scenario such as this should be avoided because it makes the IHC assay more complicated.

Aliquot Contents

Are any additives included with the antibody?

List any included preservatives, glycerol, sodium azide, the type of buffer used and the pH level.

It is useful to know all of the ingredients included with the antibody. Preservatives are commonly added to stop bacterial growth. A specific media such as glycerol is designed to aid in below zero °C storage conditions. Buffers are employed to keep the reagent within a specific pH range.

Protein Concentration

State the concentration of antibody, immunoglobulin level or total protein content.

Besides the antibody, determine if any other types of protein are present which may interfere with the staining process. It is also useful to compare protein concentration between batches to ascertain if inconsistent staining is due to batch-to-batch variations.

Lot/Serial Number

Record these data if available. Batch-to-batch variations are easier to investigate.

It is good laboratory practice to include serial numbers as a record of your experiments.

Manufacture and Expiry Dates

Consider the age of the antibody.

Some antibodies last for a very long time whereas others have a short useful shelf life. Follow the manufacturer's expiry dates and constantly survey antibody performance with appropriate control tissues.

Storage

How has the antibody been stored?

Has it been frozen with multiple freeze-thaw cycles?

Constant refrigeration at 4°C as per manufacturer's recommendations?

To get the maximum productive life of an antibody, specific storage conditions should be met as recommended by the manufacturer. Repeated freeze-thaw cycles are to be avoided. A suitable alternative is to aliquot the antibody into smaller lots. For instance, a 1 mL concentrate can be divided into 10 smaller lots, each vial containing 100 μL. One ampoule will in use whilst the other aliquots may be stored frozen until required.

Clonality and Immunoglobulin Class

Is the antibody monoclonal or polyclonal?

Is the prevalent type of immunoglobulin IgG or IgM?

The exact class and clonality are important when trying to troubleshoot suboptimal staining.

Traditionally monoclonals offer superior specificity whilst polyclonals bestow high sensitivity. Current-generation antibodies, especially rabbit monoclonals, achieve elevated levels of sensitivity and specificity.

Enrichment/Purification Process

> ***Was the antibody subjected to any other processing regimes during manufacture?***

Getting an idea of how 'pure' an antibody is may provide a useful reflection of its performance.

Visualization

> ***Choice of a fluorescence, chromogenic or metal particles such as silver or gold needs to be nominated as a label.***

The type of label to be applied for visualization needs to be decided. There are associated advantages and disadvantages of using a fluorescence signal, chromogenic stain or metal ions. The researcher must decide the most appropriate label for their IHC project.

Post-Analytical Stage

After the staining process is completed, what are the expected results? Figure 6.4 highlights the post-analytical considerations involving stain interpretation. For instance, is it a simple positive versus negative staining pattern and something that is brown or blue when DAB chromogen is used? Semi-quantitative assessments can be more complicated, especially when there is a range of intensities to which a scoring algorithm needs to be applied for reporting. Another contemplation is the need for a qualified pathologist to interpret the staining.

Localization

> ***Is the expected signal nuclear, cytoplasmic or membranous?***

This depends on where the antigen is located. Does the pattern of staining correlate to theoretical principles? For instance, nuclear transcription factors should be localized within the cell nuclei and so the IHC staining should show a nuclear localization. The family of cytokeratins, on the other hand, should be found within the cytoplasm.

Staining Pattern

> ***Is the expected pattern globular, speckled, perinuclear or dot-like?***
>
> ***Should the staining be heterogeneous versus homogeneous in the entire section?***

The amount of antigen present dictates the pattern of staining and the distribution of the signal. Naturally the low expressors would provide lighter staining intensity when compared to high expressors achieving a darker stain. The same effect is achieved when using thinner sections as opposed to thicker sections. If antigens indeed naturally occur in low amounts, the investigator may elect to amplify the signal synthetically. Various kits are available such as the tyramide signal amplification (Faget and Hnasko 2015) or CSA II biotin-free catalysed amplification (Shiogama et al. 2013). Some caution is advised here because if the signal is artificially enhanced for visual purposes and if the assay is subjected to quantitative analyses, the results achieved may not be an accurate reflection of the true antigen level.

Morphology Requirements

> ***Should normal tissue elements show positivity?***
>
> ***What is the exact pathological process to be demonstrated?***

Post-analytical

Localization	Staining pattern
Morphology requirements	

Figure 6.4 Post-analytical factors

A good question to ask is if the antibody also highlights other non-related tissue elements that may serve as internal controls. Quite often, the lineage of the cells or cellular compartments is retained in both benign and diseased situations.

Quality Control

Quality assurance measures are employed to qualify the staining and to guarantee the results achieved are in some way meaningful. Figure 6.5 examines the nature of control material to provide confidence as well as proof that the results obtained are reproducible.

Control Tissue

Is the control tissue of human origin or from some other animal such as rodent or primate?

Is adequate tissue with the disease state available for positive controls?

Are natural internal controls present in the test tissue?

Can external cell lines be used as control material?

As much as practicable, control tissue should not only contain the antigen of interest, but also closely match the test tissue in terms of fixation, processing and tissue type. In addition, it is good practice to include both negative and positive tissue controls along with the disease process concerning which the investigation is undertaken.

Tissue Source

Who is providing the control tissue?

Where did it come from?

Was it obtained from a tissue or tumour bank or derived from a diagnostic pathology archive?

Was the control tissue derived from tissue culture, specific cell lines or FFPE?

It is beneficial to know exactly where the control issue originated. Having a record of the exact source of control material and how well it matches the test tissue is important. Similar preparation and storage of both test and control tissue adds significance to the results.

Nature and Fixation

Is the control tissue fresh frozen?

Has the control tissue been through FFPE histological processing?

Has the control tissue been treated with a fixative?

What type of fixative and for how long?

Matching the control tissue to the test tissue provides a more robust IHC assay. For example, testing fresh frozen cryostat sections means that the control tissue should also be obtained from fresh frozen cryostat sections. Similarly, match the type of fixative used for the control tissue to that of the test issue. This is known as IHC validation using like-for-like conditions.

Have You Successfully Optimized a Western Blot?

Successful validation of the antibody on a Western blot does not guarantee automatic IHC success on tissue sections. There is no rhyme or reason for this to occur. The onus is on the researcher to prove the antibody can be used for IHC purposes on tissue sections.

Do You Intend to Apply Stereological Analysis?

Counting positive cells or entities demonstrated by IHC in a 2D tissue section and comparing that to a 3D structure requires careful planning. Things to consider include the thickness of sections, the unbiased and representative sampling of the 3D object and the computer software algorithms required for obtaining a precise estimate. Let's be clear about this. Using

Quality control

Control tissue	Tissue source
Nature	Fixation
Have you successfully optimized a Western blot? Yes/No	Do you intend to apply stereological analysis? Yes/No

Figure 6.5 Quality measures

computer algorithms to display quantitative data on a single section is not stereology in a classical sense because stereology requires sampling of the entire 3D structure. For example, if the principal investigation is to count the number of positive neurons in a rodent brain, stereology theory states that the entire rodent brain needs to be sampled, not just one representative section of the rodent brain. This means multiple histological sections of the rodent brain need to be prepared in order to ensure the whole brain has been sampled in the count. It is not feasible to count every neuron in the brain, therefore not every section will be used in the count. Instead, a sampling protocol of every 10th section can be used as an example. If stereological analysis is required, the thickness of the section and the sampling protocol are two critical parameters to determine (Brown 2017). This is to avoid counting the same cell or object twice within the sampling protocol.

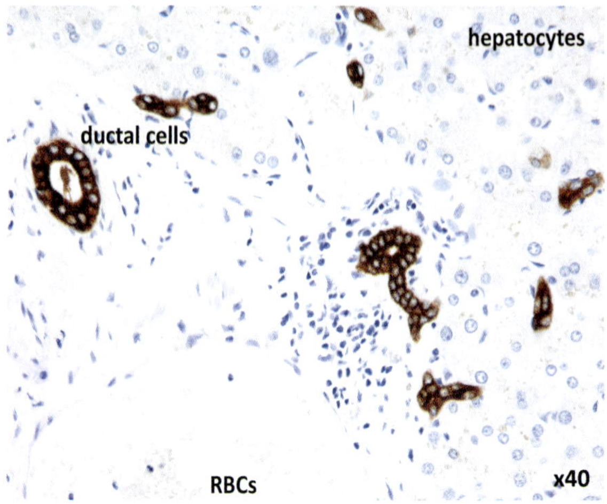

Figure 6.6 CK AE1/3 immunohistochemistry on a liver formalin-fixed paraffin-embedded section

Optimizing an Antibody for Immunohistochemistry

With so many variables to contend with within the IHC protocol, matters can get complicated quite easily when optimizing a new antibody for research. As such, it is good practice to limit as many variables as possible. Ideally, after the decision has been made on the type of visualization required, the appropriate detection system is then chosen. The detection and visualization steps relating to incubation time and temperatures should be set as standard. Whether this information comes from a manufacturer's recommendation or the protocol has been used successfully in the past, there should be no deviation from these parameters. If this is achieved, the only variables the researcher needs to contend with are the antigen retrieval and the primary antibody parameters. Tweaking these two variables is much more manageable when all the other stages are set. Figure 6.7 highlights the basic IHC assay components. It is essential each stage is well understood because they are all interconnected. It takes only one suboptimal process within the assay to lead to detrimental IHC results.

The question whether to employ automation or manual methods when optimising a new antibody is up to the researcher and the resources available. The discussion from this point onwards is directed in relation to IHC staining using a manual process. As an exercise in antibody optimization, manual methods offer easier control of the plethora of parameters encountered within the IHC assay. When an optimized protocol is found, protocol transfer to an automation platform for large batch staining of slides would be a simple task. Manual staining, although considered 'old school', is still a relevant tool to provide proof-of-concept IHC staining for verification of the antibody on tissue sections. An example of a specific and sensitive IHC assay is shown in Figure 6.6, of a pan-cytokeratin antibody on a liver FFPE section. The enzyme label chosen for this method is peroxidase, the chromogen is DAB and the counterstain is haematoxylin. Note the absence of unwanted background staining and that endogenous peroxidase activity in the red blood cells (RBCs) has been successfully blocked. The bile ducts (brown) can be easily discerned from the surrounding hepatocytes (blue). This clean and crisp stain was the result of the IHC protocol outlined in Figure 6.7

Test Material

As stated previously, the type of test tissue dictates the protocol. Fresh frozen sections do not require dewaxing whereas FFPE tissues do. The routine diagnostic FFPE IHC protocol is used as the reference protocol because it is a template suitable to be modified for research purposes. This reference protocol is reliable, robust and has been proven time and time again in real-world scenarios. To commence, a section needs to be obtained on a glass microscope slide. It is standard practice to use clean positively charged slides or

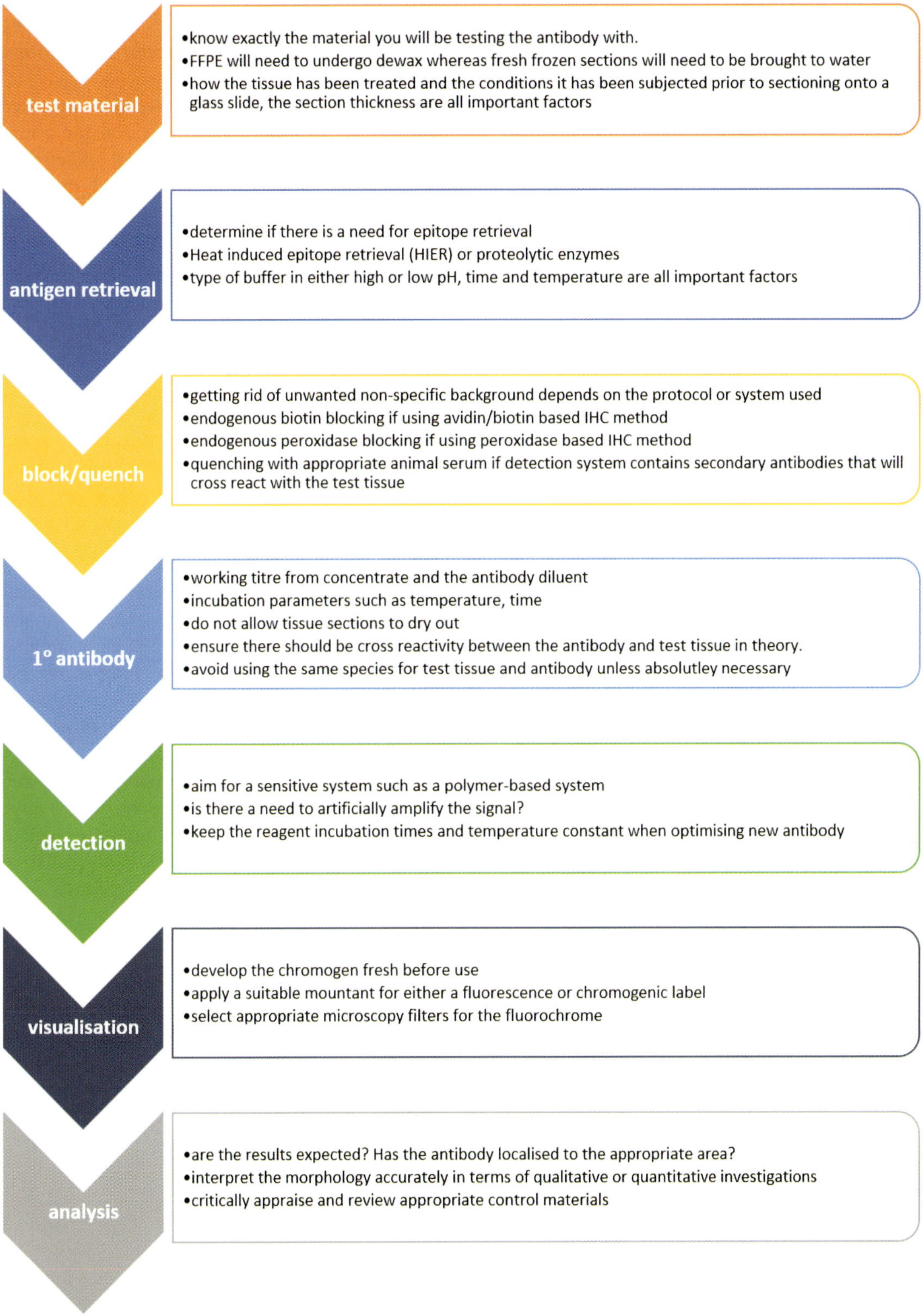

Figure 6.7 Basic flow chart of immunohistochemistry protocol steps

slides by any other means of conferring them to be 'sticky'. Using non-sticky slides would often result in lost sections during the IHC process. Ideally, a positive tissue control section is placed on the same slide as the test section. Another slide running parallel can act as the negative tissue control. Note that within a clinical diagnostic histopathology setting, negative tissue controls are routinely omitted. To replicate this practice within the research setting is entirely up to the researcher. If tissue is scarce to begin with, why waste it? On the other hand, it is useful to compare the antibody activity (if any) to the negative control. The FFPE sections always undergo dewaxing and are taken to water. Fresh frozen sections have no dewaxing requirements. Wash buffer is applied to the section officially starting the IHC assay.

Antigen Retrieval

Fresh frozen sections would not normally require retrieval. In this instance, wash buffer is applied to the section and is displaced by the next reagent in the sequence. When using wash buffer, it is important to clear as much as practicable the buffer from the slide before applying the next reagent. Failure to do so can contribute to inadvertent dilution of the following reagent. Some researchers apply ethanol or acetone to the fresh frozen section before starting the IHC process. Alcohol-based fixatives act by coagulating proteins which may stabilize proteins within the tissue before the IHC process (Grizzle et al. 2008). Whether to add or omit this step is up to the investigator. It is suggested that when optimizing the research antibody, include this step only if it enhances the IHC stain.

The FFPE sections would normally require some type of epitope retrieval. There are two main methods to achieve this. The first option is the use of proteolytic enzymes and the second is the use of heat energy. It is common practice to automatically default to heat-induced epitope retrieval (HIER) in a low-pH or high-pH buffer and decide on the maximum temperature obtained and the duration of the heating. The HIER can be somewhat destructive to certain epitopes. A gentler method of exposing antigenic-determining sites is to employ proteolytic enzymes such as proteinase K. A good analogy is a tangled ball of wool. The researcher is trying to expose the epitopes contained within this tangled mess. The wool can be placed in a pot of boiling water (HEIR) and the heat energy untangles the wool to expose the epitopes. Alternatively, using enzymes is like utilizing a pair of scissors and making precise snips within the wool to expose epitopes.

Unfortunately, there is no universally accepted protocol of performing antigen retrieval for a new antibody. As such, it is a process of trial and elimination. To make matters more complicated, there are a plethora of ways to induce heat to the test sections. The HIER can be simple exposure of the sections to boiling buffer solution, subjecting the buffer to microwave irradiation or use of high-pressure cookers, and some have even used ultrasonic energy, the latter with varying degrees of success (Leong et al. 2002). Whichever method is decided on, it is imperative that the conditions achieved during HIER are displaced evenly across the entire slide and that the process is easily reproducible for consistent results. A typical heat retrieval regime would see the temperature rise to 100°C and sustained for 10 minutes before the sections begin to cool down to room temperature. A typical protease enzyme treatment would be 10 minutes incubation at room temperature. Once again, these considerations are empirical. The onus is on the investigator to find the retrieval settings that exposes epitopes for the antibody to bind to. A typical low-pH retrieval solution would be citrate based at around pH6 whereas a high-pH retrieval solution would be Tris or EDTA based at pH9. A recipe for these retrieval buffers can be found in Table 6.1. Having access to these three main types of retrieval strategies – one enzyme and a low- and high-pH buffer – with set incubation time and temperature settings would greatly assist the optimization of antibodies for IHC. Changing the time and temperature settings is reserved for

Table 6.1 Common antigen retrieval buffers (Jackson and Blythe 2008)

Citrate buffer pH6		Tris-EDTA buffer pH9	
Citric acid anhydrous	21 g	Tris	14.4 g
Distilled water	10 L	EDTA	1.44 g
Adjust to pH6 with 1 M HCl		Distilled water	600 mL
		Tween 20	0.3 mL
		Adjust to pH9 with 1 M HCl	

occasions when unsatisfactory results are achieved with the new antibody.

Blocking and Quenching

The action of blocking, otherwise known as quenching, can be performed either before or after primary antibody incubation. It all depends on what exactly you are trying to block. If the IHC system employed is peroxidase based, then hydrogen peroxide (H_2O_2) at 3% strength is applied before the detection stage. In this instance, the blocking step can be applied either before or after the primary antibody step. The main aim of performing blocking steps is to clear away unwanted background staining. Familiarity with the enzyme's activity is helpful. For example, the alkaline phosphatase enzyme is deactivated during tissue processing to FFPE but is otherwise still active in fresh frozen sections. Blocking is therefore not required for FFPE sections in most situations. In addition, if the IHC assay is based on alkaline phosphatase, there is no need to block for endogenous peroxidase activity and vice versa. Likewise, a biotin block is required only when the IHC is based on avidin or streptavidin biotin techniques. It is not warranted when deploying non-biotin polymer technologies.

A serum block is only necessary if there is non-specific binding to the test tissue by the secondary antibody or the linker antibody is derived from an animal source that will react or bind with the test tissue. This can easily be tested by applying the detection system to the test issue whilst omitting the primary antibody step. The rest of the protocol is carried through to see if there is chromogen development. When doing this test, don't forget to include the endogenous enzyme block. Employing 3% H_2O_2 for an immunoperoxidase technique will eliminate one of the common causes of unwanted background staining. If no brown colour develops, it can be interpreted that a serum block is not required. On the other hand, if a brown colour develops and it is ascertained that it is not from endogenous enzymes, then there is a suspicion that the test tissue is reacting with the secondary antibody within the detection system. In this instance, a serum block is introduced before the detection step. There are numerous blocking agents for this. If using animal serum, match the animal of origin to that of the secondary antibody animal origin. Other blocking reagents include bovine serum albumin, casein and non-fat milk. Before embarking on this type of blocking, ensure that it is necessary. For comparison, antibodies and detection kits for diagnostic IHC settings have such a high level of specificity that a serum or protein block is not required.

Test Antibody

Commonly referred to as the primary antibody, it is commonly presented as a concentrate in research settings. The working titre is defined as the concentration of an antibody as determined by finding the highest dilution at which it is still able to cause binding of the antigen. Optimal titres need to be ascertained by experiment after the researcher has taken into consideration factors such as how it was made, storage conditions and the quantity of immunoglobulin available. Even though antibody diluent can be manufactured in house, it is recommended to use a commercially available diluent for the titrations. A 'test battery' approach is used to find the assay 'sweet spot', the highest dilution of the antibody which gives the best results in terms of staining. There is no correct way of determining this end point. It is a process of elimination.

The size of the test battery is up to the researcher. A typical first-line optimization panel may include 1:100, 1:500 and 1:1,000 dilution factors of the antibody concentrate. If using three different types of retrieval strategies, this would produce nine slides in the first line test battery. Figure 6.8 shows what this would look like. The scenario can, however, be made more manageable if multiple test sections are placed on each slide. Figure 6.9 demonstrates a reduction from an original nine-slide test battery to just three slides if the sections are small enough to allow multiple sections mounted onto a slide segregated with a wax or pap pen.

In practical terms, the actual antibody concentration is not taken literally because it is simpler to use ratios. Whatever the actual concentration is, 1 μL is sampled from the antibody concentrate and mixed with 99 μL of antibody diluent. This gives a total volume of 100 μL and a working titre of 1:100. Another way to approach it is 1 part antibody to 99 parts diluent. If a 100 μL volume was not enough and 1 mL (1,000 μL) is required, sample 10 μL of antibody concentrate to 990 μL of diluent. Figure 6.10 highlights these two titrations.

Working in ratios makes things simpler. To make a 1:500 titre, take 1 μL from the antibody concentrate and add that to 499 μL of antibody diluent and so on. Some workers simplify this further and just add the

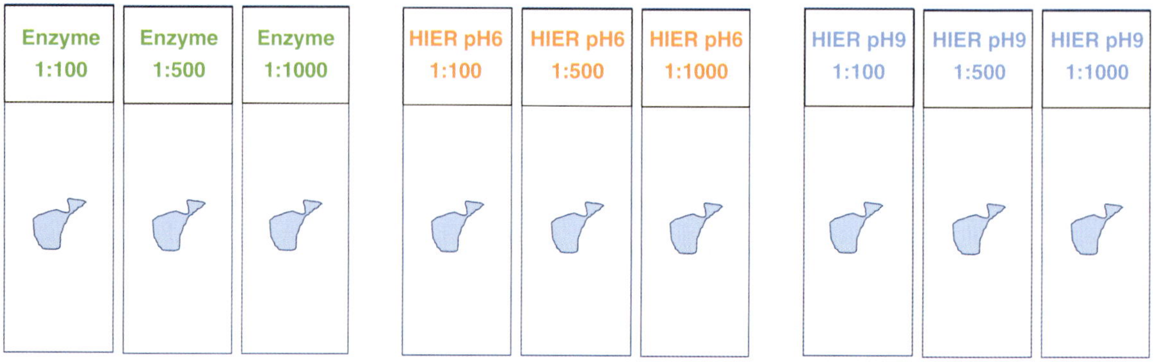

Figure 6.8 First-line test battery comprising nine slides

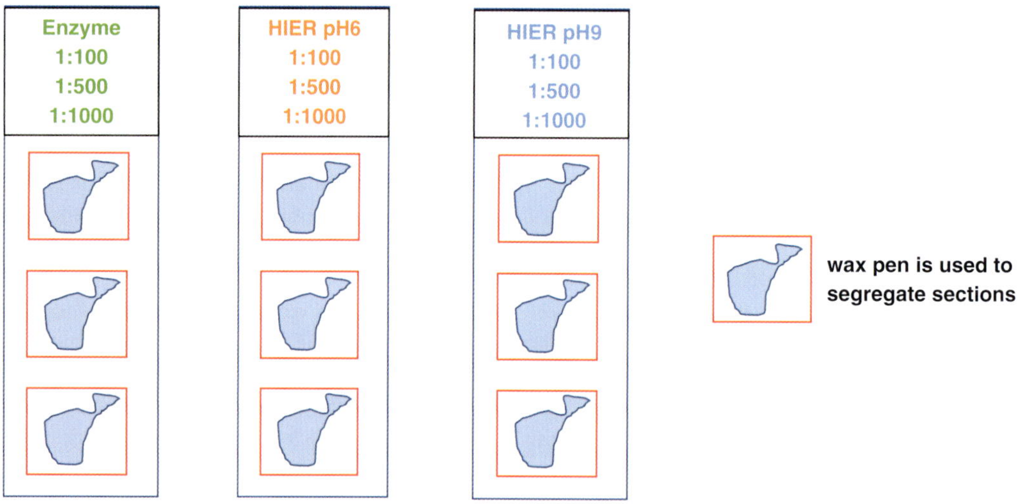

Figure 6.9 Test battery has been reduced from nine slides to three slides

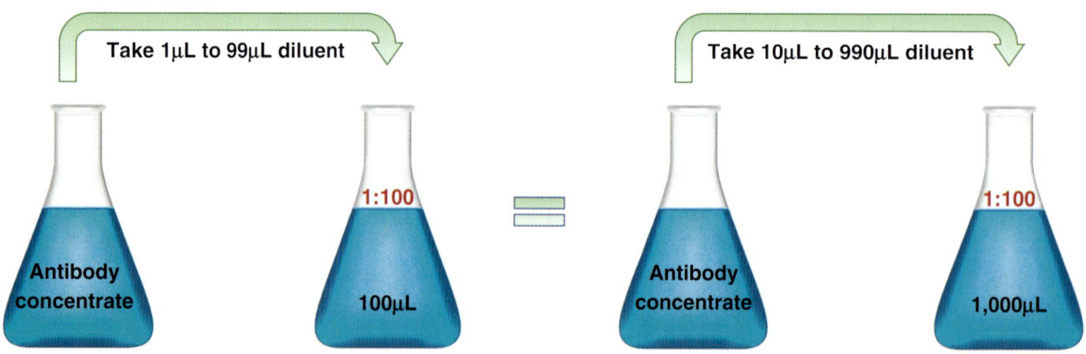

Figure 6.10 Making a 1:100 antibody titre

1 μL to 500 μL diluent and call this titre 1:500 even though the actual total volume is now 501 μL. In practical terms, ending up with either 500 μL or 501 μL is of no real concern as long as the actual method chosen for diluting out antibodies is consistently applied all the time. In other words, choose your method and stick to it! By employing ratios, whatever the actual antibody concentration is, it will be halved after a double dilution starting from 1:100 and progressing to 1:200 and so on.

It is fairly easy to employ serial dilutions, otherwise known as double dilutions. If the starting point is 1:100, the next titre would be 1:200. The one after that is 1:400, then 1:800, 1:1600 and so on. Figure 6.11 demonstrates how double dilutions are set up for the slides outlined in Figure 6.12. Keep in mind there is a total of three test sections on the slide at 1:100. Setting up for double dilutions and assuming 50 μL of primary antibody is required per test section, a total of 200 μL at 1:100 concentration is required. This is because 150 μL is required for the three sections (50 μL for each section) with 50 μL left over at 1:100.

The remaining 50 μL will be mixed with 50 μL of antibody diluent, making a total of 100 μL with a new antibody titre of 1:200. This 1:200 titre is not used. Adding a further 100 μL of antibody diluent will give you a total of 200 μL at 1:400. Once again, 150 μL will be used for three test sections at 1:400 leaving 50 μL left at 1:400. A further 50 μL antibody diluent is added, resulting in 100 μL at 1:800 antibody titre. This 1:800 titre is

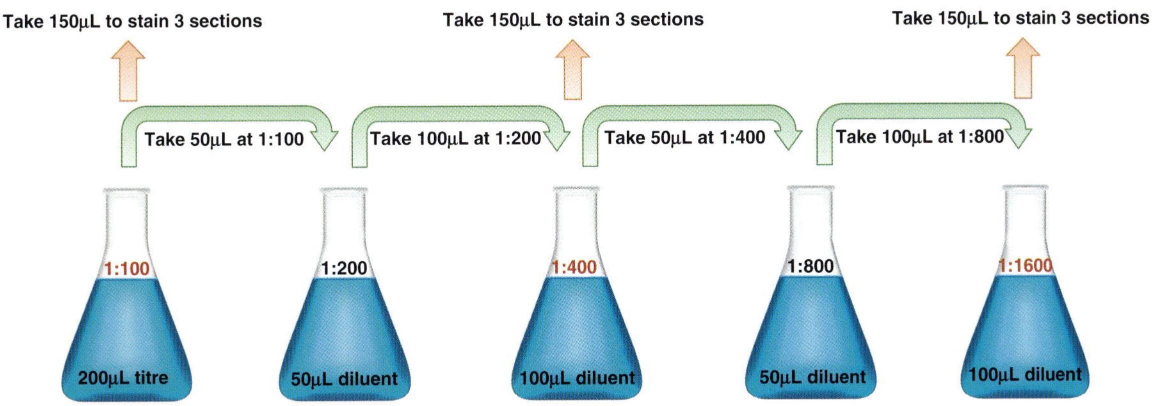

Figure 6.11 Serial (double) dilutions in theory

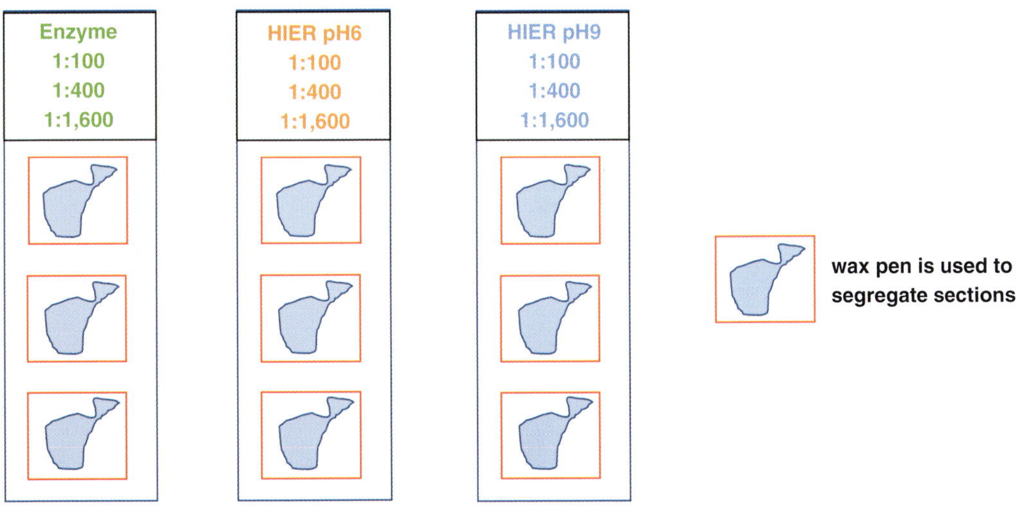

Figure 6.12 Three slides containing test sections for 1:100, 1:400 and 1:1,600 titres

not used. Adding 100 μL of antibody diluent will yield a total of 200 μL at 1:1600. So in actual fact, the three titres being tested here are 1:100, 1:400 and 1:1600. There is a big gap between 1:400 and 1:1600 titres, but in a practical sense this is a good range of antibody concentrations to get a first idea of what the antibody is capable of.

The set-up outlined in Figure 6.11 can be streamlined. Figure 6.13 shows a simplified process with exactly the same outcomes. This time only three vials are required instead of five.

Some investigators would not want to include a 1:1600 titre as a starting concentration. Fortunately, this strategy can be translated to other common, more realistic titres such as the 1:100, 1:500 and 1:1,000 combinations shown in Figure 6.15. Most workers favour this regimen because it gives a broad range of antibody concentrations as a starting point. Instead of the 1:1 ratio, which is one part working antibody titre to one part antibody diluent to result in a double dilution (1:100 to 1:200), the ratio has now changed to one part working antibody titre to four parts antibody diluent to yield a 1:100 to 1:500 dilution.

Once again, using the test battery of three slides highlighted in Figure 6.14, an initial total of 200 μL at 1:100 is required. This translates to taking 2 μL of antibody concentrate to 198 μL of antibody diluent. To stain three sections at 1:100, 150 μL is used, leaving 50 μL at 1:100 antibody concentration. Remember each section requires 50 μL.

To produce a 1:500 titre from this, add the remaining 50 μL to 200 μL of antibody diluent. This will give a total of 250 μL at 1:500 antibody concentration. A further 150 μL is used for the three sections corresponding to 1:500. This leaves 100 μL at 1:500. Then it's a simple double dilution adding the remaining 100 μL of antibody to another 100 μL of antibody diluent to make a total of 200 μL at 1:1,000 antibody titre.

Figure 6.16 shows an even more streamlined process to achieve exactly the same outcomes. This time, only one vial is required.

Performing titrations with the method outlined in Figure 6.16 is an example of an efficient use of antibody and antibody diluent. For instance, an alternative technique would be preparing three separate individual titres to stain the three slides. In doing this, a total of 4 μL of antibody concentrate and 1.7 mL of diluent is required. Remember that each slide requires 150 μL total volume to stain three sections using 50 μL each. The first dilution at 1:100 would need 2 μL antibody concentrate to make 200 μL working reagent. A further 1 μL of concentrate is required for the 1:500 titre and another 1 μL for the 1:1,000 dilution. In comparison, the serial dilution method shown in Figure 6.16 only demands 2 μL of antibody concentrate and 0.5 mL of diluent to run the three slides.

There may come a time when the researcher comes across extra-large working titres. A dilution factor reaching in the many thousands. For example, a 1:20,000 titre would logically make the investigator consider taking 1 μL antibody concentrate to 19,999 μL (20 mL) antibody diluent. This is wasteful if the investigator does not need 20 mL to stain the slides. The recommended approach to tackle a big 1:20,000 dilution is to perform two lots of dilutions. The first one could be a 1:200 and then that could be

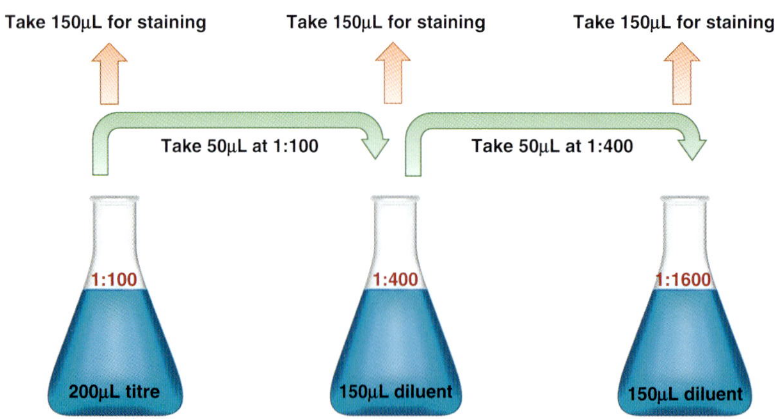

Figure 6.13 Serial (double) dilutions in practice

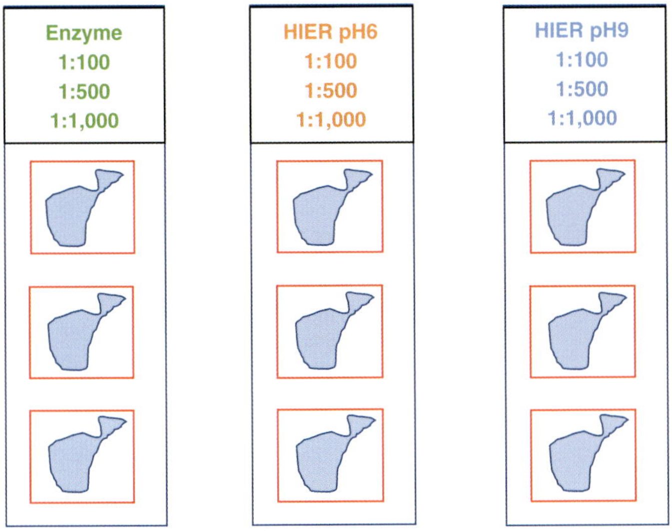

Figure 6.14 Three slides containing test sections for 1:100, 1:500 and 1:1,000 titres

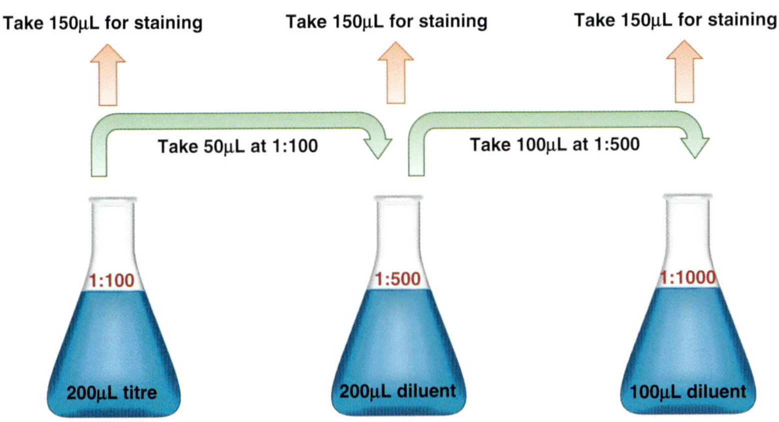

Figure 6.15 Performing serial dilutions for 1:100, 1:500 and 1:1,000

used as the 'new concentrate'. This new concentrate is diluted out a further 1:100, giving a final working titre of 1:20,000. This strategy affords the ability to make only what is required. Figure 6.17 reinforces the steps necessary to achieve a 1 mL volume of a 1:20,000 working antibody titre.

Most of the discussion up until now has centred around the primary antibody concentrate and the strategies to generate a working titre. It is now a good opportunity to consider the antibody diluent. The general recommendation is for the researcher to purchase antibody diluent from a reputable manufacturer. In the not too distant past, all manner of things were used as antibody diluents. Common to all these in-house diluents were reagents based on those used as the protein or serum block. Recipes would contain some sort of protein content, a preservative and perhaps a buffer to neutral pH.

The choice of antibody diluent is a small IHC parameter that can become more complicated than it needs to be. Investigators would need to take note of the recipe if using an alkaline phosphatase conjugated primary antibody because it is a known fact that phosphate groups interfere with the action of the alkaline phosphatase enzyme. In this situation, diluents prepared with phosphate buffered saline are not recommended. Fortunately, most primary antibodies are manufactured unconjugated nowadays, meaning

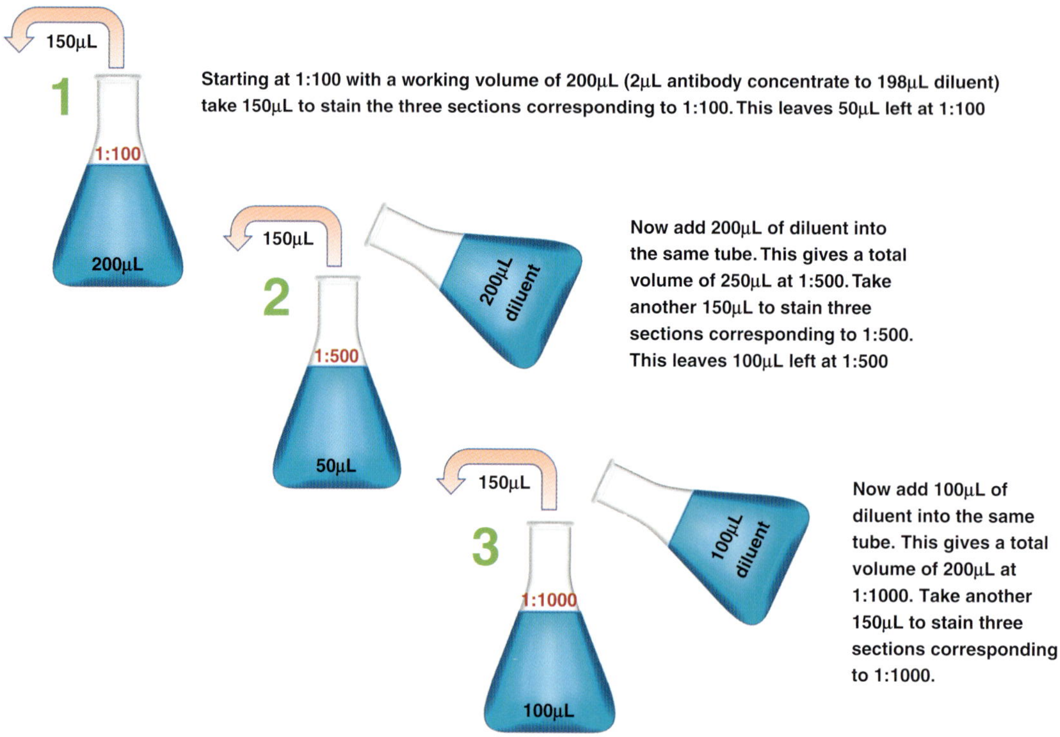

Figure 6.16 Performing serial dilutions using one vial

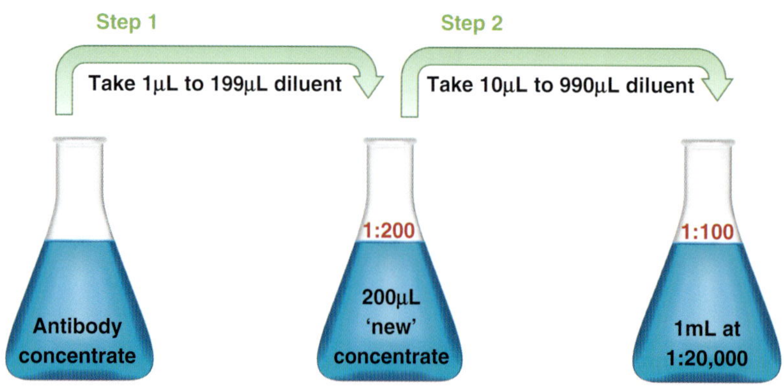

Figure 6.17 Making a 1:20,000 titre

no other substance is attached to the primary antibody. The conjugation with an enzyme or a fluorochrome, for example, occurs with the secondary or linker antibodies within the detection system. Another good reason to use unconjugated primary antibodies is the ability to enhance the signal-to-noise ratio of the IHC stain. This 'indirect' IHC method increases the sensitivity of the assay. The advice given here is to use unconjugated primary antibodies if possible and to invest in a commercially available diluent from a reputable manufacturer.

Detection System

From the earliest beginnings of the IHC assay and throughout its continued development, numerous methods have been devised to show that a primary antibody has indeed locked onto an antigen and is now awaiting visualization. Chapter 1 provides a good review of such technologies and repeating them here is unnecessary.

At the present moment, a polymer-based detection system is the recommended approach for IHC staining. Many kits are commercially available from many reputable manufacturers. The vendors which stand out are those that supply adequate information about the kit within their specification sheet. This documentation outlays important and relevant information concerning the use of the kit. Some vendors go one step further and have highly specialized application specialists who can easily be reached. One important thing to note is to ensure that the reagents that make up this detection kit has been proven to cross-react with the primary antibody – that is, a cross-reaction with the animal species from which the primary antibody is derived. Such a detection kit would normally contain a secondary antibody conjugated to the enzyme label with a polymer backbone or an equivalent technology comprising many available reaction sites to increase the signal of the antigen–antibody affinity at a specific tissue location.

For immunofluorescence, the enzyme label is replaced with a fluorochrome. As stated previously, incubation times and temperatures for these reagents should be kept constant throughout the entire optimization process. A good guide for these parameters is to use the manufacturer's recommendations. In addition, there are strategies to amplify up the staining especially if the antigen is truly low expressing. Although commercial kits are available to do this, caution should be exercised when employing the use of such amplification kits because they artificially increase the signal-to-noise ratio which in turn artificially enhances the overall staining. Achieving this for qualitative analysis is recommended if the researcher chooses to do so. For quantitative analysis however, artificially amplifying the signal may cause unwanted bias towards the end results.

Visualization

For chromogenic IHC and using the peroxidase enzyme as an example, the DAB reagent is immediately mixed with buffer before application to the test issue. Due to the hazardous nature of the DAB chromogen, it is recommended to purchase the chromogen from a vendor rather than preparing it in house. A commercial kit would typically include two reagents, one containing the DAB chromogen and the other a buffer with the substrate hydrogen peroxide. Prior to use, the two are added together at a predetermined ratio and in the presence of the peroxidase enzyme (from the detection kit), the DAB chromogen forms a brown precipitate at the precise location of the antigen–antibody binding site. The brown coloration can be enhanced by submitting the sections to metallic ions such as copper and nickel. This changes the golden-brown DAB colour to various shades of dark brown to grey and even black (Lanciego et al. 1997; Rodig 2019). To give good contrast to the DAB colour, a suitable counterstain is routinely applied to the tissue section. The choice of colour is up to the investigator just as long as it is not brown!

If using a fluorescent label, the fluorochrome would have been conjugated to the linker or secondary antibody. All that is required now is to use appropriate filters for fluorescence microscopy to visualize the signal. Hopefully, the bandwidths of light are separate and distinct when utilizing multiplex assays and there is no interference from such things as autofluorescence from tissue elements or formaldehyde-induced fluorescence in the background.

The main goal of IHC optimization is to narrow down the numerous parameters to just two. Concentrating on the type of antigen retrieval (if required) and the primary antibody titre whilst keeping washes, detection and chromogen development standard makes the trial and elimination process easier to manage. At this stage any snippet of information or clues provided by the researcher or contained within the literature can be very helpful. If somebody else has done all the hard work in working up this particular antibody, then it is a waste of time duplicating it.

Analysis

After all the hard work of optimizing an IHC protocol, an accurate analysis of the staining assay requires appropriate use of control material. In addition, there is a certain level of subjectivity when assessing the quality of the staining. As always, there are two components to look for. The first is to judge the degree of unwanted background staining (hopefully zero) and secondly, the specificity of the signal: in other words, a clean and crisp stain. A true result to any IHC assay is to achieve both high sensitivity and high specificity from the primary antibody. If this can be achieved, then the analytical process would be less difficult. If the staining achieved has low sensitivity and low specificity leading to a section that is high in unwanted background, then analysing such a section will be more cumbersome.

The easiest form of IHC evaluation is qualitative. Is a signal detected? Is there brown colour development? A negative versus a positive staining result is an example of qualitative assessment. Quantitative analysis, on the other hand, requires more considerations. Relevant questions include: Does the staining need to be categorized into low and high intensities? What objective lens should be used to perform the counting? What is the sampling regimen to be carried out? Is the signal homogeneous or heterogeneous?

An added complexity of quantitative measurement is when employing stereological principles. Counting objects of interest in only one section and deducing a total count for the entire 3D structure is not what stereology is about. The investigator will have to produce a strategy to sample the entire 3D entity. A common problem researchers encounter is what is known as the 'corpuscle problem' (de Gunst 1998). It is a description explaining that within the one tissue section, a structure such as a cell can be seen in all manners of orientation, a consequence of taking a 3D object and representing it in 2D space, which is what a tissue section as seen under the microscope is. If you happen to just nick the top of the cell within that one section, this would look vastly different if you truly did a cross-section of the cell. A good analogy to use is an orange representing a cell. We all know what an orange looks like. Take a knife and cut it in half. Notice the cut surface looks completely different to the knife just snipping the top of the orange skin only. The corpuscle principle ensures that objects such as cells are not sampled twice during the count even though they may appear as two vastly different objects. In practical terms, this is achieved by a robust sampling strategy. A simple example is if it takes 100 sections to process an entire 3D object, a suitable approach would be to use every fifth section for counting a certain object within the section. This tactic will ensure an object such as a cell cannot be counted twice because it is not big enough to span more than five sections.

Another interesting observation is that the intensity of staining does not correlate linearly to the quantity of product present. If an observation is made stating the staining appears to be twice as dense as other objects, this does not necessarily mean there is twice as much product (Weinberg 1994). A common artefact of histological processing is there may be thin and thick areas within tissue sections. Thicker areas can be observed to be 'darker stained' than thinner areas of the tissue section. This is not a natural process occurring at the cellular level. It is in fact an artificially introduced bias from the cutting of the FFPE or frozen tissue section. Be cautious when using computational image analysis software programs based on densitometry analysis. Many investigators routinely apply image analysis programs for analysis. Hopefully they understand the theory behind some of the metrics being measured and that the software is carefully calibrated to provide accurate results.

Technical Tips

Listed next are some guidelines that have been proven to aid in achieving optimal IHC assays. Arranged in no particular order, these instructions help the researcher follow good laboratory practice and should result in consistent and reliable IHC assays.

(1) Use a wax pen to restrict the amount of reagent used whilst performing a manual IHC stain. This is to use the least amount of reagent as possible so that the cost per slide is managed.

(2) Add a surfactant such as Tween 20 to reagents and wash buffers to decrease the surface tension to the glass slide. This assists the reagents to easily spread out over the glass surface preventing sections from being dried out. An added benefit is that it takes less volume for a reagent to cover a certain area of the slide.

(3) When optimizing a new antibody, do a manual proof of concept stain first. Performing the staining manually will allow you to save on reagents such as primary antibodies. If it works, then convert the manual stain to automation for big batch staining.

(4) Consider the feasibility of using tissue micro arrays (TMA) to maximize the amount of information gained per slide.

(5) Use clean slides that are either positively charged or have some other properties to make it 'sticky'. You will need all the adhesion you can get to prevent the sections sliding off the glass slide during the IHC process.

(6) Time is money. Streamline incubation times and temperatures when possible. For example, instead of incubating the primary antibody at 4° C overnight, test to see if the same results can be obtained by using a more concentrated antibody

titre at room temperature and decreasing the incubation time. As a guide, routine diagnostic IHC assays on 2–3 μm thick FFPE tissue sections are regularly completed in 2.5–3 hours.

(7) Make up fresh reagents in quantities for only what you need. Try not to be wasteful, especially with primary antibodies.

(8) Do not overcomplicate things. Do not try to alter many variables at once; be systematic instead. If the flow chart provided in Figure 6.7 is followed, then the two main areas of concern include antigen retrieval (if required) and the primary antibody working titre.

(9) Do not repeat freeze-thaw cycles of reagents, especially primary antibodies. Some are marketed and presented with glycerol added to withstand repeated freeze-thaw cycles, but this is still not a good idea. It is good laboratory practice to aliquot antibody concentrates out into smaller volumes to circumvent repeated freeze-thaw cycles.

(10) When performing washing steps, ensure the wash buffer is effectively removed before applying the next reagent. Leaving a large amount of wash buffer on the slide will effectively dilute the next reagent in the sequence. If the next reagent is the primary antibody, the risk of diluting this titre even more is a worry.

(11) Do not take the expiry date of the antibody as gospel. The additives present and the storage conditions all play a significant part in the efficacy of the antibody. Use the performance of appropriate tissue controls as a guide to the activity of the antibody. Discard antibody even if still in date when performance is erratic as dictated by the tissue controls.

(12) Largely forgotten and commonly overlooked is the need for high-quality water. A reliable supply of distilled or deionized water should be employed for use in wash buffers, epitope retrieval solutions and general reagents for IHC.

(13) Select test tissue with a high content of viable cells and low levels of necrosis. Debris from dead cells multiplies unwanted non-specific binding, causing increase background staining.

Conclusion

There is no limit when it comes to using IHC in research applications. Compared to routine diagnostic IHC assays, research protocols may seem inherently more complex even though they are based on the same technology. The basic fundamentals of employing an antibody to bind to an antigen and then developing a method to visualize the reaction is the foundation of all IHC assays. The specifics on how this is achieved is dictated by the research project. There are so many variables that it is not feasible to cover every eventuality. Take for example, the different types of labels that can be used for IHC ranging from chromogens, fluorochromes, lectins, silver ions and other metals such as gold.

A strategic approach is to categorize variables into three main groups. A system of dividing the IHC assay into pre-analytical, analytical and post-analytical stages helps to stress the importance of standardization for IHC success. All three stages are closely linked and it only takes one parameter to be suboptimal for the whole IHC assay to be affected. A prime example is under-fixation of tissues in the pre-analytical phase, causing detrimental effects on IHC staining of FFPE tissue. These dilemmas should be avoided and the most effective method to address suboptimal IHC assays is to utilize a template form. Completing the sample request documentation shown in Figure 6.1 and made available in Appendix 1 forces the researcher to pay attention to all aspects of IHC which can only lead to high-quality stains.

The majority of research endeavours would involve 'working up' a novel antibody to be applied to tissue sections. There are so many moving parts to an IHC assay that it can all seem daunting. Breaking up the protocol into smaller portions as outlined in Figure 6.7 shows a logical order that can be addressed methodically. From this, there are mainly two variables to be concerned with if the rest is kept to a standard set of conditions. Antigen retrieval (if employing FFPE tissue) and optimizing antibodies for IHC assays are the biggest challenges to successful IHC. The practical tips and recommendations offered have been taken from real laboratory experiences, proven to help achieve successful outcomes. Not all antibodies are suitable for IHC as some are incompatible with tissue sections. A Western blot is different to an IHC assay on tissue sections. It is hoped that the knowledge shared from both the theoretical and practical aspects allows the researcher to confidently ascertain this information for every antibody under investigation.

Appendix 1 Template Form

Immunohistochemistry request form for research applications

Answer the following questions accurately. Refer to guidelines overleaf. If answer is unknown, please leave blank.

Researcher details

Name	Phone
Email	Institution
Background information	

Pre-analytical

Tissue origin	Tissue source	Section thickness
Nature	Fixation	

Analytical

Antibody name	Antibody source	
Host species	Aliquot contents	
Protein concentration	Lot/serial number	Manufacture date
Expiry date	Storage	Clonality & Ig class
Enrichment/purification process	Visualization	

Post-analytical

Localisation	Staining pattern
Morphology requirements	

Quality control

Control tissue	Tissue source
Nature	Fixation
Have you successfully optimized a Western blot? Yes/No	Do you intend to apply stereological analysis? Yes/No

Researcher details

Background information: What are you trying to achieve? Have other groups worked with this antibody before?
Are there methods available with this antibody within the literature?

Pre-analytical

Tissue origin: Is the tissue to be tested human origin or some other animal such as rodent or primate?
Tissue source: Who is providing the test tissue? Where did it come from?
Was it obtained from a tissue or tumour bank? Was it taken from a diagnostic pathology archive?
Is the test tissue derived from tissue culture, specific cell lines or FFPE?
Section thickness: How thick should the sections be? Routine 2-3μm or thicker?
Nature: Is the test tissue fresh frozen? Has test tissue been through FFPE histological processing?
Fixation: Has the test tissue been treated with a fixative? What type of fixative and for how long?

Analytical

Antibody name: Include other common names the antibody is also known as within the literature.
Antibody source: Commercial vendor or obtained in-house? List specific catalogue number from manufacturer
Host species: The animal from which the antibody was derived from.
Aliquot contents: Are there any additives included with the antibody?
List any included preservatives, glycerol, sodium azide, the type of buffer used and the pH level.
Protein concentration: State the concentration of antibody, immunoglobulin level or total protein content.
Lot/serial number: Record this data if available. Batch to batch variations are easier to investigate if known.
Manufacture date: To consider the age of the antibody.
Expiry date: To consider the age and useful life of the antibody.
Storage: How has the antibody been stored? Frozen with multiple freeze/thaw cycles?
Constant refrigeration at 4°C as per manufacturer's recommendations?
Clonality and Ig class: Is the antibody monoclonal or polyclonal?
Is the type of immunoglobulin IgG or IgM?
Enrichment/purification process: Has the antibody been subjected to any other processing regimes during manufacture?
Visualization: Do you want a fluorescence or chromogenic label?

Post-analytical

Localisation: Is the expected signal nuclear, cytoplasmic or membranous?
Staining pattern: Is the expected pattern globular, speckled, peri-nuclear or dot like?
Should the staining be heterogeneous vs homogeneous in the entire section?
Morphology requirements: Should there be normal tissue elements showing positivity?
What is the exact pathological process to be demonstrated?

Quality control

Control tissue: Is the control tissue human origin or some other animal such as rodent or primate?
Is there adequate tissue with the disease state available for positive controls?
Are there natural internal controls present in the test tissue? Can external cell lines be used as control material?
Tissue source: Who is providing the control tissue? Where did it come from?
Was it obtained from a tissue or tumour bank? Was it taken from a diagnostic pathology archive?
Is the control tissue derived from tissue culture, specific cell lines or FFPE?
Nature: Is the control tissue fresh frozen? Has control tissue been through FFPE histological processing?
Fixation: Has the control tissue been treated with a fixative? What type of fixative and for how long?
Have you successfully optimized a Western blot?: Using the antibody effectively in a Western blot does not automatically guarantee success on tissue sections as there are many variables to overcome when introducing antibodies to tissue sections.
Do you intend to apply stereological analysis?: Counting positive cells or entities demonstrated by IHC in a 2D section and inferring that to a 3D structure requires careful planning. Things to consider include the thickness of sections, the unbiased and representative sampling of the 3D object and using computer software algorithms for obtaining precise estimates.

References

Brown DL 2017. Bias in image analysis and its solution: Unbiased stereology. *J Toxicol Pathol* **30**(3):183–91.

Busse D, Doughty RS, Arteaga CL 2000. HER-2/neu (erbB-2) and the cell cycle. *Semin Oncol* **27**(6 Suppl 11):3–8; discussion 92–100.

de Gunst MC, Luebeck EG 1998. A method for parametric estimation of the number and size distribution of cell clusters from observations in a section plane. *Biometrics* **54**(1):100–12.

Fabrizio FP, Trombetta D, Rossi A, Sparaneo A, Castellana S, Muscarella LA 2018. Gene code CD274/PD-L1: From molecular basis toward cancer immunotherapy. *Ther Adv Med Oncol* 7;10:1758835918815598

Faget L, Hnasko TS 2015. Tyramide signal amplification for immunofluorescent enhancement. *Methods Mol Biol* **1318**:161–72.

Fox CH, Johnson FB, Whiting J, Roller PP 1985. Formaldehyde fixation. *J Histochem Cytochem* **33**(8):845–53.

Goodpaster T, Randolph-Habecker J 2014. A flexible mouse-on-mouse immunohistochemical staining technique adaptable to biotin-free reagents, immunofluorescence, and multiple antibody staining. *J Histochem Cytochem* **62**(3):197–204.

Grizzle WE, Fredenburgh JL, Myers RB 2008. Fixation of tissues. In Bancroft JD, Gamble M, eds. *Theory and practice of histological techniques*. Churchill Livingstone Elsevier; 53–74.

Jackson P, Blythe D 2008. Immunohistochemical techniques. In Bancroft JD, Gamble M, Eds. *Theory and practice of histological techniques*. Churchill Livingstone Elsevier; 433–72.

Lanciego JL, Goede PH, Witter MP, Wouterlood FG 1997. Use of peroxidase substrate Vector VIP for multiple staining in light microscopy. *J Neurosci Methods* **74**(1):1–7.

Leong AS, Lee ES, Yin H, Kear M, Haffajee Z, Pepperall D 2002. Superheating antigen retrieval. *Appl Immunohistochem Mol Morphol* **10**(3):263–8.

Ponder BA, Wilkinson MM 1981. Inhibition of endogenous tissue alkaline phosphatase with the use of alkaline phosphatase conjugates in immunohistochemistry. *J Histochem Cytochem* **29**(8):981–4.

Rodig SJ 2019. Detecting horseradish peroxidase-labeled cells. *Cold Spring Harb Protoc Apr* **1**(4).

Shiogama K, Wongsiri T, Mizutani Y, Inada K, Tsutsumi Y 2013. High-sensitivity epidermal growth factor receptor immunostaining for colorectal carcinomas, compared with EGFR PharmDx™: A study of diagnostic accuracy. *Int J Clin Exp Pathol* **6**(1):24–30.

Weinberg DS 1994. Quantitative immunocytochemistry in pathology. In Marchevsky AM, Bartels PH, eds. *Image analysis: A primer for pathologists*. Raven Press; 235–60.

Chapter 7

Troubleshooting Immunohistochemistry

David Gan

Overview

Immunohistochemistry (IHC) is a robust staining technique employed in the study and diagnosis of disease in cells and tissue. It is a valuable analytical and research tool because consistent high-quality IHC stains are achievable. Commercial manufacture of antisera is reliable, detection reagents are produced with best practices and there is widespread knowledge of standardization requirements to achieve best outcomes. Although IHC technology is highly regarded, unfortunately, it is not infallible. Complications arise, difficulties are faced and glitches do occur. There are many 'moving parts' to an IHC assay, which is why there are numerous reasons they fail.

When problems arise, it is imperative to first have a thorough understanding of IHC fundamental processes before attempts are made to rectify the situation. The central theme of this book has been to break down the technology into three parts: pre-analytical, analytical and post-analytical. This strategy enables the worker to address IHC concepts methodically. By doing this, the intricacies and complexities of IHC are easier to comprehend, which in turn allows for successful troubleshooting.

Therefore, the topics discussed in this chapter are presented from the perspective of the IHC assay. Specifically employed for formalin-fixed paraffin-embedded (FFPE) tissues, the analytical phase involves the actual staining protocol. All events prior to staining are considered pre-analytical and all occurrences after staining are post-analytical. The challenges faced and the strategies to overcome them are presented from these viewpoints, thus keeping to the central theme of this book.

The rigors of fixation and tissue sampling technique are the principal pre-analytic areas of concern for routine IHC investigations. In this section, strategies to ensure optimal pre-analytic endeavours for successful IHC staining are explored. Overcoming these, the next set of predicaments to address belong to the analytical process. As there are many parameters to the IHC protocol, so too can there be many quandaries in which viable solutions need to be sought. Fortunately, these are easier to address because such issues are in the domain of the laboratory and therefore can be controlled and overcome if sufficient expertise is available. A commentary on the important aspects of the staining protocol and suggestions to optimize them are offered. Lastly, post-analytical problems are mainly concerned with observation and interpretation post-staining. Technical problems which manifest from the first two stages are identified when performing quality control assessments at the end. This chapter unravels the complexities which cause suboptimal IHC staining in the pre-analytical and analytical stages and offers workable resolutions. Diagnostic dilemmas and other post-analytical problems are not the focal point of these discussions.

The chapter concludes with a presentation of common problems encountered in a typical diagnostic histology laboratory and directions on how to address them. When operating within the confines of IHC processes, solutions may be found not only for day-to-day problems which may arise, but also for bizarre situations requiring technicians to 'think outside the square'. Many of these challenges will occur in both manual and automated IHC and it is important to understand that there are multiple pathways to solve a problem. It is not the intention of this chapter to cover every possible predicament. It is hoped that the issues highlighted can assist laboratory workers to develop skills and concepts to deal with common obstacles encountered in IHC practice. An astute mind is required to use the tools available and to understand the limitations of IHC so a favourable outcome can be reached.

Pre-analytical Problems

Events which occur prior to IHC staining are termed 'pre-analytical incidents' and include tissue sampling, initial fixation and delivery to the anatomical pathology laboratory. Some of the most common reasons for failed IHC staining can be traced back to errors made during tissue fixation, subjecting samples to a prolonged ischaemic time and introduced artefacts from tissue cauterization. As these actions are outside of the laboratory's direct control, problems which arise from external forces can be difficult to manage sufficiently.

Initial Tissue Fixation

Tissue fixation is the backbone of successful histology technique. It allows morphological assessment, special stains, molecular studies and, of course, IHC. Suboptimal tissue fixation therefore affects the entire gamut of histological analysis. The question herein is, why is such an important aspect of anatomical pathology out of the control of the laboratory? The reasons are multifaceted. For instance, procurement of specimens can arise from GP clinics, outpatient departments, day procedure centres, under imaging guidance in hospital and in operating theatres. It is not feasible for histology staff to be present at sample collection in order to ensure best tissue sampling practices. A compromise must be sought and usually involves the supply of formalin and suitable containers to collection areas so tissues can be placed into fixative so as to 'arrest' putrefaction and autolytic processes. The 'real' fixation starts when the sample is formally accepted into the laboratory.

Being a chemical process, 6–72 hours tissue fixation using 10% formalin is the general recommendation (Wolff et al. 2014). This guideline should be interpreted in context because such a wide range of time intervals is given. The highly variable nature of specimens submitted for histological analysis is the primary reason. A large anterior resection of bowel has significantly different fixation requirements when compared to a 3 mm endoscopic biopsy. The type of tissue, component makeup, thickness and size all determine the volume and duration of formalin required for optimal fixation. Notice the fixation front in Figure 7.1 of a splenectomy specimen subjected to 10% neutral buffered formalin for seven days. The brown tissue represents 'fixed' tissue whereas the red portion is 'unfixed' tissue. As the spleen is a 'solid' organ, the penetration rate is slow compared to that of less dense tissues. Even after being sliced in order to maximize surface area, minimal fixation occurs due to the thickness of the tissue and the ratio of specimen to fixative.

Immunohistochemical staining is adversely affected by poorly fixed tissue manifesting in uneven, patchy or total loss of staining. This is a common observation especially with nuclear antigens as highlighted in Figure 7.2 showing ERG IHC staining from a metastatic angiosarcoma. Notice the strong nuclear staining at the edges of the tissue section compared to a much weaker signal in the deeper aspect. Unfortunately, these effects are irreversible. Some antigens may be more resilient to poor fixation, in which case it is not detrimental to the overall IHC assay. In instances where there is an adverse effect, the

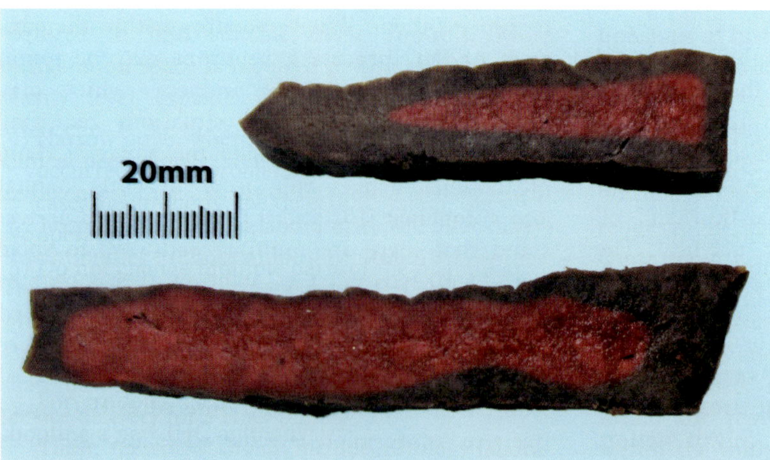

Figure 7.1 Demonstration of a clear demarcation fixation front in spleen

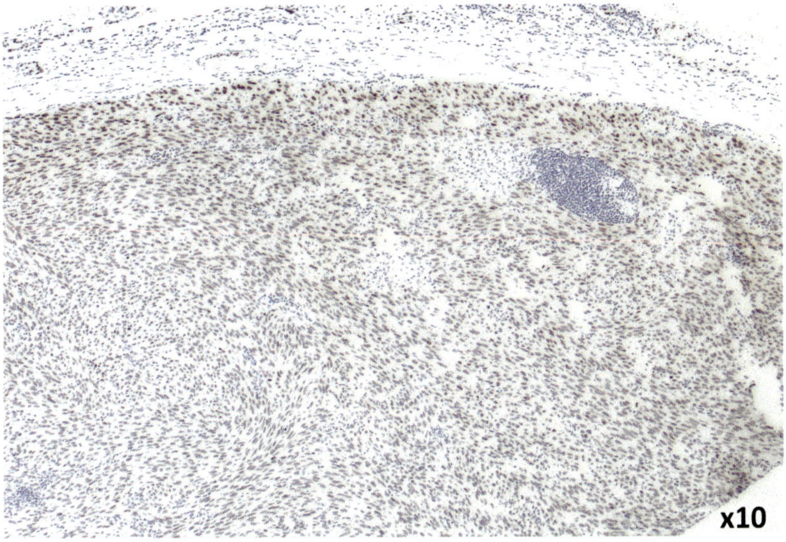

Figure 7.2 ERG immunohistochemical stain in poorly fixed tissue

only suitable workaround is to try a different clone in the hope that better staining is achieved. Conversely, prolonged fixation may also impact the IHC assay, causing false negative staining due to excessive cross-linking of proteins. This is often rectified by extending the heat or enzyme unmasking step.

Cold Ischaemic Time

Cold ischaemic time is defined as the time interval from when tissue is removed from the patient to when it is first placed into fixative. A delay in this important endeavour certainly affects IHC staining. It is recommended that the cold ischaemic time be kept to a minimum – no longer than one hour at room temperature – otherwise tissue epitopes may be irreversibly affected (Hammond et al. 2010). Once again this recommendation requires some context. Imagine a small 3 mm endoscopic biopsy without fixation after one hour. The tissue would have dried out, resulting in detrimental damage to the specimen. Now imagine a large breast mastectomy specimen under the same conditions. The tissue would not have dried out to the same extent as the endoscopic biopsy. Larger specimens are better at withstanding a one-hour cold ischaemic time compared to smaller delicate biopsies. This all depends again on the type of tissue, how robust the epitopes are and the nature of the antibodies employed in the IHC assay. Although some studies (Li et al. 2013; Yoo et al. 2014) show significant long ischaemic times may not have adverse effects on immunoreactivity of some antigens, the general consensus and best practice for standardized IHC is to keep cold ischaemic time as low as possible and for large specimens such as breast resections, limited to less than one hour (Yildiz-Aktas et al. 2012).

Cauterization

Another irreversible pre-analytical problem is the result of a surgical technique known as cauterization. In this procedure, the surgeon employs intense heat to remove tissue and reduce bleeding during the operation. 'Burning tissue', in order to remove, it creates an area of false negative staining at the cauterized margin highlighted in Figure 7.3. The antibody is P504 (racemase) employed to the prostate adenocarcinoma workup in transurethral resection of prostate (TURPs) 'chips'. Severe morphological disruption is often concurrently seen. Care should always be taken when interpreting results gathered from the peripheries of these specimens.

As problems involving tissue sampling and initial fixation often occur before the specimen arrives in the laboratory, it would be easy to dismiss them as someone else's problem. In reality, the anatomical pathology laboratory is the custodian of patients' tissue samples and therefore a concerted effort is required to consult with those collecting and transporting the specimens so adverse incidents are minimized. To

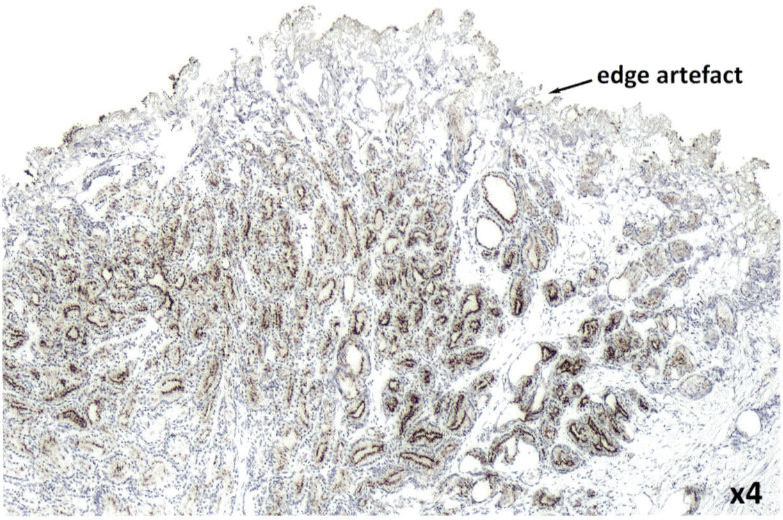

Figure 7.3 P504 immunohistochemistry with cauterization effect

facilitate best practices, the laboratory should provide suitable containers of different sizes to cater for all types of expected specimens. In addition, a supply of pre-dilute ready to use 10% formalin should be made available to those responsible for sample collection. Multiple regular specimen pickups and deliveries to the laboratory during the day ensures the samples are attended to in a timely manner. Finally, the laboratory quality manual should be updated regularly and contain clear instructions for collection staff to follow. The language should be written in a style which is easily disseminated to key stakeholders. The main points to cover include:

- The facility's operating hours and the steps to follow for tissue collection out of hours.
- Instances when the tissue needs to be kept fresh.
- Minimum requirements for the labelling and identification of specimens.
- Provision of a suitable patient clinical history.
- Special instructions for specific tissue requirements.
- Selection of a suitable size container with an adequate volume of fixative for the submitted tissue.
- Contact details of the laboratory for enquiries.

Further Fixation and Tissue Processing

At a rough approximation, 10% formalin penetrates tissue at a rate of 1 mm per hour at room temperature (Medawar 1941). To aid fixation, large specimens should be sliced prior to the macro 'cut-up' in order to expose the most amount of surface area possible and blocks selected for paraffin processing should be submitted at a thickness of 3–4 mm. The volume of fixative used should be at least 10 times the volume of tissue to be fixed. Although not always practicable from a tissue collection perspective, if this ratio cannot be met, at least it is a suitable starting point for the laboratory to continue.

If an IHC stain has been affected by extended ischaemic time, staining intensity will decrease. This is an irreversible problem most often seen in specimens received fresh in the laboratory. Therefore the transit time from operating theatre to laboratory must be immediate and specimens which are received fresh should be acted upon as soon as possible. Careful thought is needed when fresh tissue is received because ancillary tests may be necessitated. Microbiology culture and sensitivity require viable organisms (if present) to grow in a petri dish. Likewise flow cytometry and karyotype analyses cannot be performed on formalin-fixed tissue. Breast excisions received fresh in the laboratory and subjected to prolonged ischaemic time may compromise the 'true' hormone receptor score. A false decrease in the intensity of the oestrogen or progesterone receptor influences the treatment of the patient. Core biopsies from the same lesions may give a superior result as the specimen is usually placed in fixative immediately after removal.

As discussed previously, fresh specimens should be attended to as soon as possible because poor fixation and processing lead to suboptimal staining and morphology or tissue adherence to the microscope glass slide. After initial examination, margin inking and slicing if required, the specimen should be presented in a manner that facilitates maximum fixative penetration (RCPA Guidelines 2020). Prompt fixation and a suitable processing schedule for the size of the tissue are of equal importance.

Small, urgent biopsies may require only a two-hour processing schedule while extremely large pieces of tissue may take several days to process well. It is important to optimize the IHC protocol to suit these processing conditions. Small specimens with minimal fixation will require less antigen unmasking than tissue fixed for an extended time. Currently, the most powerful retrieval strategy uses heat energy and a high-pH buffer. When optimizing an antibody, try to use validation tissue that mimics the expected target tissue and choose the most robust protocol that will work on a wide range of situations. This is very important if the laboratory receives tissue from external sources such as research or consultation facilities with a variety of fixation regimes.

High temperatures during processing and embedding may cause a reduction in the immunoreactivity of some antigens, and it is recommended that molten paraffin is kept below 60°C (Boenisch et al. 2001) or 63°C (Grizzle et al. 2001). Regardless, tissue should not be immersed in molten wax for extended periods in a processor nor an embedding centre.

Decalcification

A regular conundrum in histology is the judicious use of decalcification agents for bone and other calcified tissue. First and foremost, it is imperative to achieve high-quality tissue morphology with the hematoxylin and eosin (H&E) stain. For bone tissue, this invariably means elimination of calcium within FFPE tissue via treatment with acids or chelating agents to facilitate optimal sectioning. Figure 7.4 demonstrates the results of a poorly decalcified femur FFPE unstained (A) and stained section (B). Laboratories often apply surface decalcification to the FFPE block just before sectioning in order to facilitate optimal sectioning. Unfortunately, some antigen sites will be destroyed by the process of decalcification (Athanasou et al. 1987), either before tissue processing or before sectioning. To add a degree of difficulty, a judgement needs to be made whether to subject the tissue to decalcification without knowing if IHC is required later because most decalcification procedures are carried out before tissue is processed to paraffin wax.

Strong and fast-acting decalcification involving the use of hydrochloric acid may damage DNA and RNA. Detrimental for molecular sequencing assays, this practice also leads to weaker or false negative IHC staining of some antigens. A far gentler alternative to acid decalcification methods employ calcium chelation agents such as ethylenediaminetetraacetic acid (EDTA). Ethylenediaminetetraacetic acid is recommended for FFPE tissue requiring molecular analysis and IHC. Unfortunately, EDTA decalcification is very slow and it may take several weeks to decalcify large bone specimens. For a busy diagnostic laboratory, this delay to diagnosis is simply unacceptable. Therefore a compromise may be required. Areas of non-calcified tissue may be harvested and submitted separately for IHC staining and molecular studies. Alternative acids such as formic acid and acetic acid solutions will decalcify tissue faster than EDTA and may preserve the antigenicity better than hydrochloric acid decalcification (Matthews and Mason 1984). Regardless, it is important to keep any decalcifying time to a minimum so as to reduce tissue disruption. Although methods are available to section undecalcified bone (Goldschlager et al. 2010; Lars et al. 1991), they require specific resin-embedding media and specialized equipment, rendering histology on undecalcified bone out of reach for most diagnostic facilities. In the event a FFPE block contains a small amount of calcium, it may be possible to achieve a section for IHC without decalcification if the suboptimal section quality does not interfere with the interpretation of the slide. For the sole purpose of IHC, sometimes morphology is not as important as achieving a signal. Figure 7.5 shows CD68 IHC staining where there is disruption to the bone fragment morphology including 'thick and thin chattering' artefact, but the diagnostic portion has stained well, allowing successful interpretation.

Other difficult-to-section tissues may contain keratin or dense fibrous and muscle tissue. These may be softened by a Tween- or detergent-based solution after careful 'facing' of the FFPE block. Solutions such as IHC wash buffers may also work well as softeners and are readily available in the laboratory. Unlike acid decalcification solutions, there is minimal disruption to IHC staining using these gentle reagents.

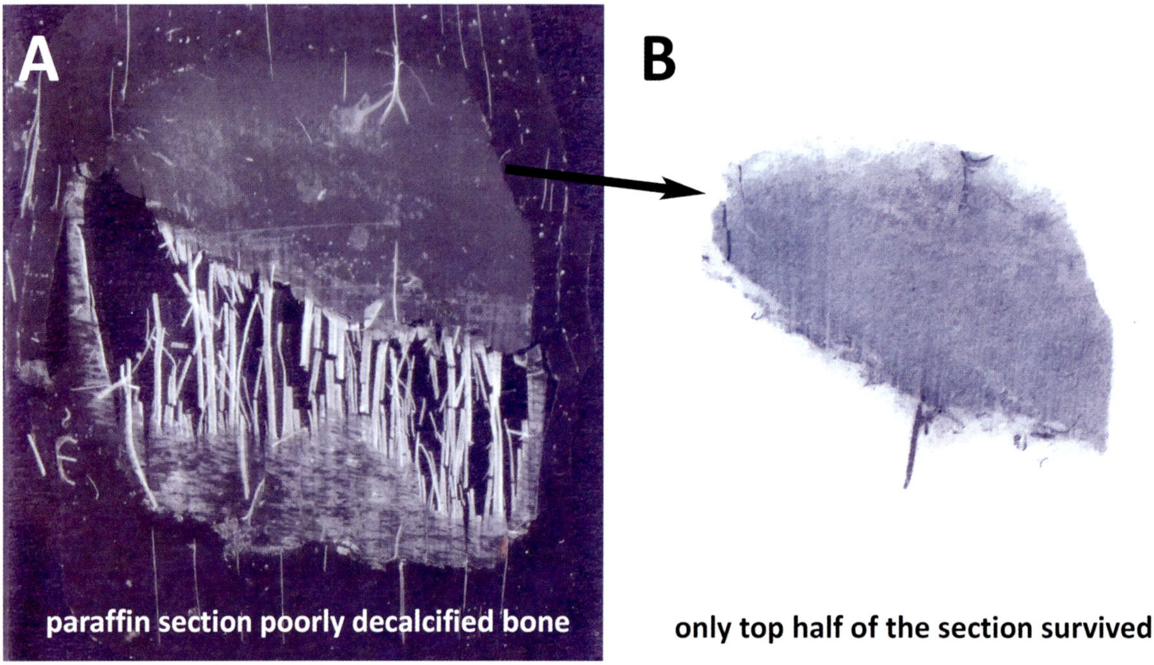

Figure 7.4 Calcified formalin-fixed paraffin-embedded tissue

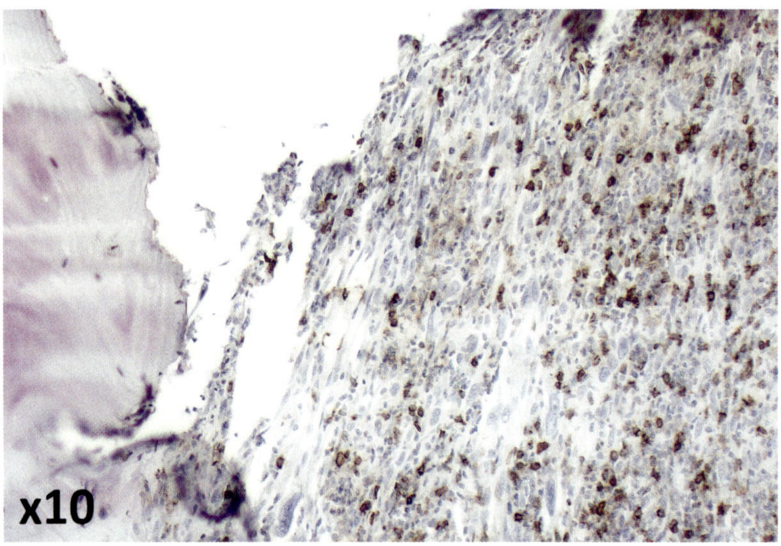

Figure 7.5 CD68 immunohistochemical-stained section of bone tissue

Sectioning

The IHC can be performed on FFPE sections that are cut at a variety of section thicknesses. A typical histological section is 2–4 μm thick. It all depends on what must be demonstrated. The laboratory will mandate a preferential section thickness for all blocks, and it is important to validate IHC protocols at this required thickness. Also, the same conditions must be applied to both the test and the control sections consistently. If the section is too thick, it may be difficult to identify specific structures and cell types such as lymphocytes. They harbour cells that are on top of each other, giving the appearance of overstaining or an increase in background staining. Thick sections can also cause tissue lifting off from the slide during staining protocols and can be the perpetrator of insufficient dewaxing. Conversely, thin sections may lead to decreased staining intensity because there is less material to stain and can even lead to false negative results.

Another common sectioning artefact is the lodgement of bubbles between the microscope glass surface and under the tissue section, causing morphology disruption and staining issues. Air bubbles will trigger the tissue in the immediate area to partially lift from the slide, capturing reagents under the surface. Figure 7.6 shows a gastrointestinal stromal tumour stained with CD117 with a large air bubble under the section. This may lead to localized, non-specific staining under the tissue, commonly referred to as 'trapped DAB'. Poor tissue adherence will occur if bubbles of water are left under the section after drying. These problems will not manifest if good sectioning practices are adhered to by ensuring all excess water is removed before drying and dewaxing.

The choice and type of glass slides used for IHC are very important and are critical for high-quality staining. Whether using an automated platform or manual staining, follow the recommendations of the supplier. Optimal slides for IHC should possess hydrophilic properties to enable uniform spread of IHC reagents over the entire glass surface. In addition, there must be excellent tissue adherence to withstand the harsh conditions of the IHC assay. Only a small amount of tissue may remain on the slide if routine 'non-sticky' microscope slides are used. Therefore standard practice for IHC is to employ 'sticky' slides either coated with a suitable reagent or electrostatically charged. Furthermore, slides may lose their tissue adherence qualities if they are stored in the open or at the wrong temperature, dipped in water multiple times or used after expiry. Unexplained, weak and non-specific background staining may be an indicator of poor slide choice for IHC purposes. Although a huge range of slides is available for IHC, most laboratories will choose slides which give the most consistent performance according to their experiences.

Additives in the water bath may also lead to background staining. Standard practice of using good-quality slides will negate the need for anything other than clean, warm water in the water bath. Ensure the water bath is not harbouring organisms and is free from contaminants because IHC may magnify any carryover picked up from the water bath or dirty slides. A common problem is the shedding of the worker's squamous cells from skin epithelium. These contaminants will stain with a broad-spectrum keratin such as CK

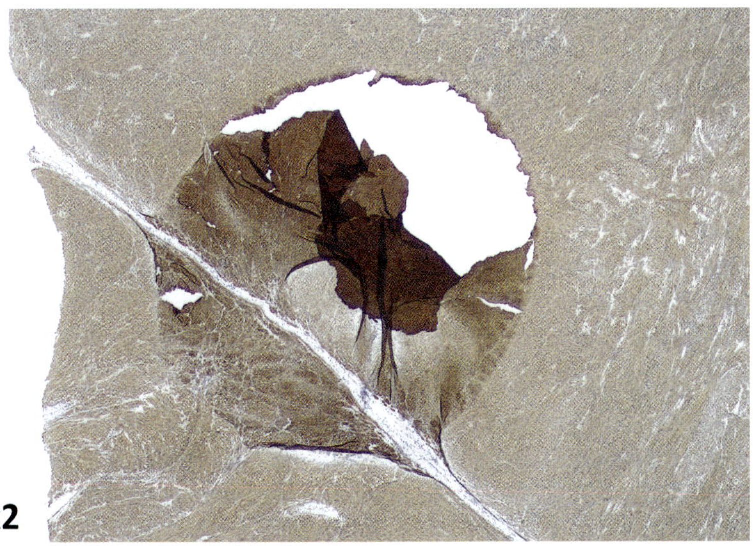

x2

Figure 7.6 CD117 with bubble artefact

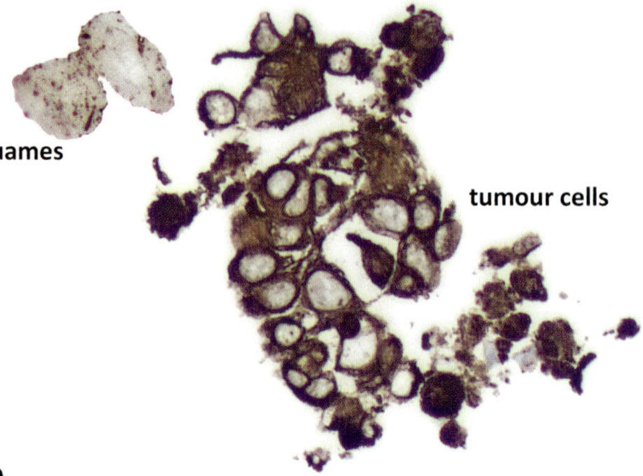

Figure 7.7 Contaminant squames inadvertently labelled by CK AE1/3

AE1/3 as seen in Figure 7.7. This image was taken from a cell block preparation of a lung fine needle aspiration (FNA) sample diagnosed as non-small cell carcinoma. Interpretation of the section can be difficult, especially in cytological preparations. Similar to routine sectioning, ensure the temperature of the water bath is kept to about 45°C without huge fluctuations. This will reduce tissue destruction (blowing apart) as well as keep the water bath clean.

Drying of the slides after sectioning may be performed at a wide range of temperatures. Williams and colleagues (1997) found that some antigens may be affected by extreme heat and recommended to dry slides for IHC at no higher than 60°C for up to four hours. Standard practice nowadays allows the regular drying of slides for 10–15 minutes. When using an oven at high temperatures it is good practice to dry IHC stains for the minimal time it takes to remove water and obtain good tissue adherence. Increases in non-specific staining and decreases in staining intensities have been noted in some IHC stains even when dried at 60°C. If time permits, air-drying at room temperature or 37°C may reduce these issues. Drying slides in an area of increased air circulation such as near extraction vents in dissection or staining areas will speed up the drying time without affecting staining. Drying slides in these conditions may be reduced to 15 minutes but, as always, ensure no water is present under or around the section before staining and use good-quality slides.

Analytical Problems of the Immunohistochemical Assay

When the specimen is formally received in the laboratory, the sample is under direct control of histology staff. A robust quality system should be in place outlining standard procedures to reduce variables which may affect IHC staining. Some facilities invest in a laboratory tracking system to follow the specimen from accessioning to reporting, recording what was done, when it was done and the staff member who performed the operation. The accumulated data may also highlight opportunities for improvement regarding IHC quality and turnaround staining times. The following dissertation is only centred around the IHC assay, leaving problems associated with other analytical processes within histology such as H&E, special stains and molecular studies out of the discussion.

Controls

It is standard laboratory practice to include control sections with all IHC test cases. The usefulness of negative controls is questionable and may be of limited value in many instances (CAP 2013). Most laboratories do not routinely use negative controls for both financial and practical reasons. However, specific clones or tissue types that are prone to increased amounts of non-specific background staining should include negative controls to aid in the interpretation of results. Positive controls are critical during the validation and routine staining of an antibody. An ideal control block should include known high, low and negative expressors of the target antigen, especially important when observing staining intensities and scoring the percentage of positive cell staining such as oestrogen receptor status in breast cancers via IHC.

Tissue controls should be from the same species as the test tissue and processed in a manner that is as close as possible to the test (Torlakovic et al. 2015). In particular, the parameters of fixation, processing and decalcification discussed previously need to match the test tissue. Consult the antibody supplier's recommendations for the most appropriate control tissue type. Ideally, this is tissue that is readily available and offers consistent performance. Be cautious of using certain tumours for controls, especially if there is a pattern of heterogenic expression of the antigen. Normal tissue expressing the antigen may be easier to source and produce more consistent staining. Immunoreactivity of an antigen may be affected if the time between sectioning and staining is prolonged. If tissue, especially controls, are pre-cut on slides for speed and convenience, a decrease in staining intensity may be seen even within 24 hours of sectioning. This applies to a number of antibodies and may be improved by storing the cut sections in an airtight container at 4°C (Economou et al. 2014) or even at −20°C. Due to a potential loss of antigenicity, caution must be taken when staining pre-cut archival slides regardless of how long they have been stored. As always, internal positive controls, if present, should be used to carefully assess the stained slide.

Dewaxing

Often dismissed as a simple irrelevance, the dewaxing step of FFPE sections is critical before staining. All excess paraffin needs to be removed before sections are hydrated because wax will not allow optimal tissue penetration of reagents if it is still present. Thicker sections will require an extended time for sufficient dewaxing. Problems due to insufficient dewaxing may be masked to a certain extent if a heat pretreatment step is used in the protocol. This high-temperature solution may remove a large percentage of remaining wax and make it difficult to pinpoint the real cause of suboptimal dewaxing protocols.

Reagent Application

It is important to apply reagents quickly and evenly to the slide. Poor staining will be achieved if the tissue is allowed to dry out during the staining process. This is more common with manual staining techniques but may also be a problem during longer incubations on automated platforms, especially if the instrument has not been maintained correctly. The key criteria when applying reagents is to ensure even coverage over all of the tissue; otherwise staining intensity may vary. For both automation and manual protocols, ensure the slides are flat and level to avoid staining gradients. Good laboratory technique is needed to remove excess wash buffer from the slide in between reagents so subsequent solutions are not diluted affecting the result. Also, the ability to apply sufficient reagent to cover the slide end to end and side to side will improve staining quality.

Catastrophic results will follow if the wrong reagent is applied in the incorrect order during the staining process. If diluting antibodies from concentrates, ensure correct clone and diluent are selected. For example, a common mistake is using CD20 instead of CK20 antibody. When making up any reagent, good manufacturing principles should be followed to record lot numbers, dilution volumes, when it was made, nominated expiry dates and the person who made the solution. Troubleshooting will be easier if a mistake occurs. It is also beneficial to have a second person check the dilution if they are available. Always check that the correct solutions are used when making up bulk reagents or filling instruments. When staining manually, always read the bottle before applying any reagent. Store all reagents as per the supplier's recommendations. The use of expired reagents is not ideal but sometimes unavoidable. Most chromogens are best used fresh and may leave a precipitate on the slide if old or stored poorly as seen in Figure 7.8. This artefact hindered the investigation for *H. pylori* organisms and required a repeat stain.

Pretreatment

The majority of IHC for diagnostic purposes is performed on FFPE tissue. It is well known that formalin as well as other fixatives will affect the immunoreactivity of many antigens. A small percentage of antibodies will not require any pretreatment at all for optimal staining. In these instances, staining protocols will be much shorter, allowing the morphology to be optimal. Care should be taken when validating these antibodies to ensure all elements are demonstrated especially if the tissue has been fixed for an extended period.

The pretreatment process, also known as antigen retrieval (AR) and epitope unmasking, is critical to the

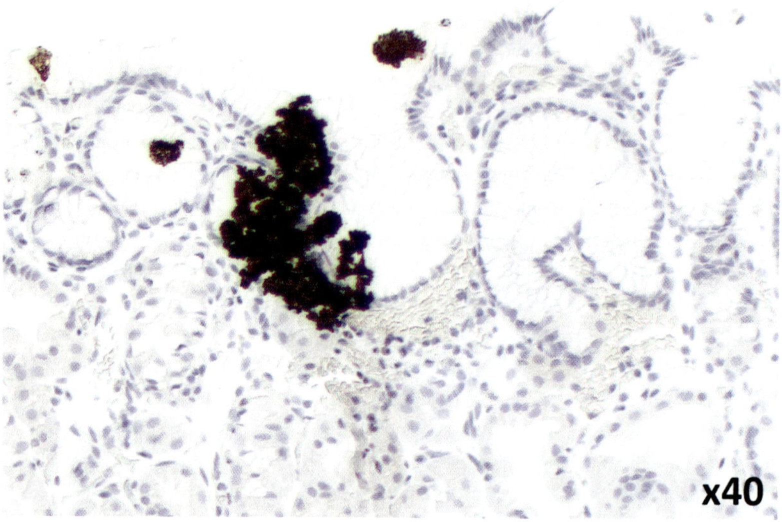

Figure 7.8 Diaminobenzidine precipitate on an *H. pylori*–stained slide

majority of IHC staining. Enzyme-induced epitope retrieval (EIER) and heat-induced epitope retrieval (HIER) are routinely employed to improve the immunoreactivity of the antigens. The aim of an AR regimen is to enable epitopes within tissue to be more accessible to the antibody by either physically breaking crosslinks formed by formalin fixation with heat energy or using enzymes to make tissue more permeable for the antibody. Unfortunately, there is not one universal pretreatment method which works for all antibodies. The laboratory worker needs to find the most suitable approach for each antibody clone.

Antibody manufacturers will usually recommend a certain pretreatment scheme for each of their antibodies. This is an excellent starting point when validating a new antibody. Unfortunately, the recommended pretreatment may not always be suitable for each individual laboratory, possibly due to variations in fixation or individual requirements. The IHC facility needs to find this out. Many different pretreatments are available from commercial vendors and produced in house by the laboratory. Automated platforms will usually have a small range of proprietary enzyme dilutions and heat pretreatments. More 'open' systems and manual methods have many more AR solutions available. Common enzymes deployed for AR include protease, chymotrypsin, pepsin and ficin. Citrate, Tris- and Tris-EDTA–based buffers ranging between pH6 and pH10 are used for HIER.

Enzyme-induced epitope retrieval is usually carried out at temperatures between ambient and 37°C. Times will vary depending on the antibody and the fixation time. Unfortunately, optimal enzyme AR is difficult to achieve if the tissue has been fixed poorly. Morphology and tissue structures will be disrupted if the tissue has not been fixed long enough. Figure 7.9 shows a comparison of applying enzyme retrieval methods on the same poorly fixed tissue. The epidermal zone is intact with no retrieval for CD34. Notice the disruption of the epidermis as enzyme digestion is introduced for S100 and F13a antibodies in varying incubation times.

Saving the morphology by reducing the time or concentration of the enzyme may lead to failed IHC staining. Optimal tissue fixation and processing is therefore the most important factor for successful IHC. Conversely, weak or false negative staining may also occur if the tissue has been fixed for too long. This problem is somewhat easier to overcome by increasing the time or concentration of the enzyme. These scenarios are not ideal, and many issues arise due to the lack of standardized protocols. The inherent nature of anatomical pathology specimens being of various sizes can be accommodated if there is a concerted effort to fix and process tissue optimally.

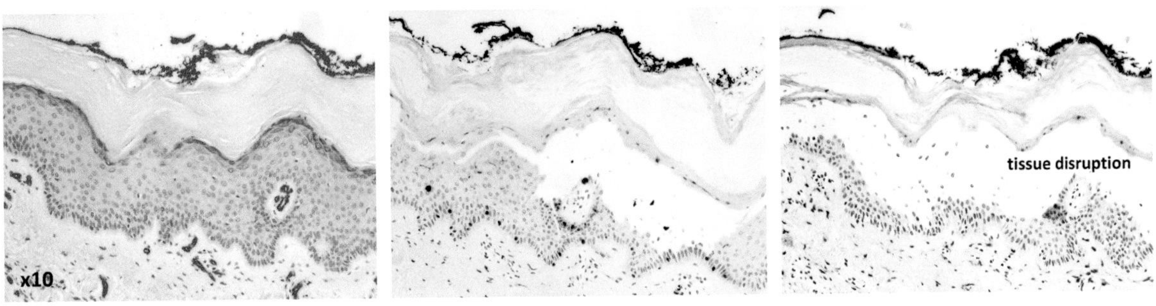

Figure 7.9 Tissue disruption from enzyme digestion on poorly fixed skin

Heat-induced epitope retrieval is the most common pretreatment strategy in most laboratories. Ready-to-use (RTU) solutions and concentrates may be purchased from many suppliers and recipes are available to manufacture in-house solutions using readily available reagents. Heat-induced epitope retrieval has been successfully performed in a pressure cooker, using a hotplate, in a microwave oven, in an autoclave or on an automated platform just to name a few. The choice of HIER will depend on what is available and the specific antibody. Automated platforms may be restricted to a couple of different solutions covering a range of pH levels. It is recommended to use a pH close to neutral (6–8) if possible, in order to reduce morphological changes and non-specific staining. Some antibodies will require HIER at a more extreme pH for adequate staining. If these solutions are not available, an increase in incubation time and/or temperature of the solution may improve staining. The temperature must be carefully controlled, especially during longer incubations at high pH, so as to eliminate variations in staining intensity as well as morphological changes. In addition, the molarity of an HIER solution may also affect IHC results. Preference is given to HIER if there is a choice between enzyme or heat for AR. Some IHC protocols require the exclusive use of EIER for optimal staining and so must be followed. If given a preference, HIER is recommended over EIER because protocols are generally more resistant to variations in fixation and processing. Be mindful that excessive HIER may have a catastrophic effect on even well-fixed tissue.

Primary Antibody

One of the most important decisions to make when validating a new antibody is choosing the optimal primary antibody clone. There are instances where many different clones are available to demonstrate a particular antigen. Doing some research before purchasing one could save a great deal of time and money. Make sure the antibody is suitable for IHC as well as for FFPE tissue if that is the intended use. Check that the antibody will be suitable for the facility's existing IHC set-up by searching for published protocols. This endeavour may save a great deal of time, so check online for quality assurance programs or enquire with other laboratories before starting from scratch. Check the sensitivity and specificity of the antibody and try to purchase it from a reputable supplier who has tested each new batch of antibody and can transport it to the IHC facility in optimal condition. If sourcing antibodies from other institutions such as research facilities, ensure consistency between batches and a solid supply chain before deciding to commit on the clone. Choose the best incubation temperature settings for the antibody as variations on staining may be observed at ambient temperature or at 37°C. Common incubation temperatures are 4°C, ambient room temperature and 37°C. A close relationship to temperature is incubation time and this will depend on the concentration of the antibody, the desired intensity and the time constraints of the laboratory.

When finding the optimal working titre for an antibody, aim for the strongest and cleanest demonstration of the antigen with the least non-specific staining. Choose the most dilute concentration that will offer this, but be aware that reactivity may decrease over time and ensure the IHC protocol will adequately demonstrate low expressors of the antigen.

The choice of antibody diluent may also be critical for optimal IHC staining. Most antibodies will perform well using any antibody diluent while others require specific diluents. Figure 7.10 shows the result of using a diluent of the wrong pH or ionic strength,

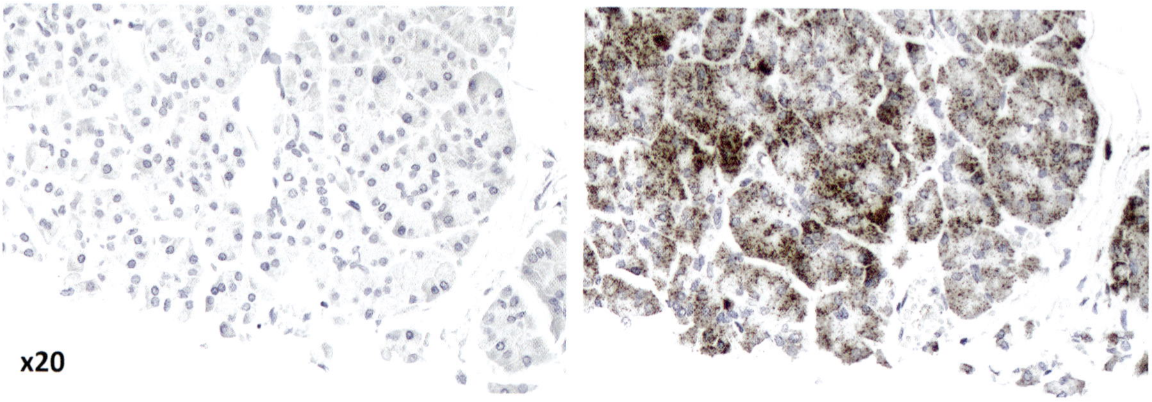

Figure 7.10 BRAF antibody diluted with two types of diluents on normal pancreas

causing false positive BRAF IHC staining of pancreas. The expected result is zero staining in normal pancreas, but this can be manipulated if the concentrate is diluted with an inappropriate antibody diluent.

When diluting antibodies for IHC, ensure clean laboratory practices are observed in order to reduce the chance of bacterial or fungal growth in the solution. Sodium azide or other additives to arrest microbial growth in the antibody solution or diluent will not always stop these growths. Figure 7.11 shows a Gram stain performed on an *H. pylori* primary antibody reagent, highlighting the presence of actinomyces and bacterial growth in the solution. The growths will multiply quickly if the antibody is left at room temperature or above for extended periods of time. These actions may attribute to poor antibody performance as dispensers can be blocked, affecting the overall instrumentation. Figure 7.12 shows a comparison of assay performance using the contaminated antibody in Figure 7.11 and a fresh aliquot. Note the decrease in staining intensity compared to the fresh antibody. Although the intensity and the number of organisms stained has decreased, the stain still appears acceptable in this instance. False negative results may easily be reported in other occasions.

Another parameter to test is the resilience factor of the antibody. Some antibodies are more 'robust' and have a longer 'shelf life' compared to others after being diluted out and stored in similar conditions. The variation in antibody performance may be similar to Figure 7.12. A likely explanation is that antibodies may not arrive in the laboratory under optimal conditions even when excellent efforts are practiced by the supplier. Quality assurance initiatives such as staining a control slide for each new antibody batch will help identify issues caused by external factors such as failed batches or poor transportation conditions. Another important parameter is the change of protein concentration sometimes observed between batches of antibody, which may produce the observed variation in stains.

Detection System

A main contributor to the mass confusion surrounding IHC technology is the wide range of detection systems available for IHC assays. Vendors have tried to limit these options by locking detection kits to particular automated platforms, but there are no limitations when performing IHC manually. Therefore it is important to choose detection kits wisely to achieve best outcomes. First, ensure the detection system is suitable for all of the antibodies and tissues in the IHC laboratory. Most clinical laboratories will limit primary antibodies obtained from either mouse or rabbit hosts. Therefore, secondary 'linker' antibodies only need to match these two species, cutting down the complexities of introducing additional serum blocking steps as a consequence of using antisera from other animals. If an unusual 'exotic' host species was used for the production of the primary antibody, a detection system designed specifically for this species will be required. Immunohistochemical technology is flexible and most techniques may be adapted to suit an individual's own general methods, including automation.

Huge technological advances have been made in the available detection systems. The main improvement has been an increase in sensitivity, leading to stronger staining, higher antibody dilutions and reduced staining

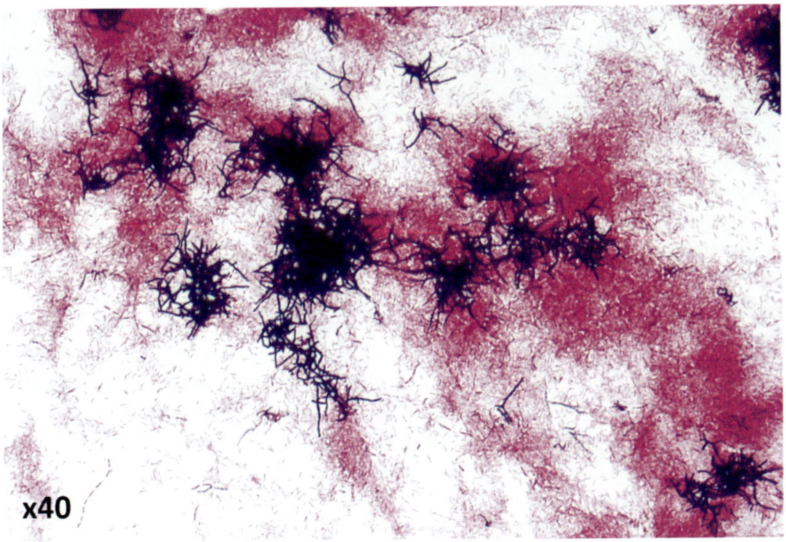

Figure 7.11 Gram stain showing microbial growth inside an *H. pylori* antibody reagent

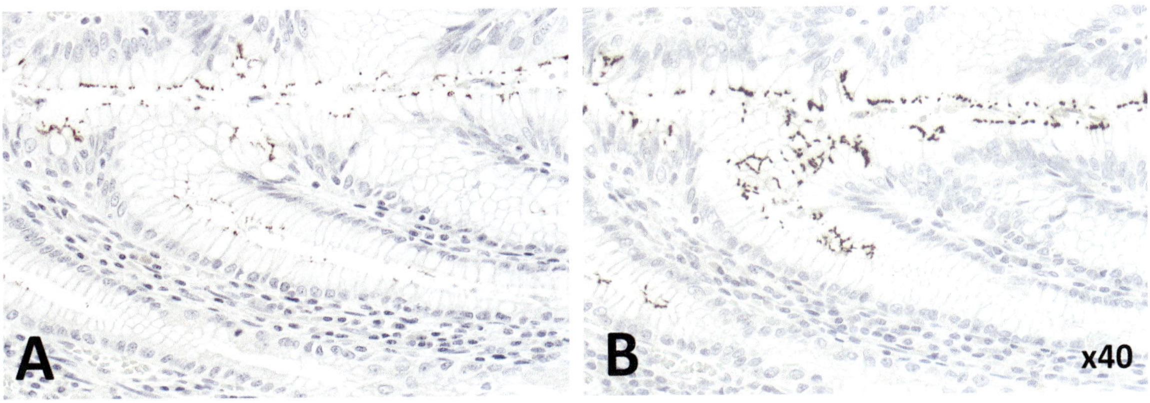

Figure 7.12 *H. pylori* with contaminated antibody (A) vs. new freshly prepared aliquot (B)

times. Unfortunately, extremely sensitive detection systems with their 'amplification' protocols may interfere with interpretation, making it more difficult to comment objectively the intensity of staining. Take, for example, the reporting of oestrogen receptor. Shown in Figure 7.13 is a validated oestrogen receptor protocol on invasive ductal carcinoma (IDC) from a breast specimen (A) and the same method but using a more sensitive detection system (B). This resulted in a stronger signal, which may lead to false positive reporting. Staff involved with interpreting IHC should be aware of changes made to the detection system. Sometimes modifications to protocols are put into effect too hastily in an effort to keep the staining consistent. Unintended consequences may arise, typically affecting extremely 'low expressors' observed as being negative originally and suddenly appearing positive. Interpretation is therefore difficult in deciding whether this is 'true' staining or artificially amplified.

The shift away from using biotinylated primary or secondary antibodies has alleviated the need for a biotin-blocking step when staining biotin-rich tissues such as liver and kidney. When using a peroxidase-based chromogen such as 3,3' diaminobenzidine (DAB), ensure there is sufficient blocking of endogenous peroxidase activity with hydrogen peroxide (H_2O_2). Actively seen in red blood cells, insufficient blocking will lead to unwanted staining of endogenous peroxidase activity

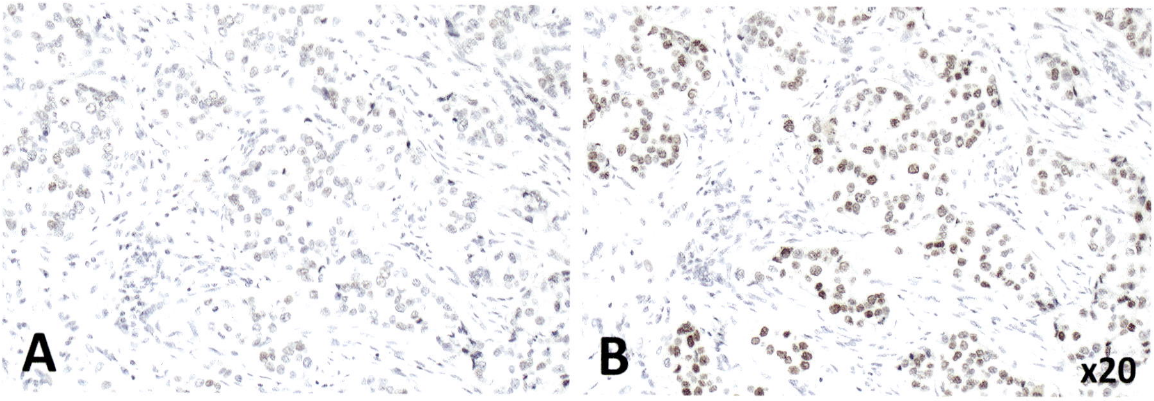

Figure 7.13 ER immunohistochemistry staining with the same primary antibody in two different detection systems

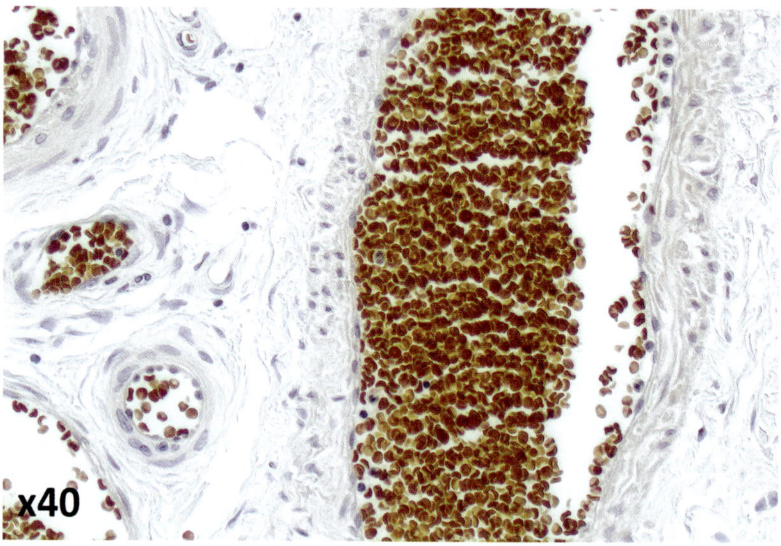

Figure 7.14 Diaminobenzidine-labelled red blood cells due to omission of endogenous peroxidase block

within these areas as shown in Figure 7.14. Variations in staining of some antibodies may occur depending on the nature of the diluent used to achieve the H_2O_2 working solution. Common diluents include methanol, phosphate-buffered saline and distilled water. In addition, the timing of the blocking step can also cause staining differences. Some antibodies produce better results when the peroxidase block is performed after the primary antibody incubation.

Chromogen

Leaving other labels such as fluorophores and heavy metals out of consideration, many different chromogens are still available to use. Diaminobenzidine is the most utilized because it is easy to use, clean, strong and robust. Unfortunately, it is also hazardous and should be neutralized before disposal (Lunn and Sansone 1991). Switching to a red chromogen for both peroxidase or alkaline phosphatase IHC systems can be done if the tissue is heavily pigmented with melanin, which may be mistaken for a true DAB signal. Whichever chromogen is used, follow the recommendations of the manufacturer during and after staining. Most suppliers recommend making the chromogen fresh each time to reduce the possibility of precipitate being deposited on top of the tissue and slide. Poor storage conditions of the chromogen may also lead to this problem. Automated IHC instruments will usually mix the chromogen on the slide or just before use. Some chromogens may be affected by alcohol and xylene and leach out or fade from the target areas. Carefully read the data sheets of the detection system and chromogen to be aware of the limitations of the product. Find a chromogen that suits the methods and tissue routinely being used. Avoid long protocols and colours that are difficult to interpret.

Counterstain

The most common counterstain used for IHC is haematoxylin. The most logical explanation is that it is readily available in histology laboratories and complements both brown and red chromogens well. The intensity of the counterstain is crucial – if it is too weak, it may be difficult to identify which cells are expressing the antigen and where they are located in the tissue. If the counterstain is too strong, IHC staining may be masked, especially when targeting nuclear antigens as highlighted in Figure 7.15. Lowly expressed oestrogen receptor signal with standard haematoxylin (A) is easier to observe than in an extended haematoxylin protocol (B). The counterstain should be fresh and filtered in order to ensure clean and reproducible staining. However, the choice of an optimal counterstain is decided on individual preferences.

Double Staining

The demonstration of multiple antigens on one slide is not uncommon. A double stain is often used to assist in the diagnosis of prostatic adenocarcinoma, but there are endless possibilities for the use of two or more antibodies. Most commonly, these protocols use two separate detection systems and their respective chromogens develop in a 'simultaneous' or 'sequential' fashion. It is also possible to use the same chromogen for two different antibodies as long as the epitopes are localized in different areas of the tissue or cell – for example, the nucleus and the cell membrane. The chosen method will mainly depend on what is available, especially if using an automated IHC system. Most automated systems have the capability to perform at least a double stain. It is also possible to perform part of the protocol on an automated stainer and the remainder manually.

The important thing to remember when optimizing a double-stain IHC protocol is compatibility. Firstly, the pretreatments should be similar. Using antibodies with vastly different pretreatments – for example, HIER and EIER – is very difficult. At least one of the antibodies will be suboptimal. The staining of the antibodies should complement each other. Staining intensities should be similar and areas of co-localization clean and obvious. This may be achieved by modifying concentrations or incubation times. If using DAB and a red chromogen, crisper staining may be achieved if the red chromogen is used for cytoplasmic staining and DAB for nuclear or membranous. Extra wash steps in the protocol may be required to reduce background noise or non-specific staining. If designing a protocol from the ground up, ensure there is no cross-reactivity between any of the steps. These same principles may be used if optimizing triple or more staining methods.

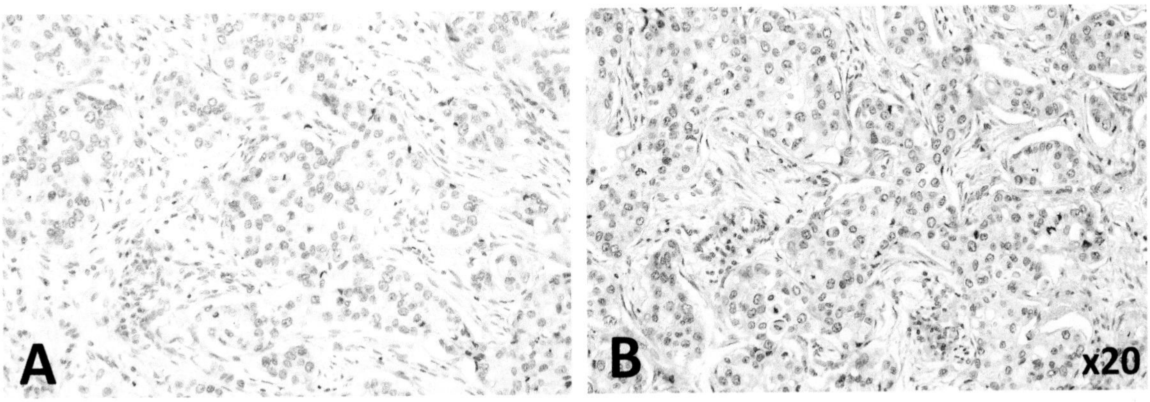

Figure 7.15 A comparison of two counterstaining protocols for ER immunohistochemical staining

Pigments

Pigments are a common occurrence in histology. Many endogenous and exogenous forms exist as described by Churukian (2008). Two common pigments which were a problem in the past are derived from formaldehyde and mercury. The use of buffered formalin should eliminate the first, and the widespread cessation of using mercury due to toxicity fears has eradicated the second. Presently, a pigment that has a high capacity to interfere with diagnostic IHC is melanin. It is seen in normal and abnormal tissue appearing brown to black in colour and often associated with melanoma.

Unfortunately, melanin pigment can mimic DAB chromogen, the most common chromogen in IHC, thus making it difficult to interpret the slide. There are many ways to combat this problem; the easiest is to employ a different chromogen. Most automated platforms have a choice of chromogens that can be used on the instrument. A red chromogen is usually available and will generally fix the problem. A downside is that some red detection systems are not as sensitive as DAB protocols. Rectification leads to extended run times to combat weaker staining. New protocols will need to be validated for each antibody and a different set of reagents is required. If the detection system is rarely used, reagents may expire before all of the tests are used in the kit, wasting the laboratory's resources. A suitable alternative is trying to bleach the melanin pigment out of the section or to stain the melanin a different colour. These methods will make interpretation easier whilst making use of the facility's existing routine IHC reagents.

The standard practice to bleach melanin from a tissue section is to use potassium permanganate ($KMnO_4$) followed by oxalic acid. Unfortunately, this may affect some antigens or disrupt the tissue itself as can be seen in Figure 7.16. The H&E shows a very low-power view of metastatic melanoma with pigmentation (A) and the bleaching has destroyed the area of interest on the corresponding IHC stain (B).

Alternative bleaching methods are much gentler for both the antigens and the tissue. Trichloroisocyanuric acid (TCCA) may be used to bleach melanin pigment either before or after IHC staining (Shen and Wu 2015). It is not a common chemical routinely used in a histopathology laboratory but may easily be sourced via a distributor of laboratory chemicals. Satisfactory melanin bleaching with minor disruption to tissue morphology and staining intensity may be achieved by treating the slide with 1% aqueous TCCA for 30 minutes after the chromogen step. Figure 7.17 shows routine Ki67 IHC stain in a heavily pigmented metastatic melanoma section (A). Bleaching with TCCA enables easier interpretation (B). An increase in time for the counterstain may be required for optimal nuclear staining. A drawback for this method is the strong chlorine smell of TCCA.

H_2O_2 may also be used to bleach melanin pigment from tissue sections and is readily available to the laboratory (Li et al. 1999). Optimal results may be achieved by bleaching with 1% aqueous H_2O_2 for

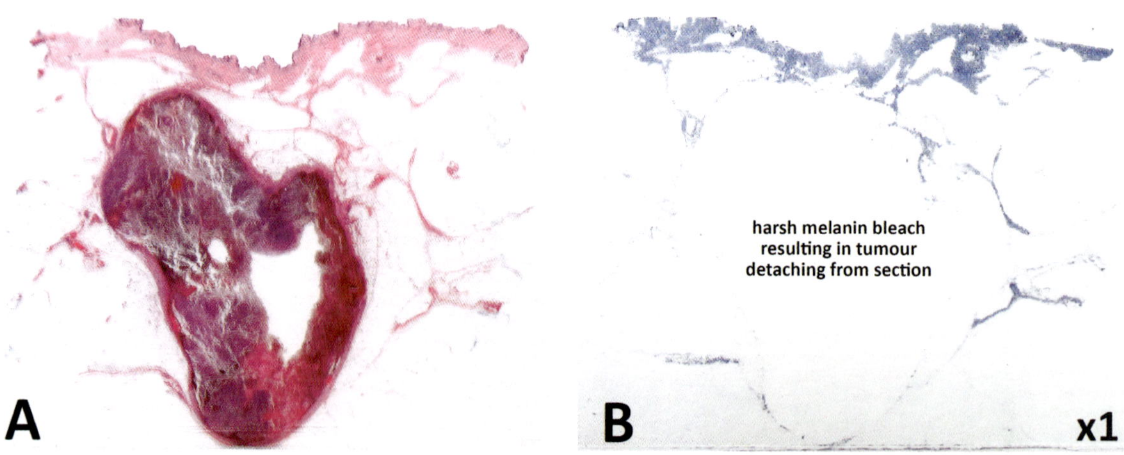

Figure 7.16 Harsh treatments to clear away pigments can destroy sections.

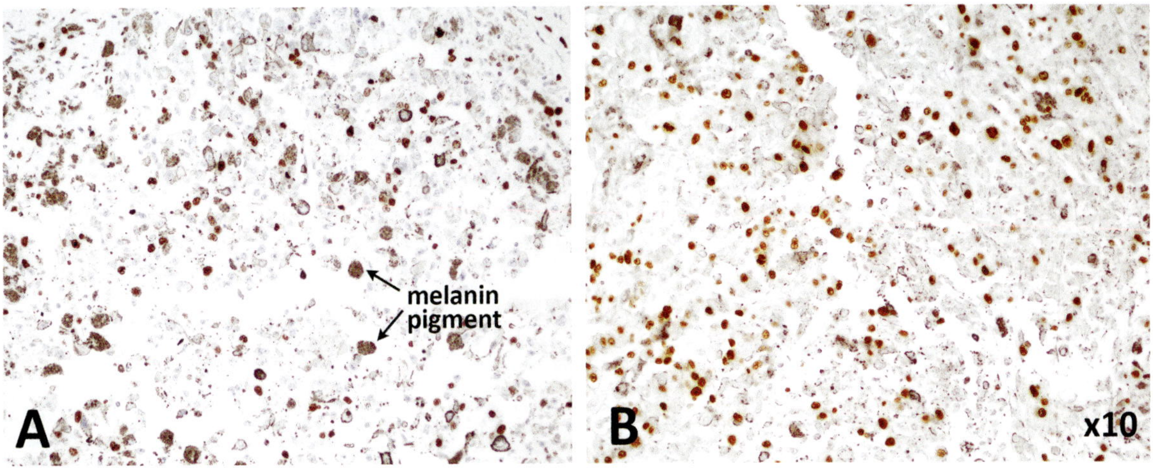

Figure 7.17 Ki67 immunohistochemistry before (A) and after melanin bleach (B) with trichloroisocyanuric acid

90 minutes at 55°C before any pretreatment. Alternatively, bleach duration can be shortened to 10 minutes if the slide is placed in 3% H_2O_2 diluted with phosphate-buffered saline and heated to 70°C in a laboratory grade microwave oven. Figure 7.18 shows both strategies work equally well when stained with Ki67. Note strong nuclear staining with no melanin pigment remaining in both images. Great care must be taken when microwaving H_2O_2 even at low concentrations. It is possible to use H_2O_2 to bleach the melanin after IHC staining, but this will affect the tissue morphology more than employing it pre-IHC staining. If only one pre-stained slide is available and melanin pigment is making interpretation of the IHC slide difficult, TCCA or H_2O_2 may be used to assist after the section has been brought back down to water.

Possibly the easiest way to negate the effects of melanin pigment in an IHC section is to stain the pigment a different colour to the chromogen. Melanin pigment may be stained a different colour with Azure B (Kamino and Tam 1991) or Giemsa solution. Figure 7.19 shows Ki67 counterstained with azure B for 90 minutes before dehydration in absolute ethanol, clearing in xylene and coverslipping. The melanin pigment has changed from a brown to a greenish blue. Using Giemsa stain for 4 minutes, the melanin is also stained greenish blue. Both of these dyes have the added bonus of staining nuclei as well, negating the need to counterstain with haematoxylin. The use of Giemsa solution is much faster than Azure B but may leave a slight tinge of pink in other tissue elements.

Post-analytical Problems

The majority of errors occurring in IHC are first noticed at the post-analytical stage. This is where each stained slide is scrutinized for staining quality, controls are examined and assurances are given that the correct block has been cut and the right antibody applied. Not only is there a need to identify problems in staining, but technical staff are also expected to be able to offer suitable remedies.

Hints for Troubleshooting

Solving problems for IHC staining can become very messy. A good strategy to employ is to differentiate problems into two broad groups: failed IHC stains which have been validated and proven to work in the past and protocols for antibodies which are newly acquired and undergoing validation.

For problems encountered in a validated IHC procedure that has been working previously:

(1) Do not try to overthink the problem. Look for the simple answers first. Has anything been done differently to usual? Is there anything out of the ordinary?
(2) Work out if this is the first time the problem has occurred. Has this happened before? Is it slowly getting worse? Has there always been a problem with this particular antibody clone?
(3) The concern may be specific to the tissue. Has the test tissue been treated differently? Are internal controls staining appropriately in the test?

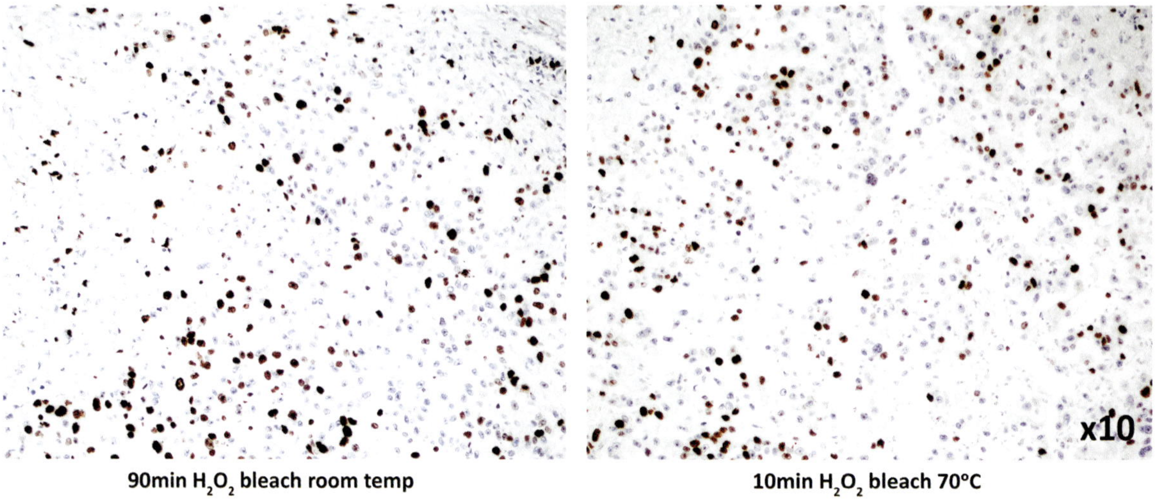

Figure 7.18 Ki67 immunohistochemical staining with two acceptable melanin bleaching methods using H_2O_2

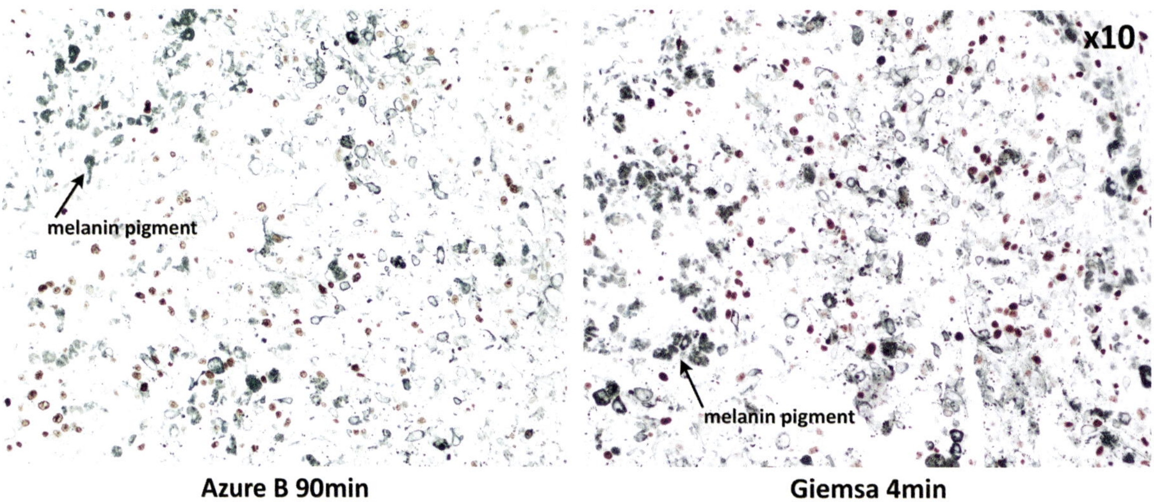

Figure 7.19 Ki67 with Azure B and Giemsa counterstain to change the colour of melanin pigment

(4) Narrow down where the problem may have occurred. Is the problem specific to the slide, the case, the antibody, the detection system, the operator/instrument?

(5) Do not change multiple parts of the method at once. Be methodical. Otherwise you may not be able to work out what part of the procedure has failed.

For troubles faced when validating or troubleshooting a new IHC antibody:

(1) Choose the best antibody for the specific need. Before committing to purchase, take time to research the different clones available and how they perform under existing methods. Does the clone work with routine protocols or existing instrumentation? Check journal papers, quality assurance programs or other laboratories to certify if the clone has been validated previously.

(2) The antibody should be readily available. Is it easy to acquire and delivered in optimal condition and in a timely manner? Will the antibody be cost-effective?

(3) Have a validation plan for the antibody covering situations it will be used in. Why is this clone

needed? What appropriate controls and key performance indicators are required to validate the test? Is there adequate control material to validate the antibody?

(4) Start trials using the supplier's or a peer laboratory's recommendations. Try not to reinvent the wheel, although what may work elsewhere may not be optimal in another unique situation.

(5) When deciding on a final protocol, ensure it is robust. Will the protocol work for all tissue for which it is required? Will the staining be suitable when the antibody and reagents are close to expiry?

Addressing these simple questions are sometimes all that is required to treat suboptimal IHC staining. At other times, technical staff may need to get creative to offer suitable workaround strategies and the ability to think outside the square.

Thinking outside the Square

Many steps can go wrong during IHC staining. It may seem like a very difficult and finicky, technique but most available methods are quite robust and adaptable to a laboratory's specific requirements without the need for major modifications. The remainder of this chapter focuses on adaptations which may be helpful in unusual situations. An in-depth knowledge of general histological techniques will be necessary to attempt these in-house modifications. Always validate the method and use appropriate controls for analytical IHC techniques.

Manual versus Automated Methods

Routine manual methods for IHC staining allow easy modifications applied to protocols as the need to address unusual situations arise. Simply, this may include a new retrieval solution or method of retrieval – for example, swapping out a microwave oven for a pressure cooker. Other alternatives may include using a different secondary antibody or a different detection system and chromogen. Whatever changes are made, try to keep it as close to the original standard protocol as possible. This will help in daily workflow and create fewer opportunities for errors. It will also reduce the number of different reagents and equipment accumulating in the laboratory as well as keep operational costs down.

Automated IHC staining has many advantages in reproducibility and freeing up staff members for other duties. Unfortunately, it comes at a cost both financially and in terms of flexibility. When choosing an automated system, work out the likely different scenarios and decide on the most suitable instrument. Some IHC machines are more 'open' than others, and this should be taken into consideration when sourcing a suitable instrument for the needs of the facility. If there is still a need to manually stain, the output efficiency will be reduced. For example, when testing non-human tissue or using primary antibodies from uncommon hosts, make sure there is a compatible detection system or secondary antibody that can be used on the automated instrument. If this is a rare occurrence, it may be possible to stain the slide manually using reagents already available in the laboratory.

Consider this scenario. A lymph node was received from a rabbit with a suspected lymphoma. The primary antibody was of rabbit origin, but the routine automated detection system for this indirect IHC method the laboratory routinely used contained a cocktail of secondary antibodies directed against rabbit and mouse antibodies. If this kit was used, the entire tissue would stain non-specifically because the anti-rabbit secondary antibodies would bind to the endogenous host (rabbit) immunoglobulins as well as to the primary (rabbit) antibody. Fortunately, the laboratory had purchased a different monoclonal mouse primary antibody that came with its own manual detection system which included a secondary antibody directed against mouse immunoglobulins. This was used on the case with great success as illustrated in Figure 7.20, using CD79a to stain the B-cell lymphoma and CD3 highlighting the normal T cell lymphocytes. Internal controls were used in this instance because of the lack of rabbit-derived control tissue.

If the laboratory intends to perform IHC on non-human tissue, it is important to ensure the antibody chosen will react with the test species. Many antibodies employed to stain human tissue will also cross-react with other mammalian species and some bird, fish or reptile species. This needs to be confirmed from the data sheet or via experimentation. Multiple trials may be needed to find a suitable antibody and procedure. Some clones will work well while other clones, although being the same antibody, will not. In the case of the rabbit lymphoma from Figure 7.20, the laboratory's regular B-cell marker CD20 did not stain rabbit B-cell lymphocytes but a specific CD79a clone did. This same CD79a clone was also used to stain dog

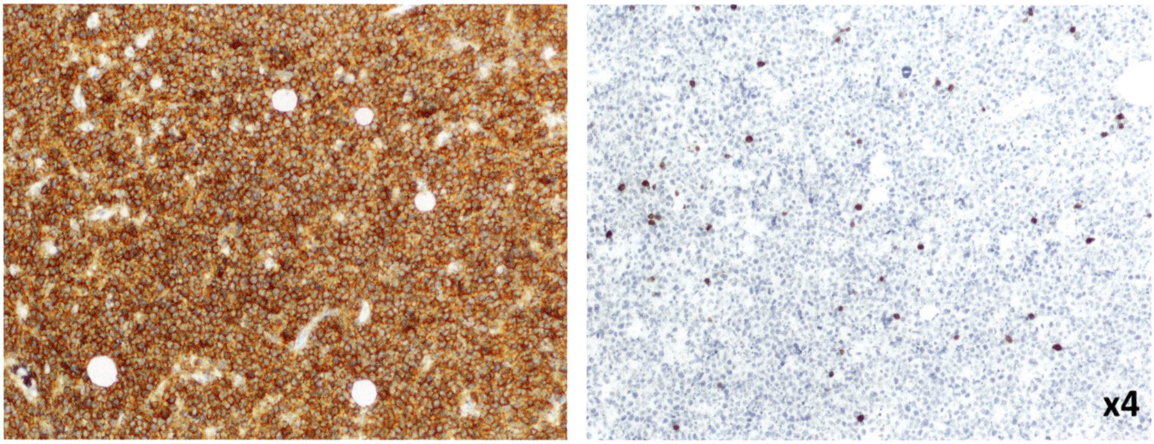

CD79a IHC stain CD3 IHC stain

Figure 7.20 Immunohistochemistry using a primary antibody and detection kit suitable for rabbit tissue

and cat tissue with great success. The CD3 clone was the laboratory's routine antibody for human tissue.

Making the Most of a Specimen

There are instances when multiple tests are required from a very small specimen sample. The tissue from the paraffin block may have been exhausted before all of the required assays are completed. Unfortunately, this is a common dilemma encountered in both diagnostic and research or clinical trials where not enough paraffin tissue is available. In what follows are a number of strategies to make the most out of a specimen for IHC.

Restaining

It is possible to restain a slide with an IHC stain. There may be no relevant tissue left in the FFPE block, but IHC is still required to reach a diagnosis. If a spare H&E is available, it may be possible to restain it after taking the coverslip off and bringing the section back down to water. A caveat is that this will only work well if the tissue was initially mounted onto a charged or coated slide; otherwise there is a risk of the section falling off during IHC staining. The IHC pretreatment step should decolourize the tissue sufficiently. If not, the tissue may be treated with acid alcohol briefly before starting IHC protocols. Restaining is also suitable for cytological and haematological smears.

It is also possible to restain a negative IHC test slide with a different antibody stain. This method works best when both pretreatments are similar, and staining may be improved with a second reduced pretreatment step before the subsequent IHC stain. If possible, experiment with these methods before using them on real test tissue and use slides that are surplus to requirements. Retention of critical tissue is important for the archives, and there should be no risk of histology material being lost forever if the method fails. Internal controls are the best way of assessing if these unorthodox methods have worked. Figure 7.21 shows a broad spectrum cytokeratin AE1/AE3 applied to a tumour initially thought of as epithelial in origin. When a negative result was achieved, the same section was used again for HMB45, a marker for melanoma.

Hidden Sections

A slight modification of these methods is to partially restain a slide with serial sections while keeping one section with the original stain intact. This is possible by 'hiding' some tissue on the slide and restaining the remainder of the tissue (Kubier and Miller 2002). The coverslip and mounting media are removed before a small amount of new mounting media is dried onto the section that is to be kept in its original state. Figure 7.22 shows three consecutive serial sections of a prostate core biopsy on a slide. One core is hidden from subsequent IHC staining and the other two exposed cores will be subjected to IHC staining (A). When IHC staining is finished, the mounting media is then dissolved and the entire slide coverslipped. Notice the original H&E section has survived while the other two sections have been restained for CK5/6 (B). This method may not be suitable for all automated instruments as the mounting media may disrupt the staining.

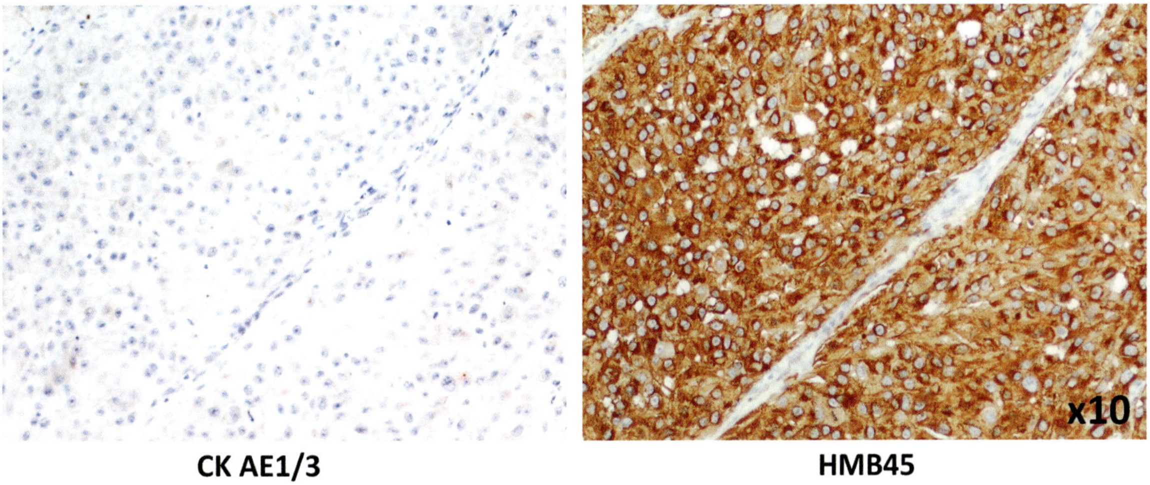

Figure 7.21 Section of melanoma stained for CK AE1/3 first then the same section stained for HMB45

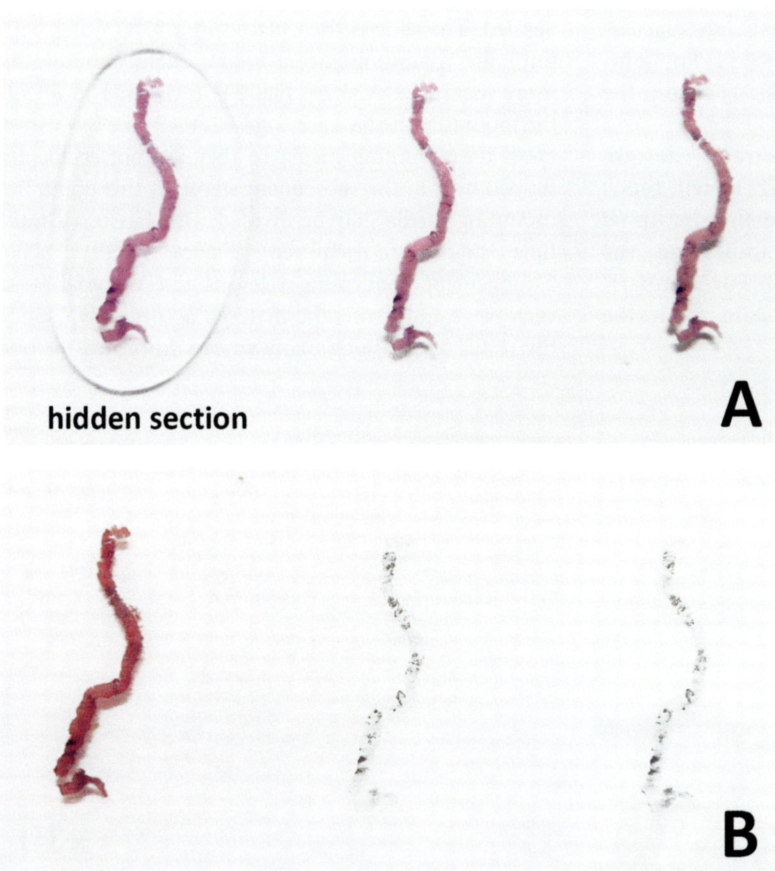

Figure 7.22 Keeping one hematoxylin and eosin section whilst immunohistochemically staining others on the same slide

Creating Cell Blocks

If only one slide is available and multiple stains are required, it is possible to scrape the tissue off the slide with a sharp blade and manufacture a cell block with it. This is achieved by first removing the coverslip and any residual mounting media before bringing the slide to water via graded ethanols, carefully scraping the tissue off of the slide and into deionized water. Routine cell-blocking methods using agar or thrombin may be used to create the cell block of the tissue. A microtomy 'feather' blade is ideal for the scraping step because of its long, flat blade. Creating a cell block from a tissue section allows the tissue to be available for a huge number of IHC stains if required. Unfortunately, morphology and the original tissue structure may be lost. Figure 7.23 shows CD117 IHC sectioned from a cell block made from tissue scraped off an H&E slide of a gastrointestinal stromal tumour (GIST) (A). This scenario is required when the original histology block has been cut to extinction. The morphology has been severely affected but the IHC has successfully demonstrated a CD117 positive GIST. For comparison, this is a slide stained with CD117 from the original paraffin block (B).

Likewise, Figure 7.24 demonstrates desmin IHC sectioned from the same GIST cell block scraping from a H&E slide. Notice the disrupted morphology is still diagnostic, indicating the tumour is not of muscle origin (A). For comparison, see a routine desmin IHC stain from the original paraffin block (B).

Lifting Sections

Another avenue to 'do more with less' is to lift sections or smears from one slide and transfer parts of them to other slides for IHC (Jimenez and Gangi 1986). This scenario is most useful with sections mounted on routine 'non-sticky' microscope slides or when multiple IHC stains are required from only a single cytology or blood smear. This is technically difficult to imagine and to perfect, but still possible using materials found in a histology laboratory. Commercial vendors such as Newcomer Supply (www.newcomersupply.com) markets 'Mount-Quick mounting media' for tissue transfer purposes. The coverslip and mounting media are removed before fresh mounting media are applied to the area to be 'lifted off'.

Figure 7.25 shows a Diff Quik stain from a dog lymph node aspiration suspected of lymphoma (A). Mounting media are applied and dried in an oven until the mounting media hardens. Any mounting media may be used. The drying time will vary depending on the type of mounting media and the amount applied. The slide is then placed in a 37°C water bath until the mounting media soften slightly, becoming more malleable. A sharp blade is then used to lift off the mounting media, carrying with them the test tissue. Label the mounting media so they are not accidently flipped over in the subsequent steps. At this point, the mounting media may be divided with scissors if multiple stains are required (Figure 7.25B). Make a judgement confirming relevant test material is in each piece and divide the material accordingly. Notice the result of obtaining many smears from just the one

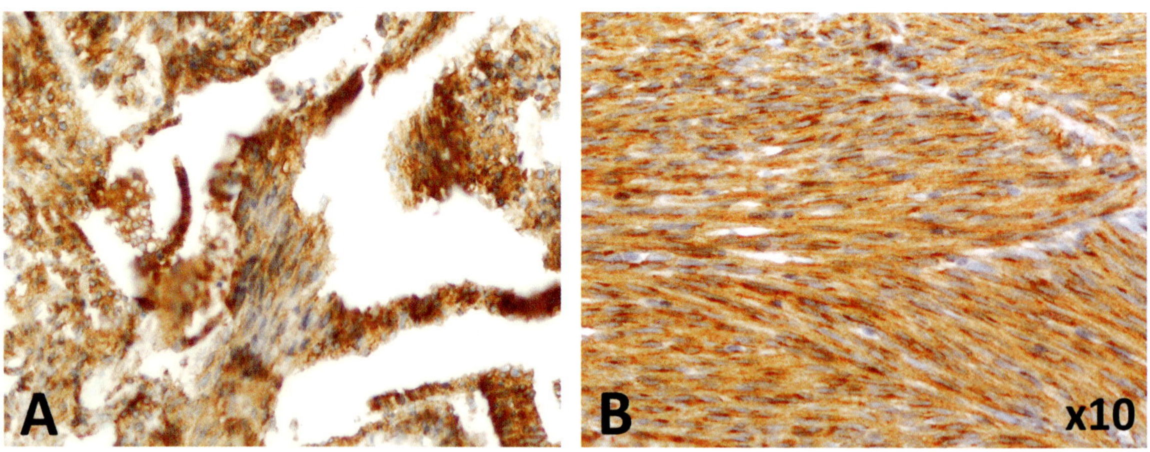

Figure 7.23 CD117 immunohistochemical stain on a cell block made from scraping the original hematoxylin and eosin section (A) vs. routine paraffin section (B)

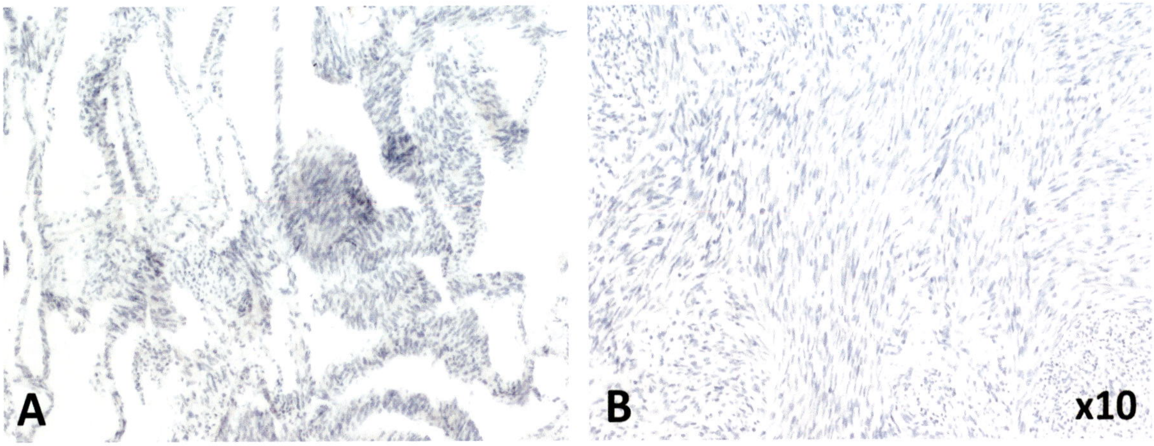

Figure 7.24 Desmin immunohistochemistry on the same cell block preparation (A) as Figure 7.23 and the original block (B)

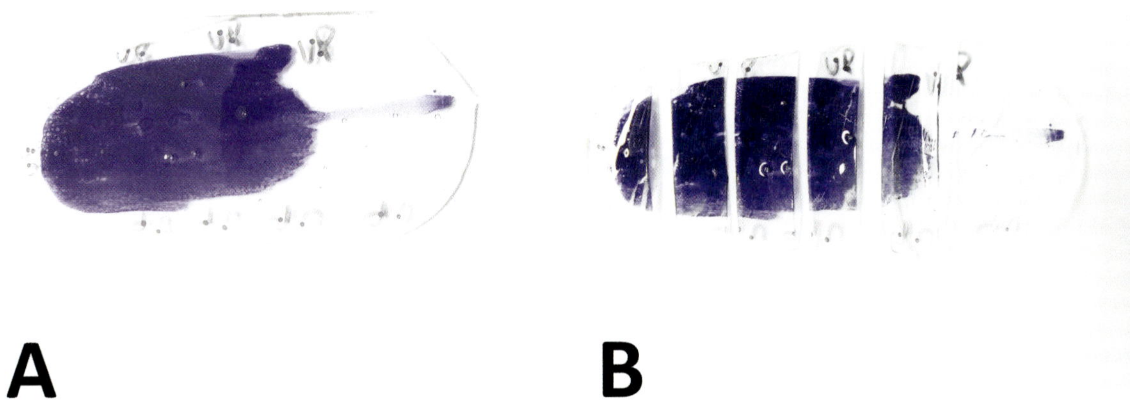

Figure 7.25 Obtaining multiple immunohistochemical assays from one cytology smear

original smear. Each piece may then be pushed firmly onto separate slides for IHC, making sure the piece is not flipped over. This slide is then dried in an oven in order to improve adherence. The mounting media are dissolved by the laboratory's routine reagents, leaving the cells on the slide to be stained. The slide may then be brought to water and used for routine IHC protocols.

Figure 7.26 shows a PAX5 (A) and CD3 (B) IHC stain on lifted cells staining the B-cell lymphoma and T-cell lymphocytes, respectively. As always, practice and validate the method with tissue or smears before using the technique routinely. Internal positive controls are necessary to check if the stain has worked.

Another successful demonstration of 'lifting' an H&E section and restaining it for IHC in order to investigate cutaneous Paget's disease is shown in Figure 7.27. This situation arose from exhausting all diagnostic tissue in the FFPE block after obtaining the initial H&E levels and seeing that the original H&E slide was not mounted onto a 'sticky' slide. A successful demonstration of this 'lifting' technique was performed and then IHC stained with CK7 whilst

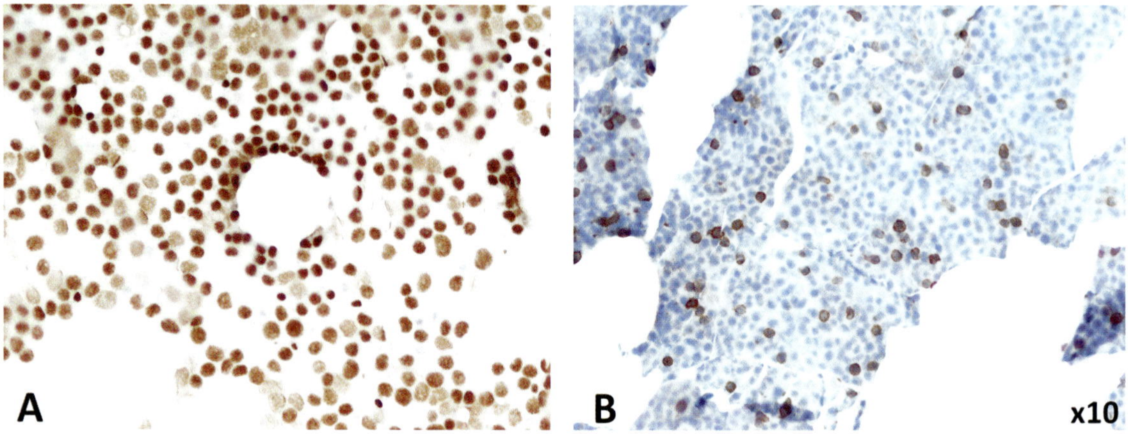

Figure 7.26 PAX5 (A) and CD3 (B) immunohistochemical stains on cytology smear sections created from Figure 7.25

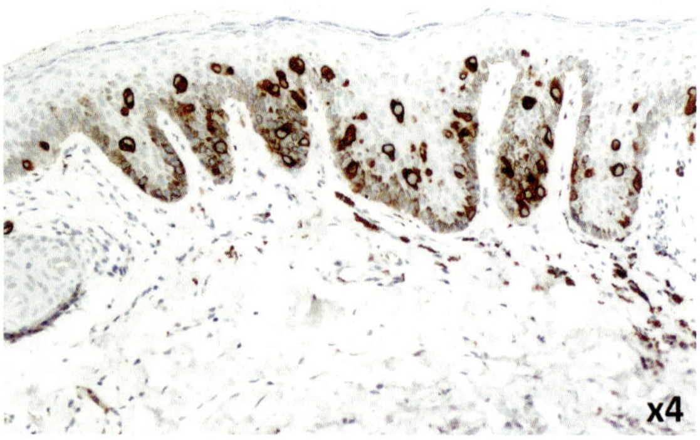

Figure 7.27 CK7 immunohistochemical stain from a 'lifted' hematoxylin and eosin section

retaining tissue morphology. A detailed protocol and tips about lifting sections can be found in Appendix 1.

Double Staining with a Difference

Double staining in this context does not mean using multiple antibodies for multiplex IHC assays. This discussion is based on combining the IHC assay with another histological technique such as a special stain or an *in situ* hybridization assay. It is possible because of the characteristics of DAB chromogen. When developed, DAB is very difficult to remove or even decrease the staining intensity. This attribute can be advantageous and may be used to couple IHC with other staining techniques. Most histochemical stains can be combined with IHC excluding methods requiring strong bleaching steps. Even dilute acids have a minimal effect on IHC stains, allowing Periodic Acid-Schiff (PAS) and trichrome stains to be combined with IHC staining.

For instance, a CD3 IHC stain followed by a PAS reaction may be helpful when investigating tubulointerstitial infiltrates within the kidney or mycosis fungoides in skin lesions. Another example is shown in Figure 7.28 involving Protein Gene Product 9.5 (PGP9.5) IHC staining nerve fibres (brown) in combination with a Gomori's trichrome to demonstrate myelin (red). This arrangement is used to demonstrate both nerves and myelin on the one slide to assist in the diagnosis of peripheral neuropathy. Image A shows myelinated sural nerves and image B demonstrates demyelination in sural nerves. In this instance, the haematoxylin counterstain was omitted, enabling the brown nerve fibres to be easily seen.

A slightly more difficult double-stain procedure involves the use of chromogen *in situ* hybridization (CISH) and traditional IHC methods. Figure 7.29 shows amplification of the *HER2* gene (black) in relation to normal chromosome 17 expression (red) in the nuclei demonstrated by CISH. The *HER2* gene is amplified to such a great extent that it has overpowered the red chromosome 17 signal. The red signals are easier to discern in the surrounding stromal cells (arrow). This finding is concordant with the Her2 IHC assay because of the accompanying strong 3+ membrane staining DAB brown. In this instance, the *in situ* hybridization was performed using a standard automated method

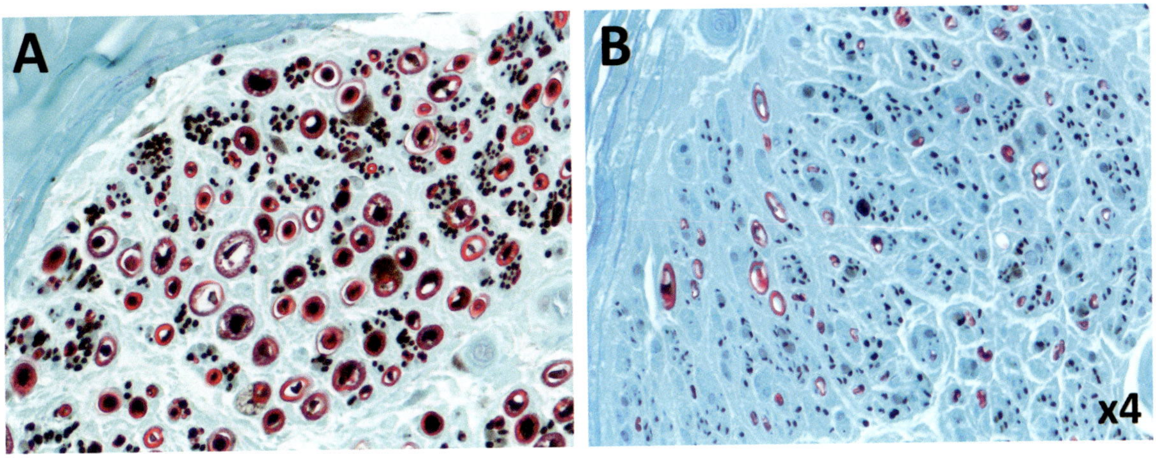

Figure 7.28 PGP9.5 immunohistochemical stain in combination with Gomori's trichrome to demonstrate myelinated (A) and demyelinated (B) nerve fibres

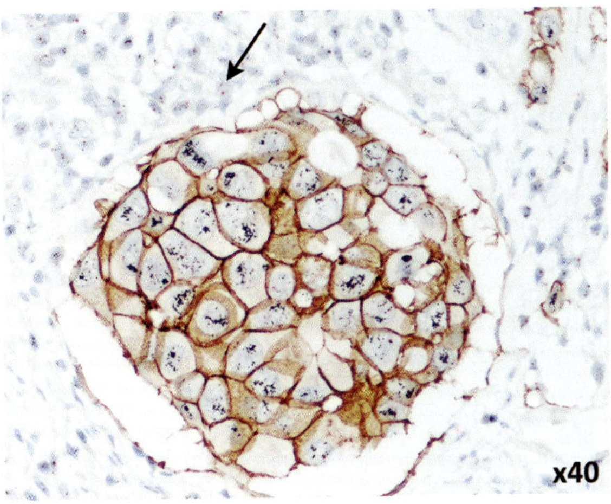

Figure 7.29 Her2 dual-label chromogen *in situ* hybridization in combination with HER2 IHC

followed by an automated IHC procedure without the need for extra pretreatment before the IHC protocol. A stronger haematoxylin counterstain was required.

These techniques are just a few different ways IHC may be used in a less traditional manner. As with all methods that are modified, try to experiment, test and validate procedures as stringently as possible before putting them into routine use. This does not mean excessive time and money must be invested to get the assays up and running. Be smart and practical about the expectations and planning. Then try to implement them using good science, sound advice and creative thinking.

Conclusion

It is hoped that this chapter has served as a treatise on why things can go awry and offered practical advice to rectify problems encountered in IHC. Classifying troubles into pre-analytical, analytical and post analytical stages helps identify the root cause of IHC problems in a methodical manner. A catalogue of every possible error and how to fix them is beyond the scope of this chapter and was not the primary intention.

By far, the most common mistakes are made at the analytical phase in any of the numerous parameters attributed to the IHC protocol. Some problems are easily solved while others require the laboratory worker to be more resourceful. What matters most is that the worker must first have a thorough grounding in basic fundamental histology and IHC principles before any attempts are made at solving predicaments.

The ability to gain the maximum amount of testing from limited samples is invaluable in diagnostic and research applications. By 'thinking outside the square', what was thought to be impossible may become possible, what was in the too hard basket is now easily achievable and what was unconventional has now become conventional. Amongst all of these new ideas, remember the backbone to all of this is that quality assurance still matters. Controls are needed to verify assays and prove the results obtained are legitimate. The IHC technology is robust and reliable in the same manner that it is also flexible and adaptable. The onus is on the laboratory worker to utilize the technology to its full potential and possess the expertise to successfully troubleshoot any problems as they arise.

Appendix 1 Lifting Section Technique

Next is a step-by-step procedure for lifting sections or smears from a slide and repurposing them for additional IHC staining. Gloves should be worn during all steps to reduce the chance of contamination with the worker's own cells.

(1) Remove coverslip and all mounting media with xylene. This may take days if the slide was coverslipped a long time ago.
(2) Do not bring the slide to water. Allow it to air-dry before placing fresh mounting media over the area you wish to lift. The dry slide allows the mounting media to remain thick, which assists during the lifting step.
(3) Dry the slide in a 60°C oven until the mounting media just hardens. This usually takes three or four hours, but will vary depending on the type of mounting media and the thickness with which they are applied. The mounting media will compress if they are not dry enough and will become more brittle if dried for too long.
(4) Remove the slide from the oven and mark the areas of interest and the 'up' side so the correct orientation may be kept.
(5) Place the slide in a 37°C deionized water bath for at least 15 minutes. This will make the mounting media more malleable when lifting.
(6) Carefully cut all of the mounting media off the slide in one piece using a sharp blade. This step is critical; a supported microtomy blade with a handle (often used in cut up) is ideal. Angle the blade at 30–45° to the slide and push firmly onto the slide and slice under the mounting media. Do not use a sawing motion and ensure all of the mounting media and tissue lift off together. More even, downward force may need to be applied if the tissue or mounting media remain on the slide. If areas of interest do remain, the slide may be taken back to step 1.
(7) Cut the mounting media that now contain the tissue into the required number of pieces, making sure relevant tissue is in each piece.
(8) Keeping the same orientation, press each piece firmly onto your standard IHC slides.
(9) Place the slides in 55°C deionized water for five minutes to soften the mounting media.
(10) Remove slides from water and press each piece very firmly onto the slide. Controls may be added to the slide at this time if required.
(11) Bake slides for 30 minutes at 60°C before removing the mounting media with xylene.
(12) Ensure all mounting media are removed from the slides before air-drying.
(13) Place slides directly into water or phosphate-buffered saline. Do not place slides in ethanol as this may cause the tissue to lift from the slide.
(14) Stain with the routine staining method, excluding the dewaxing step.

Quality control should be performed for each slide with emphasis on internal positive controls. False negative results are possible for some antibodies. There are many other techniques to lift tissue from slides, so some experimentation may be required to find the most suitable method for individual needs.

References

Athanasou NA, Quinn JMW, Heryet A, Woods CG, Mcgee JO 1987. Effect of decalcification agents on immunoreactivity of cellular antigens. *J Clin Pathol* **40**(8):874–8.

Boenisch T, Farmilo AJ, Stead RH, Key M, Welcher R, Harvey R, Atwood KN, comps. *Handbook on immunohistochemical staining methods.* 3rd edition. DAKO; 2001.

Bussolati G, Leonardo E 2008. Technical pitfalls potentially affecting diagnoses in immunohistochemistry. *J Clin Pathol* **61**(11):1184–92.

CAP 2013. *College of American Pathologists Anatomic Pathology Checklist CAP Accreditation Program.* College of American Pathologists; 35–7.

Churukian CJ 2008. Pigments and minerals. In Bancroft JD, Gamble M, eds. *Theory and practice of histological techniques.* Churchill Livingstone; 233–60.

Economou M, Schöni L, Hammer C, Galván JA, Mueller DE, Zlobec I 2014. Proper paraffin slide storage is crucial for translational research projects involving immunohistochemistry stains. *Clin Transl Med.* **17**;**3**(1): 4.

Goldschlager T, Abdelkader A, Kerr J, Boundy I, Jenkin G 2010. Undecalcified bone preparation for histology, histomorphometry and fluorochrome analysis. *JoVE* **35**(1707):1–3.

Grizzle WE, Stockard CR, Billings PE 2001. The effects of tissue processing variables other than fixation on histochemical staining and immunohistochemical detection of antigens. *J Histotechnol* **24**:213–19.

Hammond ME, Hayes DF, Dowsett M, Allred DC, Hagerty KL, Badve S, Fitzgibbons PL, Francis G, Goldstein NS, Hayes M, Hicks DG, Lester S, Love R, Mangu PB, McShane L, Miller K, Osborne CK, Paik S, Perlmutter J, Rhodes A, Sasano H, Schwartz JN, Sweep FC, Taube S, Torlakovic EE, Valenstein P, Viale G, Visscher D, Wheeler T, Williams RB, Wittliff JL, Wolff AC 2010. American Society of Clinical Oncology/College of American Pathologists guideline recommendations for immunohistochemical testing of estrogen and progesterone receptors in breast cancer. *Arch Pathol Lab Med* **134**(6):907–22.

Jimenez-Joseph D, Gangi MD 1986. Application of Diatex compound in cytology: Use in preparing multiple slides from a single routine smear. *Acta Cytol* **30**(4):446–7.

Kamino H, Tam ST 1991. Immunoperoxidase technique modified by counterstain with azure B as a diagnostic aid in evaluating heavily pigmented melanocytic neoplasms. *J Cutan Pathol* **18**(6):436–9.

Kubier P, Miller RT 2002. Tissue protection immunohistochemistry: A useful adjunct in the interpretation of prostate biopsy specimens and other selected cases in which immunostains are needed on minute lesions. *Am J Clin Pathol* **117**(2):194–8.

Lars JN, JøRgen JS, Klaus G 1991. A method for histological preparation of undecalcified bone sections containing acrylic bone cement. *Biotechnic & Histochemistry* **66**(2):82–6.

Li X, Deavers MT, Guo M, Liu P, Gong Y, Albarracin CT, Middleton LP, Huo L 2013. The effect of prolonged cold ischemia time on estrogen receptor immunohistochemistry in breast cancer. *Mod Pathol* **26**(1):71–8.

Li LX, Crotty KA, Kril JJ, Palmer AA, McCarthy SW 1999. Method of melanin bleaching in MIB1-Ki67 immunostaining of pigmented lesions: A quantitative evaluation in malignant melanomas. *Histochem J* **31** (4):237–40.

Lunn G, Sansone EB 1991. The safe disposal of diaminobenzidine. *Applied Occupational and Environmental Hygiene* **6**(1):49–53.

Matthews JB, Mason GI 1984. Influence of decalcifying agents on immunoreactivity of formalin-fixed, paraffin-embedded tissue. *Histochem J* **16**(7):771–87.

Medawar PB 1941. The rate of penetration of fixatives. *J Royal Microscopical Society* **61**:46–7.

RCPA 2020. Guideline subject: Fixation of Tissues (online). Available at www.rcpa.edu.au/getattachment/d6f7f095-e8b7-45eb-8dcb-6a9d9bd5a88a/Fixation-of-Tissues.aspx# (Accessed 1 November 2020).

Shen H, Wu W 2015. Study of melanin bleaching after immunohistochemistry of melanin-containing tissues. *Appl Immunohistochem Mol Morphol* **23**(4):303–7.

Torlakovic EE, Nielsen S, Vyberg M, Taylor CR 2015. Getting controls under control: The time is now for immunohistochemistry. *J Clin Pathol* **68** (11):879–82.

Williams JH, Mepham BL, Wright DH 1997. Tissue preparation for immunocytochemistry. *J Clin Pathol* **50** (5):422–8.

Wolff AC, Hammond ME, Hicks DG, Dowsett M, McShane LM, Allison KH, Allred DC, Bartlett JM, Bilous M, Fitzgibbons P, Hanna W, Jenkins RB, Mangu PB, Paik S, Perez EA, Press MF, Spears PA, Vance GH, Viale G, Hayes DF 2014. Recommendations for human epidermal growth factor receptor 2 testing in breast cancer: American Society of Clinical Oncology/College of American Pathologists clinical practice guideline update. *Arch Pathol Lab Med* **138** (2):241–56.

Yildiz-Aktas IZ, Dabbs DJ, Bhargava R 2012. The effect of cold ischemic time on the immunohistochemical evaluation of estrogen receptor, progesterone receptor, and HER2 expression in invasive breast carcinoma. *Mod Pathol* **25**(8):1098–1105.

Yoo TK, Moon HG, Kim J, Lee JW, Kim MK, Lee E, Kim J, Han W, Noh DY 2014. Effect of prolonged cold ischemic time on immunohistochemical testing of estrogen receptor, progesterone receptor, and HER2 expression in breast cancer. *J Clin Onco* **32**:15 suppl e11505.

Chapter 8

Current Status of Immunohistochemistry

Trung Nguyen

Overview

The continuous evolution and development of immunohistochemistry (IHC) throughout the years has culminated in a technology that is widely accepted, is considered essential and is currently applied in both diagnostic laboratories and research facilities globally. Antibodies are now more reliable, reagents for epitope retrieval consistently achieve successful outcomes and detection systems are constantly proven. The advent of robotic automation has provided precise control over incubation time and temperature conditions for the IHC assay. These factors and a concerted effort to 'standardize' IHC protocols have contributed to the evolution of the IHC assay as a medical device classified as *in vitro* diagnostic (IVD) by the Therapeutic Goods Administration (TGA) in Australia.

Before the reasons for conferring IVD status are conveyed in this chapter, a summary of common terminology relating to IHC is offered. Key words such as *assay validation*, *verification*, *sensitivity* and *specificity* are examined. These terms are often used interchangeably but there are specific differences in their meaning. Other examples include *accuracy*, *precision*, *resolution* and *resolving power*. These terms' use within an overall IHC context is explained. The contrasting nature of a predictive marker versus a prognostic one is also evaluated because understanding the nuances of IHC terminology will assist in an overall appreciation of the subject.

After key terminology concepts have been covered, the IHC facility within the broader diagnostic pathology framework and the numerous applications requiring IHC stains are discussed. A dissertation incorporating how and where IHC assays are developed, the capacity in which they are used and the occasions when they are relied upon is reviewed. Key concepts and the complex tasks to achieve IHC standardization are appraised in relation to assay protocols and antibodies.

A commentary on how IHC is employed for accurate diagnosis and predicting patient prognosis is outlined with reference to cancers of lung, bowel, breast and melanoma. A treatise on the deployment of IHC for all body systems is beyond the scope of this chapter. The 'big four' tumours selected represent the utilization of IHC as IVD assays and associated molecular techniques to find appropriate treatments for the patient in the most efficient manner. Immunohistochemical digitization and image analysis with artificial intelligence is beginning to be adopted, but has not reached mainstream acceptance. Hence digital technologies such as whole slide imaging are discussed in Chapter 9. The current status of diagnostic IHC is presented within the context of the 'what, where, how, when and why'. At the conclusion of this chapter, it is hoped that an awareness is gained of the challenges IHC laboratories face and the efforts involved in producing a clean, crisp and reliable IHC stain.

Key Terminology Concepts

Certain buzzwords or common phrases are heard when working within the field of IHC and indeed pathology. Although similar in their intended meaning, there are subtle differences, and it is incumbent on the IHC professional to select the correct word for the situation. Some of the phrases readily heard in the laboratory are listed next along with their contextual meaning.

Immunohistochemistry and *In Situ* Hybridization

IHC stands for 'immunohistochemistry', an analytical tool using antibodies to detect antigens or proteins expressed on cells, then visualized by microscopy. ISH stands for *in-situ* hybridization, the use of either DNA or RNA molecular probes to detect nucleic acid sequences contained within the cell's DNA repository and visualizing this hybridization by microscopy. *In situ* hybridization (ISH) has the ability to interrogate the mutational changes within a cell's DNA instead of proteins. In comparison, it is the lock-and-key mechanism of an antigen–antibody reaction (IHC) versus the base pairing of nucleic acids A to T and C to G (ISH) that is the difference between these two techniques. For both IHC and ISH, methods for labelling and visualization techniques can involve fluorescence or chromogenic means. At the present moment, an IHC assay is cheaper, faster and more readily available from laboratories than an ISH assay.

Sensitivity and Specificity

Sensitivity is a measure of the ability of a test assay to demonstrate the presence of the analyte, even if the analyte exists in low numbers. In terms of IHC, an antibody's sensitivity is a measure of its ability to demonstrate an antigen within a tissue section and to visualize the reaction by microscopy. An antibody with high sensitivity has reduced risk of providing a false negative result.

Specificity, on the other hand, is the ability for the antibody to discriminate between similar but different antigens. Binding to the wrong antigen (low specificity) will provide a false positive result. Antibodies for IHC ideally possess high sensitivity as well as high specificity.

Traditionally, polyclonal antibodies have higher sensitivity but lower specificity. This is due to the production of polyclonal antibodies via immunization of the host animal to result in a population of B-cells generating antibodies to different epitopes from the one antigen. Conversely, monoclonal antibodies show higher specificity but lower sensitivity because the immunoglobulins manufactured from a single B-cell and myeloma cell hybridoma are directed to just one epitope. All of the antibodies manufactured from this hybridoma cell line are identical. Fortunately, antibody production has matured to the extent that some rabbit monoclonal antibodies for FFPE IHC do, in fact, match the polyclonals for high sensitivity as well as retaining the high specificity monoclonals have always been known for.

False Positive and False Negative

A false positive result happens when the interpretation of the slide is incorrect by way of determining that an antigen–antibody binding reaction is observable as positive staining. There are numerous examples of how this can happen. False positives commonly occur when there is suboptimal blocking or quenching. The resulting 'positive staining' is not due to the presence of an antigen, but to endogenous tissue elements reacting with the chromogen.

Inappropriate reagents introduced to the IHC protocol is another cause of false positive results, especially when using mouse antibodies on mouse tissue. This occurs when using a secondary anti-mouse antibody to detect the primary mouse antibody, but in doing so, it also binds to endogenous mouse antibodies already present in the tissue, resulting in high unwanted non-specific staining.

An additional false positive causation is the presence of endogenous pigments such as melanin, lipofuscin and ferritin within tissue. These naturally occurring pigments may cause confusion when diaminobenzidine (DAB) chromogen is used because of the similar observable colour tone and be mistaken for real staining.

False negatives occur when there is a failure in detecting the antigen present in tissue – a mistaken determination of no antigen–antibody binding when in fact, there should have been. Common reasons include an inappropriate IHC protocol, a failure of reagents, including the antibody clone, suboptimal retrieval standards or misinterpretation of the IHC slide.

A simple mistake in using the incorrect antibody, such as using CD20 antibody when intending to use CK20 antibody, may lead to both false positive and false negative staining. Although CD20 stains cell membrane whereas CK20 stains cell cytoplasm, it can be difficult to distinguish the two, other than relying on morphology. Lymphocytes do not exhibit CK20 staining, and a false interpretation of positive staining will lead to a false positive result. Likewise, using CK20 antibody to label B-cells present in the tissue will not label them, even though they are present, resulting in a false negative.

Predictive Marker and Prognostic Marker

These two terms are used interchangeably. To separate the two, a predictive marker offers the ability to estimate the behaviour of a disease condition with therapy outcomes. Most often, these markers predict response behaviour towards a certain therapy regimen. For example, breast cancers ascertain oestrogen hormone receptor status because tumours expressing oestrogen are likely to respond to hormone therapy.

A prognostic marker outlines the intrinsic behaviour of the tumour itself if no treatment was afforded. For example, a high proliferation index as outlined by the Ki67 antibody suggests the cancer is highly aggressive, which means a poor prognosis. Likewise, colorectal carcinoma harbouring a BRAF mutation is associated with overall decreased survival rate (Koulis et al. 2020).

Resolution and Resolving Power

These two terms are used quite often within microscopy and image analysis. Resolution refers to the production of digital images and the number of pixels required to produce that image. In a digital context, the higher the resolution, the closer the image is to a conventional print photograph developed from film. High-resolution images contain high numbers of pixels, which, in turn, increases the number of bits used. These images contain increased levels of information and therefore ultimately increase the memory size of the image file.

Resolving power, on the other hand, pertains to a microscope's ability to separate two distinct entities. The juncture at which two points of reference merge into one is observable when the microscope is at its resolving power limit. The resolving power of an electron microscope is far superior to an optical microscope, highlighted by the fact that the optical microscope can separate two adjacent red blood cells whereas the transmission electron microscope has the ability to separate two adjacent organelles. The visible light spectrum is the physical limitation of the optical microscope. The optical microscope cannot resolve anything smaller than the wavelength of light. Electrons, on the other hand, can detect entities smaller than the wavelength of light and are thus able to resolve smaller objects.

Accuracy and Precision

Precision can be considered another word for reliability or consistency. A test assay has high precision if the result is the same after performing the test multiple times over a defined period. That is, the results have low variance and each individual result is consistently close to the one before it. Therefore, the protocol or procedure is precise because the result achieved today is the same one achieved last week, for example. In terms of IHC, the assay has high precision because it works all day, every day. Accuracy is a measure of the real value of the target. For instance, if there are 100 tumour cells in a sample, a test assay has high accuracy if the acquired result is very close to the number 100. Obtaining results with high accuracy means the testing system is unbiased or has low bias (Browne et al. 1995). An example of IHC accuracy is the reference range that 20% of all breast carcinomas are Her2 amplified (Wolff 2007). If an audit was conducted on Her2 IHC results from a laboratory and concordance was achieved with this reference range, the facility's Her2 IHC assay results can be considered accurate.

Verification and Validation

Often used interchangeably, these two terms can be separated with the use of antibodies as an example. An antibody manufacturer typically offers an antibody for sale after an extensive validation process. Within this process, the vendor will test the antibody for use in certain clinical contexts or for use under specific conditions. They will then validate the antibody against the intended purpose for use and will include this information within the reference specification sheet detailing the use of that antibody under specified conditions. For example, the Agilent pharmDx PD-L1 (clone 22C3) antibody has been verified for IVD use in determining the PD-L1 status of non-small cell lung cancers on the Agilent Dako Omnis IHC staining platform, in order to identify patients suitable for pembrolizumab (Keytruda) therapy (Roach et al. 2016). Although the antibody manufacturer has provided validation for this companion diagnostic assay, the responsibility still lies with the end user to verify the antibody is suitable for the laboratory to use within this clinical context.

The laboratory's verification process would involve staining the cell lines if they are included with the kit and to use the antibody with appropriate tissue controls known to have PD-L1 expression. Due to the fact that manufacturers often 'lock' protocols for these companion diagnostic assays, it is, in fact, an indirect measure of the laboratory's tissue fixation and processing compliance and all the other pre-analytical parameters.

On the other hand, if the laboratory chooses to use an antibody concentrate or a ready-to-use (RTU) antibody not intended for a specific IHC platform (using

Roche Ventana PD-L1 clone SP263 on a Leica Bond III, for example), the assay becomes an in-house IVD and it is the responsibility of the laboratory to perform validation processes because the laboratory is considered the 'manufacturer' of that test assay. The term *optimization* is commonly used in reference to validation and in this context, the two words mean the same thing. The validation process can be arduous. Considering both pre-analytical and analytical variables need to be accounted for, it is understandable why laboratories are moving to RTU antibodies for IHC.

To summarize, manufacturers validate and end users verify. These two terms are different from each other and both processes are required because when the vendor has given validation status to an RTU product, they have no control over the pre-analytical parameters such as fixation time and other conditions of the laboratory including in-house tissue controls. Therefore a verification process is needed from the purchasing laboratory before use on patient testing.

The Immunohistochemistry Facility within Diagnostic Pathology

A modern anatomical pathology laboratory includes histology, cytology, an IHC department and possibly a mortuary. Most laboratories incorporate IHC testing under the umbrella of anatomical pathology. Due to their complementary roles, it is rare to find an IHC facility separated from the histology laboratory. Usually anatomical pathology departments have a dedicated space for IHC purposes along with cytology and the mortuary practice. As highlighted in Figure 8.1 and reproduced from Figure 2.7, this is because IHC belongs to a process, a stage in the histology production line. The same formalin-fixed paraffin-embedded (FFPE) block used for the haematoxylin and eosin (H&E) section is also sourced for IHC. It is fortunate that IHC can be performed on the same FFPE tissue that was submitted for histology originally.

Traditional histological analyses of tissue specimens existed decades before IHC technologies arrived in the 1970s and 1980s for most laboratories. The advantages are numerous. The biggest benefits include the ability to interpret IHC results in the context of morphology. Another advantage is the convenience of using existing tissue specimens and the majority of IHC assays are performed on FFPE tissue, which is relatively stable and can be stored easily.

Although IHC can be performed at the level of individual cells (immunocytochemistry), greater information is gained from interpreting IHC in the context of a histology tissue section. For instance, Figure 8.2 shows the presence of carcinoma cells labelled with a cytokeratin antibody inside a blood vessel, indicating metastatic spread to a distant site. Labelling these cells alone does not give the full picture. Observing them within a blood vessel is the important parameter. The pathologist requests IHC stains in the same manner as ordering extra H&E levels and other special stains.

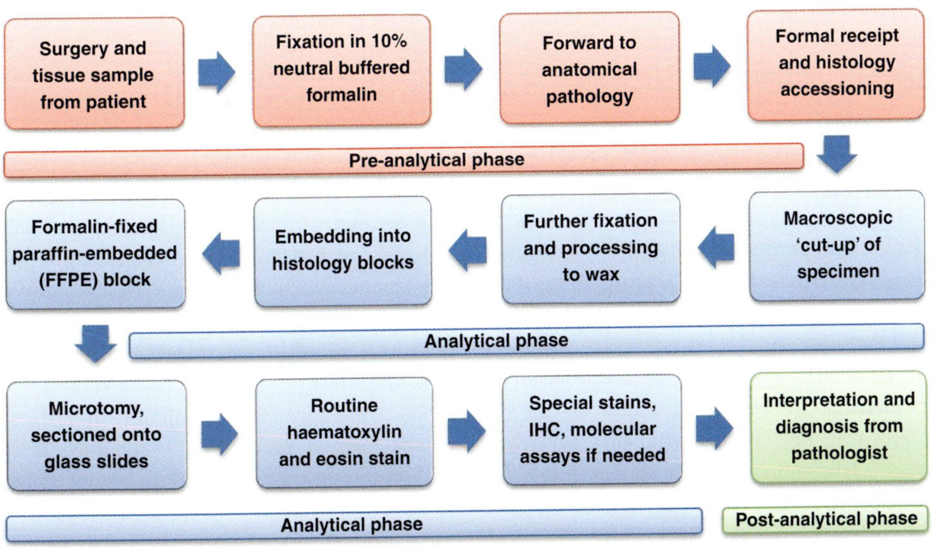

Figure 8.1 A stepwise approach to general histological analysis of tissue specimens

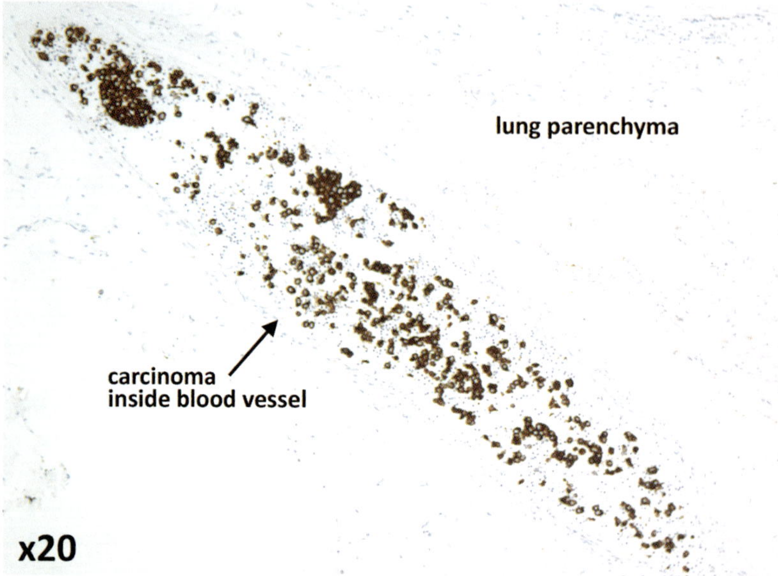

Figure 8.2 Cytokeratin immunohistochemistry stain showing tumour presence within the vasculature

Preparation of the tissue section for IHC onto a glass slide uses existing equipment already found within the histology laboratory.

Facility Requirements

The prerequisites for an IHC facility are not onerous. The main considerations can be categorized into equipment needs, reagent and consumable essentials along with adequate space provisions. Appropriately trained staff must oversee daily operations and troubleshoot problems.

Equipment and Space Essentials

The histology laboratory already possesses most of the equipment essentials for IHC. Unlike specimens for electron microscopy, for example, where fixation and processing protocols are vastly different, the majority of IHC assays are performed and compatible with the same formalin-based fixative, dehydrate and clearing regimens as well as other standard histology tissue-processing parameters. Likewise, the infrastructure for microtomes and the associated requirements for sectioning are already present. Some laboratories may set up a dedicated microtome and cutting station solely for IHC purposes. Others incorporate IHC sectioning into their routine microtomy set-up. The strategy employed depends on workflow and individual preferences. In a setting where multiple microtomes are used, the important task is to ensure all microtomes are aligned with one another and this alignment should be checked regularly. Refrigeration of IHC antibodies and other reagents is a must, and the laboratory should already have temperature monitoring at regular intervals.

Most modern laboratories will choose automation for their IHC assays due to the scale of their testing volume. There is no correct machine to choose as there are advantages and disadvantages with any model. With so many parameters to consider when choosing IHC automation (as discussed in Chapters 3, 4 and 5 of this book), the specific workflow and how the instrument complements the provision of IHC service dictates the form of automation for a laboratory. If limited numbers of cases do not justify full automation, a semi-automated or even manual IHC method is just as effective. The Sequenza marketed by Shandon is one example whereby a technician employs capillary action and gravity to manually apply reagent to tissue sections by way of cover plates. Indeed, IHC can be performed manually within a humidity chamber. If this is the scenario, it is important for the sections to not dry out during the procedure. Pretreatments for antigen retrieval are performed separately. Fully automated IHC appliances offer epitope retrieval on board within the system.

Some instruments do have a big footprint, so accommodating adequate space is always an important consideration. In addition to the physical requirements of the machine itself, storage of bulk reagents, refrigeration of antibodies and treatment of chemical waste products all need to be accounted for. All of these considerations should be easily accommodated within the existing histology facility.

For direct immunofluorescence (DIF) assays, a dedicated darkroom and specialized microscope set-up with appropriate filters for reflected microscopy and camera are required. Direct immunofluorescence techniques are similar to chromogenic IHC assays, only the label is a fluorochrome and therefore localization of the antibody is detected by a fluorescence microscope.

Reagent and Consumable Prerequisites

Acquiring tissue sections for IHC testing is identical to those for routine histology. The correct patient FFPE block is retrieved before a 2–3 µm section is cut with the microtome and placed onto a glass slide. The glass slides routinely possess an adhesive property so that the tissue section can withstand the IHC process and stay attached to the slide. A recommended practice is to place a tissue control section onto the same slide as the test section. These control sections may be pre-cut for convenience. The main reason for placing a control section and test section on the same slide is to prove that both tissue sections have been identically treated during the IHC assay. The FFPE IHC sections must be dried before dewax and 'taken to water'. Hence the consumables required for IHC to this point are common and readily available in any histology laboratory.

The reagents specific to IHC include buffers at specific pH levels, antibodies, detection and visualization reagents. Common buffers for heat-induced epitope retrieval (HIER) include Tris-based (high-pH) buffers and citrate-based (low-pH) solutions. Certain proteolytic enzymes may also be used to unmask antigenic sites. Antibodies are commonly of mouse or rabbit origin and are available in either monoclonal or polyclonal varieties. The detection reagents include the secondary antibodies, the peroxidase enzyme and the chromogen to visualize the IHC assay. Note that the type of chromogen needs to be matched to the type of enzyme label. In the case of peroxidase, the DAB chromogen is standard practice. For an alkaline phosphatase enzyme, DAB chromogen will not work. Instead, an azo dye such as Fast Red will. Similar to H&E and special stain slides, the IHC slide is mounted and coverslipped, ready for microscopy after staining. As with many reagents used in histology, the laboratory may choose to invest in RTU reagents or manufacture reagents in house from stock chemicals. For antibodies, the vendor would have RTUs to be certified as IVD or for research use only (RUO). Reagents prepared by laboratories are known as in house-IVDs and their use must be documented and notified with the appropriate authorities such as the TGA in Australia. As can be seen, offering IHC within anatomical pathology is a sensible approach. Most of the consumables, reagents and equipment are readily available to offer a reliable IHC service.

Staffing Obligations

Staffing and the qualifications required can be contentious. Some laboratories classify IHC as a subspecialty of anatomical pathology which requires a dedicated IHC senior scientist for adequate supervision. This scientist's main role is to oversee the provision of IHC obligations for the organization. Other laboratories deem IHC another type of special stain and will roster suitably trained personnel through the area. The strategy chosen depends on the complexity level of the antibodies provided. Certainly, wide-ranging and complex IHC services require a dedicated experienced scientist to manage day-to-day operations. The advantage is that there is a more intimate feel of how the antibodies are performing with the slightest deviation from optimal activity easily detected. If different people are rotated into IHC on a daily basis, it is more difficult to appreciate the subtle changes in antibody activity on the tissue sections. On the other hand, if the laboratory offers a small set of basic antibodies which are robust, reliable and easily managed, there is a good argument for enlisting different staff members working in IHC on a daily basis. Advantages include the redundancy to cover for staff absences and the accessibility of the laboratory workforce to develop IHC-specific skills.

Standardization Requirements

Laboratories may refer and request IHC assays to other institutions. There are many reasons for this. Expertise and the number of IHC requests for a particular antibody may be outside the scope of a specific facility. Antibodies are expensive, and if only a handful of assays on a particular clone is required annually, it is best practice to refer that assay to a laboratory that runs it routinely. Likewise, if a pathologist does not have the confidence to interpret the staining results, it is recommended to summon the referral laboratory to perform the IHC stain and interpret the results. Typical examples include semi-quantitative analysis for specific disease states such as ascertaining Her2 status for stomach cancer or achieving a PD-L1 score for triple-negative breast cancer. This scenario is most pertinent to referral laboratories tasked to perform IHC from tissue sections processed by a different histology facility. The reference laboratory has no control over the pre-analytical conditions attained for that tissue section or block. Therefore a reliance is made by the referral laboratory on the key aspect of standardization of histological techniques for the IHC protocol employed by one laboratory to work on tissue provided from another laboratory. Fixation, tissue processing and microtomy are specific considerations which must be closely aligned between the two histology laboratories. This is achieved by all histology facilities adopting a set of universal protocols. For instance, tissue fixation is dependent on tissue size, the nature of the fixative, the volume of fixative used, the duration of fixation and the amount of cold ischaemic time. If laboratories bring these parameters into close alignment with each other, the resulting FFPE tissue section can be successfully referred to different facilities for IHC staining.

The notion of one laboratory offering every IHC antibody available is a lost cause. It doesn't exist. New clones are available all the time. The more antibodies an institution offers, the more work is needed to verify and validate these antibodies. Increased effort is required to find suitable tissue controls. More refrigeration space is required and so on. The complexity level expands exponentially. Laboratories often choose to stock IHC antibodies according to clinical need. Small 'boutique' laboratories will have an inventory that is vastly different to a tertiary teaching hospital. Specialized laboratories will offer different antibodies to those of local community hospitals. The idea of creating a network of IHC laboratories which complement each other by offering to run assays on antibodies others don't possess or that can share tissue control blocks is crucial to overall IHC service delivery for a large population.

These 'networks' should include histology laboratories which cater to an area of specialty. For instance, a neuropathology laboratory would possess techniques and antibodies which a general histology facility may not have the expertise to perform. One such neuropathology reference service is the Victorian Neuromuscular Laboratory Service (VNLS) based at the Alfred Hospital in Melbourne, Australia. The VNLS receives muscle and nerve tissue from hospitals all over the state of Victoria. They offer routine H&E staining, special stains and IHC on formalin fixed and fresh frozen tissue in addition to Western blot protein analysis and electron microscopy. Some antibodies on offer at this facility are specialized for muscle pathology. For example, a general histology laboratory will not offer antibodies such as spectrin, dystrophin and sarcoglycan. Likewise, a specialist children's hospital will have an antibody inventory that is geared for paediatric pathology. The IHC markers for leukaemia and lymphoma, Wilm's tumour and neuroblastoma would be common in such an organization. These institutions are part of a good network of laboratories, each with its specific expertise from which other laboratories may benefit. Having this resource to refer to is a better outcome than trying to offer every single available antibody that is on the market within a single facility. For those markers that are required only a handful of times a year, it is good practice to refer them to another laboratory. This way the facility bypasses the laborious purchasing process, validation requirements and tissue control procurement activities which would have been mandatory to only use the clone a handful of times a year. Once again, it is stressed that standardization of histological processes is essential for this 'network' of laboratories to be fruitful.

Another example of the evolving professional relationships of histology organizations is when patients are referred to a different hospital for treatment. This may happen when patients have undergone surgery with their initial histology at one hospital and the oncologist refers them to a different cancer specialist hospital. Routine practice ensures the referral hospital requests the initial histology material for review. Quite often a request is made for the provision of a representative tumour block or a set of unstained sections on adhesive slides so further IHC or tests such as ISH and molecular sequencing analysis can be performed. In the past, the referral laboratory would also repeat IHC assays that were performed within the initial workup. In the present situation, more trust seems to be given to the original laboratory's IHC panel and repeat assays are not necessary. This stems from a higher degree of standardization achieved within current histology practices and includes IHC procedures as well as fixation and processing protocols. Such a level of standardization has resulted in IHC being more consistent between laboratories and allows, for instance, an external laboratory to successfully stain an antibody that they have validated themselves according to their fixation and processing regimes and apply it to successfully stain a section from another laboratory. This feat is made possible since fixation and processing of tissue is similar at both facilities.

Doing More with Less

There has been an increase in using less invasive techniques for the procurement of histology samples. If the clinical diagnostic question can be answered by a smaller biopsy, this reduces the risk of complications from major surgery or the need to do so in the first place. Neoadjuvant therapies have similar objectives for the patient. Another example is performing core biopsies for better patient outcomes in terms of recovery. Typically needle cores in the order of 10–15 mm x 2 mm are obtained. As is commonly the case, there are associated advantages and disadvantages in submitting needle core biopsies for histology. The most important consideration is sampling errors and whether a true representative sample of the lesion has been successfully obtained. More pertinent in this context is the sampling of patchy lesions otherwise known as heterogeneous tumours. For example, there have been instances where lung carcinomas show negative TTF-1 phenotype in localized areas. TTF-1 positivity is common in a lung cancer panel workup. If a needle core biopsy samples an area of TTF-1 negativity, this does not necessarily represent the entire tumour population, which may lead to confusion as to the nature of a patient's lung lesion.

Another example is in breast cancers whereby it is common to have heterogeneity in the hormone receptors within the breast tumour mass. Analysing a patient's oestrogen receptor (ER) status would be inaccurate if the needle core biopsy happens to sample an ER negative area missing the predominant areas of ER positivity. In fact, it is common practice to repeat the hormone status via IHC on the mastectomy or wide like local excision specimen even though they were previously done on the original breast needle core biopsy.

Another potential pitfall of using tissue core biopsies is the needle sampling an area of high tumour necrosis. The last thing a pathologist wants to see in a needle core sample is a prominent pattern of debris caused by necrotic cells. This makes interpretation very difficult and the IHC will typically return a slide that has very high background and non-specific staining. Being 'sticky', these necrotic fragments do not readily allow the antibodies conjugated to the detection system to be successfully washed off during the staining process. The chromogen therefore develops colouration at unsuitable sites. A tactic to reduce the risk of sampling necrotic areas is to target the periphery of the lesion because the central portion of the mass is often highly necrotic. However, there is also the possibility of the clinician missing the lesion entirely, forcing the inconvenience of a re-biopsy.

Whether it is a small needle core biopsy or a large whole organ resection, the same workup as described in Figure 8.1 has to be performed so the patient gets the best treatment possible. There is always an H&E stain followed by special stains and IHC if required. A panel of antibodies can contain anywhere from 3 to 20 antibodies and beyond. The reason IHC panels are chosen rather than just the one antibody in certain cases is because panels give a more definitive picture of the disease process under investigation. The IHC panels help in confirming a diagnostic impression by ruling out other, similar conditions. However, more tissue is required the larger the panel of antibodies chosen. In addition, the tissue core might then be subjected to further molecular-sequencing analysis. The quantity of tissue available for all of these analyses thus becomes an important consideration. A limited amount of tissue is available in core biopsies, and it is not uncommon to find there is not enough tissue or tumour yield to perform all of the required testing assays.

One way to mitigate this conundrum is to split the tissue core sample into multiple blocks. For instance, if multiple cores were sampled via multiple needle passes through the lesion, the received tissue cores for histological analysis can be processed in multiple blocks even though these cores can be easily accommodated into one FFPE block. This way an IHC tumour workup can be performed on one block whilst saving the other block for further analysis such as molecular pathology if required. All FFPE blocks will still have to be cut and H&E stained of course, and it is the reporting pathologist who ascertains if tumour is representative in both blocks. This is one method to save precious tissue. If all of the tissue cores are processed in one block, each successive sectioning of the block gets thinner and thinner and the tissue within that block diminishes. This strategy works very well for epithelial lesions such as carcinomas. Lymphomas, on the other hand, can be tricky, and so there is a preference from the pathologist to analyse the entire sample. This means every tissue core would need to be submitted for IHC analysis, a simple task if all cores are in the same FFPE block. Imagine if the sample was split into multiple blocks. The lymphoma panel, which is usually quite large anyway, would need to be performed multiple times because every block needs to be examined. Clearly some thought is required on whether to process tissue core samples in a single block or separately in multiple blocks. Provision of accurate clinical history from the clinician would aid this decision.

The demand for IHC is increasing more than ever before. This is seen not only in lymphoid pathology, but also in the area of what is collectively called soft tissue tumours. Most notable are the ones with spindle-type cells, requiring IHC to determine the lineage of the tumour. The main driver for this increase is the expansion in tumour subtypes recognized in various classification systems. All of these subtypes may have prognostic and treatment differences. The revolution in personalized medicine and tailored treatment regimens requires not only accurate diagnoses, but also prognostic and predictive information for targeted therapies.

The Various Roles Immunohistochemical Assays Serve

Immunohistochemistry has become ubiquitous. It is now considered an essential service to the anatomical pathology laboratory because it enables more accurate diagnoses. Assays are run every day and night in big, busy facilities long after the laboratory staff have gone home. Regarded as another cog in a plethora of histology techniques, it is often a second-line analytical tool called upon at the later stages of the histological process. A classic example is when IHC is tasked to classify an undifferentiated tumour into a particular cellular lineage, classifying the tumour as epithelial or mesenchymal and so on. Some tumours look remarkably similar at the morphology level, but IHC enables them to be distinguished for prognostic and treatment considerations.

In all cases, the corresponding H&E is required to ascertain the pathological condition within a morphological landscape. However, there are also instances when the IHC assay can be a stand-alone test performed concurrently to the H&E or used exclusively for diagnostic purposes. To add another level of complexity, the IHC assay must be applied to all tissue samples within anatomical pathology, a feat that is easier said than done, especially with bone and other heavily calcified samples. Debate still rages about the relationship of IHC and the traditional special stains. Is IHC just another special stain? The answer depends on one's perspective and it is time for an in-depth discussion.

Complementing the Hematoxylin and Eosin Stain

As highlighted in Figure 8.3, a pathologist examines the H&E section before requesting IHC markers. The gold standard stain in histology is the H&E stain. Pathologists and technical staff have been trained to interpret the subtle nuances and revelations from the combination of these two dyes. The aim is to extract and dissect morphological details from the H&E section at the specific moment in time when the tissue was removed from the patient. For such a simple stain, the amount of information contained within the H&E section is phenomenal.

The 'H' in H&E stands for haematoxylin, a naturally occurring dye derived from the *Haematoxylum campechianum* tree. The oxidized form of haematoxylin is called haematein, the active component of the dye, and when this is combined with a mordant, it forms the haematoxylin reagent used mostly for cell nuclei staining. Workers have exploited the versatility of this dye to fulfil different roles just by varying the type of mordant chosen. Most notably, Mallory used tungsten to stain striated muscle fibres and Verhoeff used iron to stain elastic fibres. Formulations are available for mucin staining and identification of calcium deposits in tissue. By far, the main use of haematoxylin is to stain cell nuclei and to contrast that with eosin. This is the 'E' portion of H&E and is also known as tetrabromofluorescein, a synthetic dye staining various shades of pink to red in cell cytoplasm and surrounding matrix. The combination of these two dyes allows interpretation of cellular processes occurring as a snapshot in time. Immunohistochemistry and, to an extent, other

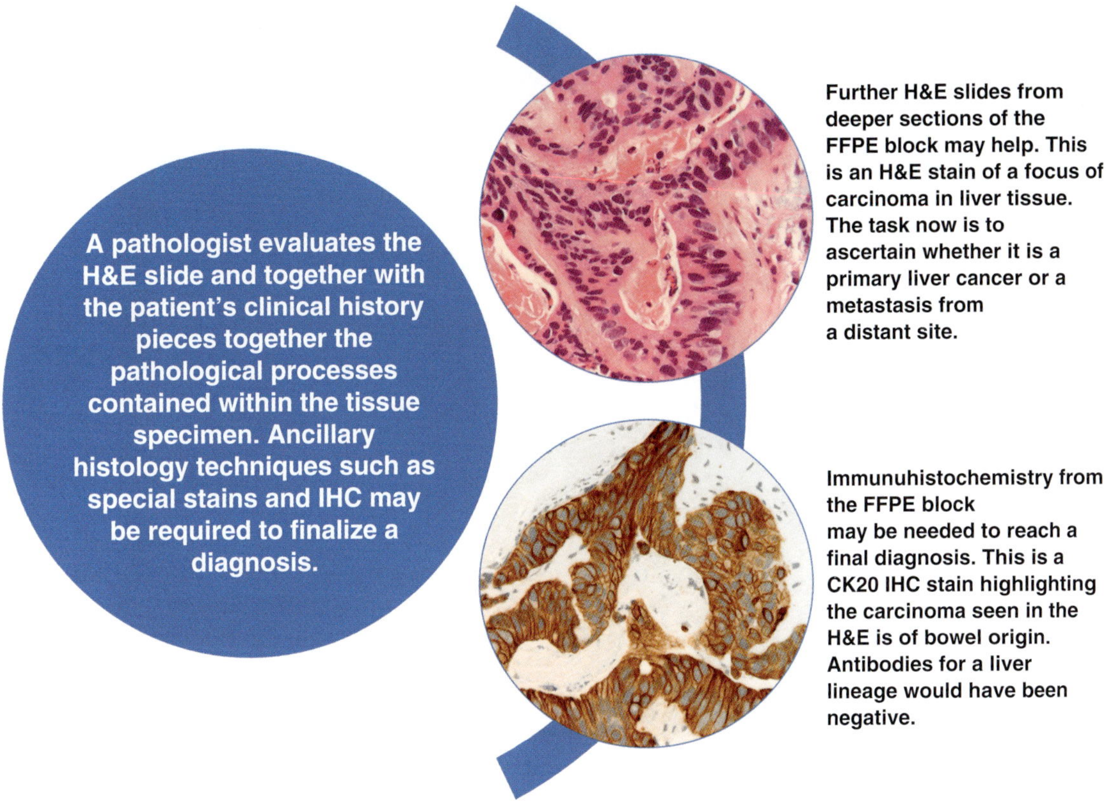

Figure 8.3 Immunohistochemistry comes towards the later stage of the histological workup

special stains offer an extra layer of information. To effectively manage the use of IHC in a clinical diagnostic context, the H&E stain is critical.

Front-Line Diagnostic Technique

Usually IHC ordering happens after assessment of the H&E morphology, but this adds more time to reach a definitive diagnosis. In cases of clinical urgency, both IHC and histology can run concurrently when there is high certainty that tissue used for IHC is representative. For example, a panel of ER, progesterone (PR), Her2 and Ki67 antibodies is routinely used for breast cancer IHC workups. The ER and PR assays are used to ascertain hormone receptor status, Her2 is employed to find the amplification status of the Her2 gene, and Ki67 determines the tumour proliferation index. Some laboratories nominate a particular block for these IHC assays when dissecting the breast tissue at the macroscopic 'cut up'. When the FFPE block is sectioned for routine H&E stain, the corresponding IHC markers can be sectioned at the same time. The IHC assays can be run and the stained slides given to the pathologist on the same day as the H&E stain. This achieves a faster turnaround time for diagnosis and prognosis, benefitting the patient. The clinician can then initiate appropriate treatment and management.

Another example of when IHC is concurrently run with the H&E stain is for investigations of skin-blistering diseases such as bullous pemphigoid lesions. The current protocol for investigating these skin lesions involves performing DIF on fresh frozen skin punch biopsies and scanning specifically for immunoglobulin and/or complement deposits within the dermal area of the skin. Figure 8.4 shows deposition of complement C3 along the dermal epidermal junction commonly seen in bullous lesions.

Direct immunofluorescence is a straightforward procedure. In this instance, a fluorochrome is directly conjugated to the antibody. The reaction depicted in Figure 8.4 uses fluorescein isothiocyanate (FITC)–conjugated antibodies applied to fresh frozen sections for 30 minutes at room temperature. The sections are then washed and mounted with an aqueous mountant

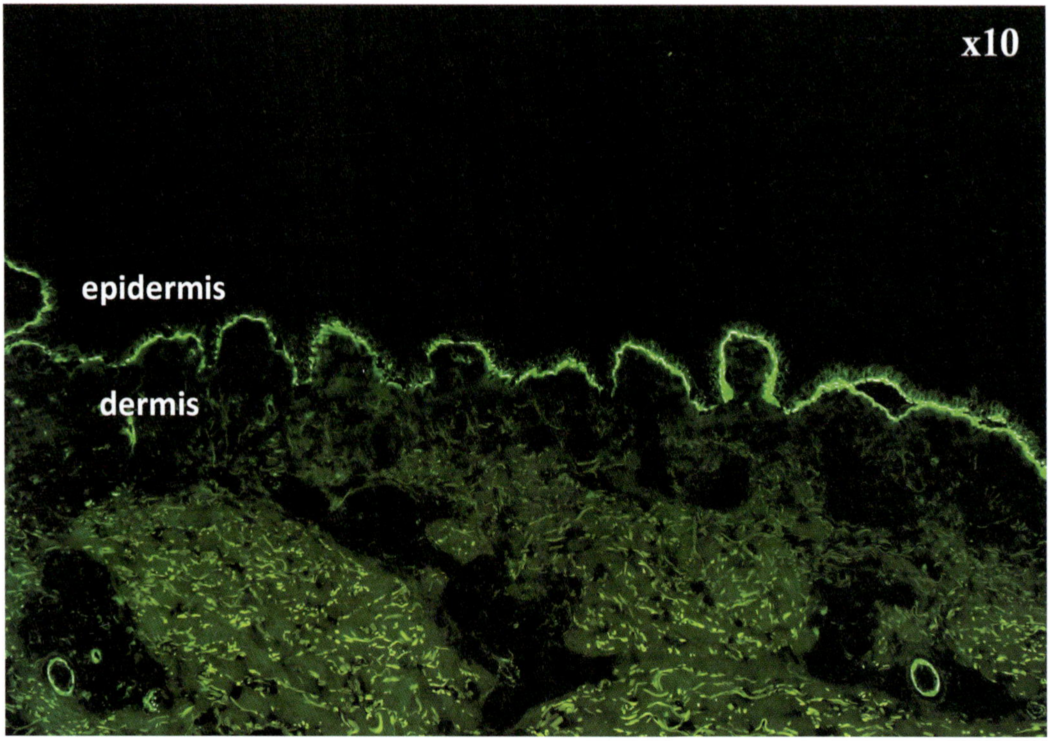

Figure 8.4 Direct immunofluorescence of fluorescein isothiocyanate–labelled C3c deposition within the epidermal/dermal junction

containing anti-fade properties. A fluorescence microscope set-up with appropriate filters for FITC is required. A different concept to transmitted optical light microscopy, fluorescence microscopy focuses wavelengths of light in the ultraviolet spectrum onto the specimen and the photons of light reflected off of the specimen are passed through appropriate filters for detection. To observe the fluorescence signal, a dark room is required, and it is common practice to capture images for record-keeping as the fluorescence signal fades over time. The science of fluorescence microscopy has major applications in medical research because it is possible to acquire different light wavelengths for multiplex studies. *In situ* hybridization assays can also utilize fluorescence (FISH) in both research and diagnostic settings. In a similar fashion in which IHC complements morphology for certain clinical situations, DIF and FISH techniques can supplement the H&E findings.

Some laboratories have tried rapid IHC assays on fresh frozen sections. The term 'frozen section' is used when a tissue section is acquired from a cryostat. This piece of equipment is essentially a microtome housed inside a cabinet kept at temperatures below 0°C, designed to section fresh unfixed frozen tissue. The cutting temperature of the cabinet is commonly set at −20°C. Terata and colleagues (2017) have described a rapid IHC protocol using a pan-cytokeratin antibody on frozen sections to determine both micro and macro metastasis within sentinel lymph node biopsies with a turnaround time of 20 minutes. At present, the importance of sentinel lymph node pathology in breast cancers has declined. The presence of micro metastasis has been shown to have little to no impact on patient outcome in terms of axillary dissection (Galimberti et al. 2013). Although most diagnostic histology laboratories shy away from routinely performing IHC on fresh frozen sections, perhaps there will be a clinical need in the near future. Current IHC technology certainly makes it possible.

Deployed after Tissue Decalcification

Calcified tissue is notoriously difficult to section without prior treatment to render the tissue soft enough for sectioning. There are two main ways to treat calcified tissue; via reagents containing acid, or the use of a calcium sequester such as ethylenediamine tetra-acetic acid (EDTA). The use of acids is the first line of treating very hard bone tissue in a comparatively short amount of time because turnaround time to diagnosis is tremendously important in a diagnostic setting. Most laboratories will automatically default to the use of hydrochloric acid, nitric acid or formic acid within a decalcification mixture. This strategy has proven reliable for subsequent morphology studies using H&E staining and special stains.

At certain times, IHC is required after a specimen has gone through the decalcification process. This is needed when there is suspicion of a metastasis into bony tissue, for example. What is becoming more evident now is that the use of acids can have a detrimental effect on subsequent IHC and molecular studies. Indeed, a gentler approach to preserve proteins and nucleic acids is preferred, but this strategy is also much slower. Not every antibody shows the same degree of decreased activity. What is the laboratory to do in this situation? There is an element of predicting the future of what is required even before the H&E is evaluated. This is because the tissue fixation, decalcification and processing steps are implemented before IHC is contemplated.

When it comes to the stage of sectioning and IHC, the fixation and processing regime cannot be undone. Keeping this in mind, most laboratories will decide on the most appropriate decalcification regimen on a case-by-case basis. For instance, since EDTA is slow acting, it can be used on small bony core issue or fragments such as bone reamings. To increase the rate of calcium sequestration, a small amount of heat can be applied during incubation and a 37°C oven is ideal. For larger specimens such as femoral heads, it is common practice to use acid-based decalcifying reagents because it would take weeks for EDTA to render that much bone suitable for sectioning. The most important factor to consider is that the tissue is well fixed before submitting it to any form of decalcification and to wash the block well in running water, especially after the acid decalcification process has finished. When it comes time for IHC, fortunately there are antibodies which complement each other and if one marker is adversely affected by acid decalcification, hopefully there is another suitable clone to enlist in the panel. For example, CD79a can be substituted for CD20 if the decalcification has negatively impacted the CD20 assay.

The dilemma faced here is that to perform IHC, a decent section on a slide is a requirement. Decalcification of hard bone tissue is therefore necessary. In a similar context, degraded DNA for molecular studies is akin to suboptimal fixation for histology. The recommendation is to avoid using acid as a form of decalcification in order to preserve DNA integrity. One may ask why this is so as molecular technologies such as next-generation sequencing (NGS) do not necessarily need 'perfect' sections. The sample is homogenized during the DNA extraction process anyway. The key point to understand here is that the integrity of the DNA is of utmost important in this situation. Acid treatment is known to degrade DNA, and it also hinders the reliance on complimentary base pairing for ISH assays using molecular probes. Although there are technical difficulties faced by IHC and indeed molecular assays, more often than not, satisfactory diagnosis of metastasis within bone samples via IHC and NGS assays is routinely performed on a day-to-day basis.

Immunohistochemistry and the Special Stains

The relationship between special stains and IHC is worthwhile to visit. Debate still rages whether IHC is just another special stain or something that deserves its own special area within the science of histology. To answer this tricky question, we must first define what a special stain really is. In the context of histology, a special stain is defined as any stain that is not H&E. Therefore, special stains are diverse and eclectic, including techniques of simple selective dye uptake, histochemical reactions, silver impregnation methods, metachromatic phenomena and enzyme histochemistry. Perls' Prussian blue, periodic acid Schiff (PAS), Masson's trichrome and Stokes Congo red for amyloid are examples of what histologists refer to as special stains.

Immunohistochemistry on FFPE tissue with DAB chromogen relies on enzyme histochemistry principles. The peroxidase enzyme facilitates the reaction of hydrogen peroxide, oxidizing DAB to a brown insoluble compound. It is logical to consider IHC another special stain in this context. But in addition to the peroxidase enzyme, antibodies have been introduced to bind tissue antigens. Some would argue that the technology behind this antigen–antibody complex goes beyond what has historically been considered special staining. The contention is that the production of antibodies, whether polyclonal or monoclonal, from various host animals makes IHC more than just a special stain.

Immunohistochemistry can be positioned as a special stain when differentiating certain tissue structures. Muscle tissue can be identified with common antibodies such as desmin and smooth muscle actin. Nerve tissue can be tagged with S100 protein or glial fibrillary acid protein. The demonstration of muscle and nerve tissue can also be achieved with traditional trichrome stain or silver impregnation techniques. Likewise, Helicobacter pylori infestation within gastric biopsies can be investigated with simple dye-based staining such as Giemsa and other azure eosinates, diff quick and Romanowski type stains. Metachromatic dyes are just as effective. Toluidine blue is one such example. Figure 8.5 shows two staining methods of *H. pylori* located within the glandular structures (red triangles) as a comparison. A diff quick takes less than one minute to perform, but the bacteria is difficult to differentiate from the background (A). Vartanian and colleagues (1998) overcame this issue by using alcian yellow with toluidine blue to add contrast to the blue organisms, making them easier to observe within the pale-yellow background of the glands. A specific antibody for *H. pylori* is available and provides a better view of the organisms (B). However, the assay takes two and a half hours and costs more.

The use of silver stains in the Warthin Starry or Steiner techniques is more complex but produces stunning results if performed optimally. Indeed, a good H&E section can also demonstrate *H. pylori*, especially when there are high numbers of infestation. Antibody markers for *H. pylori* are available for IHC and have shown to be highly sensitive and specific, but the protocol is longer than the special stain techniques highlighted. Some special stain techniques are preferred. For instance, a succinate dehydrogenase on fresh frozen tissue is the gold standard to observe mitochondria in a muscle stains panel. Equally so is the acetlycholinesterase reaction for Hirschsprung's disease in infants. Laboratories continue to rely on a special stains panel of FFPE liver biopsies. Ultimately the pathologist determines the demonstration technique in each clinical setting. The laboratory continues to offer both special stains and IHC assays. Certainly there is no clear delineation between the two and there is no doubt that IHC has crept into the special stains sphere, but each serves a specific purpose under the umbrella of anatomical pathology.

In this context IHC can be accepted as a special stain technique. On the other hand, when IHC is used to tailor treatment, to predict response to therapy or to enlist patients into clinical trials, it has changed from being a special stain to a technology with higher responsibilities. Markers for PD-L1, ROS1 and ALK status highlight the versatility of IHC because it is employed in many diagnostic applications. In addition to differential tissue staining, IHC is reliant for micro-organism identification, determination of tumour cell lineage and the classification and staging of cancers.

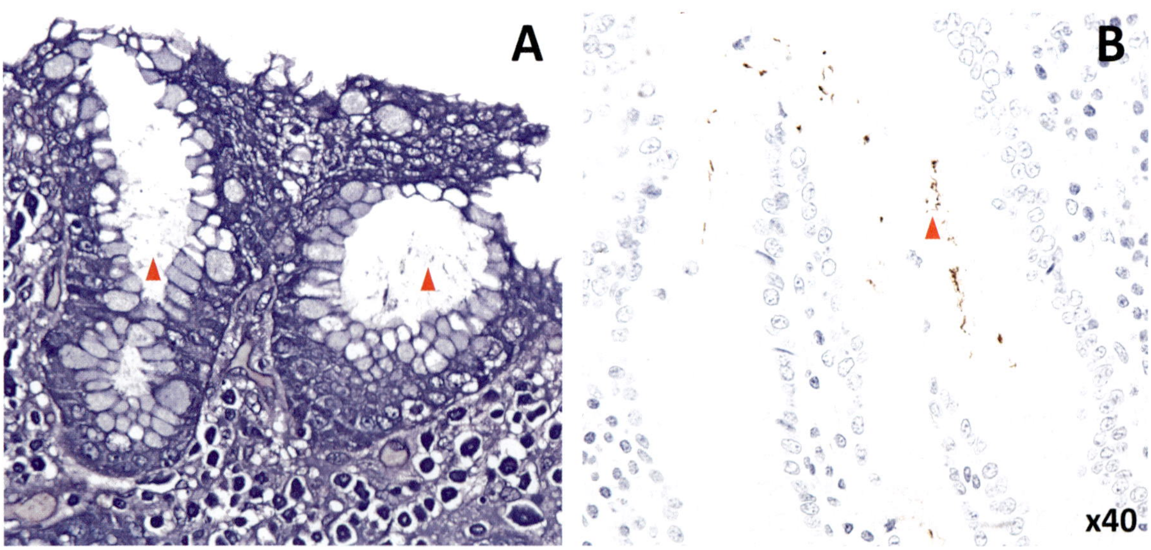

Figure 8.5 *H. pylori* demonstration with diff quick stain (A) and immunohistochemical stain (B)

Tailoring treatment according to a patient's IHC profile is a rapidly evolving and expanding field.

There are instances when IHC has become preferred to special stains. This is especially the case with silver impregnation techniques. The 'silver stains' are notorious for being capricious and difficult to optimize for inexperienced technicians. These methods rely on the impregnation of silver deposits onto sensitized tissue components similar to the old-style black-and-white photography developing prints. It doesn't take much to get suboptimal results. In the past, silver impregnation techniques were utilized for investigations of neuroendocrine tumours and commonly known carcinoid tumours. Nowadays, robust antibodies such as synaptophysin and chromogranin A demonstrate neuroendocrine differentiation. Moving forward, newer antibodies such as syntaxin are available (Kővári et al. 2020).

Quantitative and Qualitative Analyses

Another trend that is being seen within IHC is the increasing need for quantification, particularly for providing prognostic rather than diagnostic information. In these situations the assessment of staining now requires not only if there is staining, but also how much is present. A quantitative measurement may include the intensity of the signal as well as the proportion of positives within a cell population. Pathologists are traditionally trained to observe and interpret morphological changes in cellular processes and the added responsibility of counting cells can be attempted, but the questions of accuracy, precision, reproducibility and reliability of the process must be addressed. Although pathologists are highly skilled in interpreting what they see under the microscope in terms of pattern recognition, there is still a certain amount of inherent subjectivity. Inter- and intra-observer variability is influenced by the level of experience, the degree of training and the obtained skills of the pathologist. The quality of the H&E stain with its associated special stains and IHC also contributes significantly to an overall successful diagnosis.

One example of a quantitative measurement commonly required is the analysis of the proliferation index of tumours. This is a measure of the current state of mitotic activity the cells are in and can be taken as an indirect measure of how aggressive the cancer is. Proliferation indices are given as a percentage from an estimation obtained at best, but which may seem like an 'eye balling' exercise with Ki67 expression via an antibody such as MIB1 clone. Pathologists are trained to consistently use established methods on where to count and the number of cells to count, but there are limitations to this strategy. The biggest one is using a representative section to determine a quantitative measure of an entire cell population. To this end, the use of digital Ki67 counting with computer software is also limited. To really count cells under a microscope, one must employ sound stereological principles.

Most will not be familiar with the discipline of stereology. In essence, stereological principles state that to accurately count entities such as cells, the entire population – in this case the specimen – needs to be examined. By sampling the entire specimen, a truly accurate estimate of cell numbers can be achieved because the object is a 3D structure. A pathologist commonly only assesses one tissue section of Ki67 IHC stain for the overall proliferation index of the tumour. This is only a rough guess as the entire specimen has not been assessed. An assumption by default is that the tumour is homogeneous in nature, but this may not be the case for every specimen. Another possible area of concern is the variability amongst individual pathologists. When a collection of pathologists is asked to provide a score for an antibody, there should be a reasonable level of concordance within the group. In addition, if an individual pathologist is asked to ascertain a cut-off value of a tumour on a Monday, the same individual should provide the same results on a Friday afternoon when looking at the IHC slide again. The same answer is hopefully achieved six months down the track and so on and so on. As histology assessment continues to expand beyond diagnosis into providing clinical prognostic information, it seems the request to quantify IHC staining and provide meaningful quantitative data to determine if a patient is suitable for certain therapeutic agents will only increase into the future.

Standardization and Other Key Concepts

The aim of standardization is to look at processes with the intention of conforming to a standard. Whatever the 'standard' is, it needs to be widely disseminated so the objectives are realized. The importance of standardization has been raised in this book, especially in the context of pre-analytical, analytical and post-analytical variables. Optimal tissue fixation, appropriate use of controls and defined automation parameters have evolved the IHC assay to a 'standardized' platform which enables the exchange and staining of IHC slides between external institutions. This achievement would not be possible if laboratories were fixing and processing tissues in vastly different manners. In addition to standardization efforts directly affecting the IHC assay, there have also been attempts at using conventions when naming antibodies and their clones. Multiple names exist for one antibody and the question posed is why this is so. Related to this theme is the choice of chromogen label for the assays. What are the indicators that make a laboratory choose a specific chromogen over an alternative?

Tissue Fixation and Processing

The most important consideration for IHC on FFPE is the tissue fixation and processing. Suboptimal fixation due to delays, low volumes or time being too short is deleterious to morphology interpretation and H&E outcomes. For most laboratories, the default fixative is formaldehyde based and the most common is 10% neutral buffered formalin. Formaldehyde is a gas in its natural state and exists as a 40% concentrate weight per volume (w/v) aqueous solution. This 40% 'strength' reagent is known as 'concentrated' formaldehyde solution. The concentrate is then further diluted 1:10 – that is, one part concentrate to nine parts water – to produce a working reagent commonly referred to as '10% formalin'. Note the actual formaldehyde content is 4% from the concentrate. To avoid formalin pigment development in acidic environments, most laboratories buffer the 10% formalin to neutral pH. Thus it is now known as 10% neutral buffered formalin (10% NBF).

Some laboratories have established slight variations to this fixative. Some routinely do not buffer the fixative to neutral pH. Perhaps they do not regularly work with highly vascular organs or they achieve such a fast turnaround time from surgery to diagnosis there is a very low chance of formalin pigment occurring. As a safety net, formalin pigment can be removed with alcoholic picric acid treatment of the tissue sections prior to H&E staining. Some laboratories add sodium chloride to the fixative in order to simulate favourable osmolarity conditions for cell membrane integrity. Regardless, the choice of fixative and processing regimen must produce optimal tissue histology and morphology. Each individual laboratory chooses its fixation protocol for this objective.

Not only is a choice of fixative important, but so is the length of fixation and the volume of fixative employed. An adequate amount of fixative required is relative to the size of the tissue and should be at least 20 times (20x) the volume of the specimen (Rolls 2021). Fixing tissues and rendering them resistant to putrefaction and autolysis requires time. The process of fixation is like cooking food; it is a physical penetrative procedure. An adequate investment in time and volume is needed for the protein cross-linkages to transpire. At room temperature, 10% NBF penetrates 1 mm per hour into solid tissue such as muscle. Loose tissues that are easily penetrated into will be fixed the fastest whereas solid organs and fatty tissues will take longer for the fixative to penetrate.

Most laboratories are well versed in these two important factors of time and volume when it comes to tissue fixation. However, there are additional factors to consider. Often forgotten is the time taken to first fixation. This is what is meant by 'cold ischemic' time and is defined as the time interval from removal of tissue from a patient to the first drop of fixative applied to that issue. In an ideal situation, the cold ischemic time is measured in seconds and the length of fixation, with appropriate volume, is measured in hours. Figure 8.6 shows a spleen cut surface subjected to 10% NBF after two hours at room temperature before slicing. The black arrows indicate the brown discoloration in the periphery and around vessels signifying tissue that is fixed. The fixation front is clearly delineated with the majority red coloration designating 'raw' unfixed tissue.

Another factor to consider is to direct the fixative to the tissue in a manner that is most effective. There are plenty of examples where laboratories employ specific strategies to achieve this. Large, solid organs such as the spleen should be serially sliced in a 'bread loaf' pattern so as to expose the fixative to an increased surface area. Tubular specimens such as bowel resections are opened and cleaned for the fixative to penetrate both the mucosal and adventitial surfaces. Lung resections are 'inflated' and perfused with formalin. Hysterectomy specimens are sliced so that the endometrial cavity is exposed to the fixative. Urothelial tissue in cystectomies is fixed by introducing the fixative via catheter. Specimens are pinned onto a cork board if preservation of shape and orientation is important.

One other consideration often neglected is the temperature effects of fixation. Routine standard

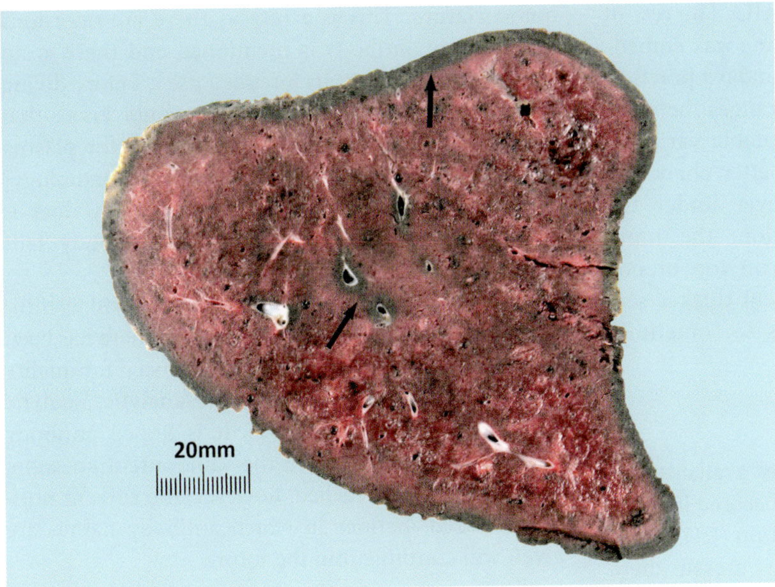

Figure 8.6 Spleen fixation after two hours at room temperature before slicing

FFPE fixation is performed at room ambient temperature. Increase the temperature and the rate of fixation increases; lower the temperature and the rate of fixation decreases. There is no need to place histology specimens fixing in 10% NBF into the 4°C fridge overnight after the anatomical pathology facility has closed. This occurs when overnight pathology specimen reception staff are not educated that this practice actually prevents optimal fixation. Another point to make is that fixing specimens at room temperature overnight will be undermined if the heating is turned off overnight. Especially in the middle of winter, the ambient temperature drops and so does the fixation rate. Taking into account all of the highlighted factors and using the ancillary techniques mentioned for specific specimens should ensure optimal fixation and gives every chance of IHC success.

To clearly demonstrate this point, analysis of microsatellite instability status of bowel tumours can be referenced. Endoscopic specimens are typically 2–3 mm in size and are placed directly into fixative as soon as the biopsy is taken. The cold ischemic time being measured in seconds, an appropriate volume of fixative being applied and the time duration of fixation all being appropriate will engender an optimal MMR IHC assay. Compare these characteristics to a big specimen such as anterior resection of the bowel and the fixation challenges start to mount up. The most important area to target fixation is the epithelial mucosal lining of the bowel. The laboratory has to 'open' bowel resections and clean and dispose faecal contents so optimal fixation can occur. Some laboratories routinely pin them out flat onto a cork board for the best fixation. The time interval between resection and the laboratory cleaning and opening the bowel has to be as short as possible. High-performing organizations keep this time to an absolute minimum. When comparing the staining results of an optimally fixed endoscopy biopsy versus a large resection, you can appreciate the difference in IHC results between properly fixed tissue and one that is suboptimally fixed.

Once the tissue is adequately fixed in formalin, tissue processing continues with dehydrating alcohols, whose primary focus is to displace water content from the tissue blocks. An additional benefit of using ethanol is the secondary fixation property of these reagents and that alcohol is not detrimental to IHC studies. Most laboratories after dehydration will clear with a solvent such as xylene in order to prepare tissue for wax infiltration. Historically, the term 'clearing' reagent was coined because the tissue blocks actually appeared clear when observed macroscopically after adequate solvent treatment. Some laboratories have become 'xylene free' and found that isopropanol can be used as a dehydrating agent as well as a clearing agent with no ill consequences for IHC. The rest of the FFPE histological process involving wax embedding and microtome sectioning is standard practice. Routine tissue section thickness ranges between 2 µm to 4 µm, and this is an acceptable variation for IHC. Thinner sections offer a better chance to view individual cells as a monolayer under the microscope. The thicker the section, the more chance that cells are seen stacked on top of one another. Technically, it is easier to cut thicker sections than it is to cut thin sections so sometimes a compromise is made.

Nomenclature

Given the vast catalogue of antibodies available, the nomenclature of antibodies has now become important. There is the cluster of differentiation (CD) number system for cell surface markers. At present there are CD numbers from 1 up to the high 300s (Engel et al. 2015) and calling the antibody via this CD number is 'loosely' followed. For example, many clones are available to identify the cell surface marker CD20 to isolate B cells within a lymphoid population. Convention states that the exact clone can only be ascertained through direct enquiry. The name 'CD20' does not offer information on whether it is polyclonal or monoclonal, from mouse or rabbit etc. In this scenario it is not important to know. In contrast, the PD-L1 antibody is also known as CD274, but the clone is important to identify because certain therapeutics are linked to specific clones of PD-L1.

There is no adopted convention by which antibodies are given their names. CD15 is equally called by its clone name of Leu-M1, CD117 is generally called c-KIT and CD45 is known as leucocyte common antigen (LCA). Similarly, the family of cytokeratins have been grouped and given numbers according to their acidic or alkaline properties known as Moll numbers (Moll et al. 1982). Antibodies such as CK7 and CK20 are commonly used to classify epithelial tumours without knowing exactly the clone used. Some years later, Schweizer and colleagues (2006) proposed an extension to the Moll system to accommodate the growing number of keratins being discovered. They also proposed to drop the 'C' in 'CK', so CK7 is now known as K7. Such is the strength of historic conventions still existing today that many laboratories have not adopted this new nomenclature. Excluding CD and Moll numbers, there is no widespread standardization in antibody nomenclature. This is a pity as there are occasions when a new antibody is mentioned and there is no way of knowing what its intended use is before diving into the specification sheet. Who would know that syndecan 1 is actually CD138, a marker for plasma cells? Or that PAX5 is used for lymphoid pathology? Sometimes working out what the antibody does is straightforward. Androgen receptor antibody tells you exactly its target antigen.

Perhaps IHC antibody nomenclature will eventually conform to a standardized format. There has been a monumental effort to recognize the need for quality standards in IHC in terms of pre-analytic, analytic and post-analytic parameters; it is hoped antibody nomenclature will receive the same attention soon. Until that time is reached, however, the current non-standardized manner in which antibody names are given will continue into the future.

Detection System and Chromogen Choice

As a tool, IHC is quite flexible in its use and applications. There is no one size fits all in regard to how a particular histology laboratory uses IHC. Currently, at the beginning of the third decade of the 2000s, most histology laboratories offering diagnostic IHC prefer polymer-based technologies and detection systems. They are available from many manufacturers, each marketing its own 'brand name' differently. Leica calls it the 'Refine detection system', Roche Ventana names it the 'OptiView detection system' and Agilent Dako refers to it as their 'EnVision Flex system'.

Older and superseded technologies such as avidin-biotin are considered inferior to a polymer-based IHC system for routine use. Amplification kits, unless absolutely necessary, are not endorsed as these kits synthetically overemphasize the true nature of the antigens within tissue. Artificially enhancing 'low-expressing' antigens for a visually acceptable threshold may introduce unwanted bias when quantification or semi-quantification applications are required. It interferes with the accuracy and precision of the IHC assay. Current routine diagnostic IHC protocols, the quality of antibodies available and the current generation of polymer-based detection systems provide satisfactory results most of the time. Protocols invoking amplification kits not only add cost to the IHC assay but also prolong staining times, which may be counter-intuitive in a diagnostic environment.

Amplification kits may be more appropriate in a research setting. Most laboratories also prefer the use of automation achieving staining times of two and a half to three and a half hours per slide. Add the advantages of batch staining, 'set and walk away' protocols and the benefit of overnight staining when staff have left the laboratory, and it is little wonder automated IHC has been firmly embedded into routine histopathology practice.

Deciding on the type of chromogen used to visualize the labelling of cellular components is not set in stone. In Australia the DAB chromogen is the default choice for routine FFPE sections. Its ability to discretely localize the antigen–antibody bonding with high specificity and sensitivity are the properties which make it a routine choice for IHC. The peroxidase enzyme is sourced from the horseradish plant and acts as a catalyst on the hydrogen peroxide substrate to oxidize the colourless DAB chromogen into a brown precipitate. This simple histochemical reaction requires fresh preparation before each use. Other laboratories may prefer a red chromogen for both peroxidase and alkaline phosphatase immunoenzyme methods. There is no right or wrong choice, and it is up to the individual laboratories to choose the most appropriate chromogen for each clinical setting. For instance, there are many situations where the brown DAB is hard to discern from naturally occurring brown pigments within tissue structures such as melanin, lipofuschin and ferritin pigments, which may lead to a false positive result. In such situations, a red chromogen compatible with peroxidase label is recommended. Similarly, haemopoietic cells such as granulocytes with very high levels of endogenous peroxidase activity most often cannot be effectively blocked or quenched. Introducing a peroxidase-based system for IHC is a recipe for false positive results. A simple solution for this situation is to deploy alkaline phosphatase as the enzyme label instead of peroxidase and use a suitable azo dye such as Fast Red for the chromogen.

Current Status of the Immunohistochemistry Protocol

The IHC protocol for diagnostic histopathology has achieved a certain degree of standardization even though there are many 'moving parts', and it includes parameters which can influence the end result. The actual IHC process can be summarized in six steps:

(1) Dewax tissue sections and take to water.
(2) Antigen retrieval, if required using either protease enzymes or buffers at low or high pH.
(3) Block and quench endogenous enzyme activity.
(4) Apply primary antibody.
(5) Employ secondary antibodies and the detection system, including chromogen development.
(6) Counterstain (usually with haematoxylin), dehydrate and coverslip.

The importance of using clean, high-quality water cannot be overemphasized. Wash and retrieval buffers are often prepared from concentrate, and it is important to always use the best-quality water possible for IHC.

Wax pens are popular to create a boundary around the tissue section concentrating the reagent onto the section and not the entire slide. This is a cost-saving exercise to use the least amount of reagent possible. These wax pens are most suitable when employing manual IHC methods. Current-generation automation platforms achieve frugal use of reagents without the need for wax pens. They aspirate 100–50 μL of reagent to achieve total slide coverage. Each manufacturer has devised different solutions to achieve this. Leica employs cover plates for the Bond III, Roche uses liquid coverslip for the BenchMark ULTRA and Dako endorses dynamic gap technology for the Omnis. Incorporating robotics for IHC is quite affordable in the current climate of precision medicine. Most laboratories have calculated a favourable 'cost per slide' when building a business case for automation and come to a decision that an investment in some form of automation for the IHC is a sound one. The convenience of reproducibility and reliability with IHC assays are the major determinants.

Epitope Retrieval

There is a preference for using high-pH buffers for HIER whereas in the recent past, more consideration was paid to both citrate low-pH and tris/EDTA high-pH retrieval solutions. The laboratory needed to find the optimal retrieval pH buffer for the antibody during validation. The default retrieval buffer now seems to be the high-pH solution.

The HIER methods are now more standardized with precise temperature control afforded by advanced automation platforms. The application of uniform heat energy to the entire tissue section for antigen retrieval purposes was questionable in the past. For instance, microwave ovens inherently have 'cold spots', which not only compromises the capacity to distribute heat evenly over the entire slide, but also reduces the high degree of reproducibility required for IHC. Current technology deployed via automation achieves this routinely. Enzymes are still utilized as an alternative form of retrieval, and it is important to remember that some antibodies are incompatible with HIER methods. Many laboratories nominate one enzyme for routine retrieval with Proteinase K popular as an RTU reagent.

Blocking and Quenching

The use of blocking steps to remove unwanted staining has been a long-standing necessity in the development of IHC assays. The exact blocking or quenching strategy depends on the IHC protocol. To keep things simple, diagnostic immunoperoxidase laboratories employing 'polymer' technology on FFPE tissue currently utilize only one blocking step. The application of 3% hydrogen peroxide aqueous is required to quench endogenous peroxidase activity within the tissue section. This chemical reaction produces water and oxygen as by-products. The oxygen is liberated as a gas, and if this process is automated, give some thought as to whether these oxygen bubbles may interfere with subsequent staining steps. Some laboratories prefer to do this blocking step manually on a staining rack, the theory being that the generation of oxygen 'bubbles' interferes with the uniform spread of subsequent reagents onto the tissue section, especially if there is application of some form of cover plate trapping the bubbles, preventing them from being liberated.

Biotin blocking is only necessary for avidin-biotin IHC techniques. These assays were quite popular in the 1980s and 1990s, but the minimum standard for IHC should be the current 'polymer' technology in the various forms marketed by manufacturers. Each vendor refers to its polymer technology differently. Leica has the 'Refine' kit whereas Dako has the 'EnVision Flex' series and Roche promotes the 'UltraView and OptiView' reagents. Application of a serum block and matching that to the species of origin of the secondary antibody is not required because in routine diagnostic human pathology laboratories, the primary antibodies are either mouse or rabbit origin. The secondary antibody, also referred to as the linker antibody, is manufactured and incorporated into detection kits to cross-react with mouse or rabbit primary antibodies. The species from which the anti-mouse or anti-rabbit antibody conjugated to the polymer is sometimes not communicated by the manufacturer. Leica, for example, employs a rabbit anti-mouse linker but does not mention the host species for the anti-rabbit conjugated polymer (Leica 2019). Dako employs a polymer derived with goat immunoglobulins to bind the mouse or rabbit secondary antibodies (Dako 2020). Ventana substitutes the polymer entirely with a hapten-based detection technology.

Sticking to either mouse or rabbit primary antibodies enables a form of standardization that manufacturers can work with for diagnostic purposes. For research purposes, however, this may not apply, especially if the primary antibody is not murine or rodent origin. It is therefore incumbent on researchers to diligently find the exact nature of the primary antibodies they are using, but also the detection reagents to be utilized. Chapter 6 explains these concepts in more detail. In any situation, unnecessary steps that can be left out to make the IHC assay simpler and decrease protocol time is most welcomed.

Personal Preferences

There seems to be a bias towards the IHC stain being over-stained or overemphasized. Somewhat a subjective and personal choice, the default position of IHC staining is to end up with a nice dark stain for interpretation. Technical staff have adopted a preference of increased sensitivity sometimes to the detriment of decreased specificity. Some operators are ignorant to naturally low-expressing antigens because under the microscope they do not give a picture that is as appealing as high-expressing markers. When these low-expressing antigens are encountered, the first reaction is to artificially amplify the signal in order to achieve a nice dark stain. This practice can be counterproductive for diagnostic purposes. Take for example the CD10 antibody. Figure 8.7 shows a very strong intensity in renal tissue (A), but equally important, it is also positive in the lymph node follicles albeit to a lesser extent (B). Careful deliberations must be made when considering amplification steps for quantitative IHC because unwanted bias towards the end result may ensue.

Pathologists would agree more trust and reliance are placed upon IHC now than in the past. The technology has matured sufficiently regarding reliability and dependability because of increasingly standardized IHC methods. However, the gold standard of histology is always morphology with H&E stains, and it could be argued that the H&E slide can still sway interpretation if special stains and IHC prove equivocal. For instance, there has always been and will always be S100 negative melanomas. Remember 'tumours do not read textbooks'. Fortunately, a growing list of antibodies are available that can assist in these ambiguous diagnostic dilemmas. This, however, can be a double-edged sword because with more choice there is more responsibility and potentially more avenues for things to go wrong. It is easy to overcomplicate matters when there are more antibodies to choose from. An unintended consequence of having more markers available is that IHC panels are becoming larger and larger as more tumour subtypes are discovered and more prognostic information is expected by clinicians. This not only adds extra costs to the testing regime, but can also introduce more confusion for the reporting pathologist. Classification of lymphoma subtypes can result in a panel of up to 20 antibodies, for example.

Interpreting Immunohistochemical Assays

A clean, crisp and optimized IHC assay only requires a few moments to interpret under the microscope. There are essentially three main patterns of staining depending on the area of antigen localization. Figure 8.8 shows an example of a nuclear (A), cytoplasmic (B) and membranous staining pattern (C). Sometimes an antibody may localize in both nuclei and cytoplasm (D). Knowledge of theoretical principles of the protein to be demonstrated is important because it can serve as a type of inherent control when assessing IHC stains. For example, transcription factors such as TTF-1, SOX10 and Pax5 should show nuclear staining because these proteins are found inside the cell nucleus. A membranous or cytoplasmic localization for transcription factors means the IHC assay warrants further investigation because something is wrong. Likewise, the cadherin family of proteins is found on cell membranes, which should imply a membranous pattern.

Cytoplasmic staining pattern can be further categorized as demonstrated in Figure 8.9. Hepatocyte-specific antigen is described as speckled (A) and glial fibrillary acid protein exhibits a granular appearance (B).

Vimentin stains most tissue elements and is therefore a good antibody to use to check the health of the entire IHC system. Used as a surrogate IHC assay control, variable staining will result when there are problems with automation calibration. It is standard practice to validate new instruments by batch-loading vimentin slides in each slide staining position to test the consistency parameters of the new machine. If optimally calibrated, the new machine should stain each vimentin slide with matching intensity. If performed regularly, the state of detection kits, chromogen performance and other errors within the assay can

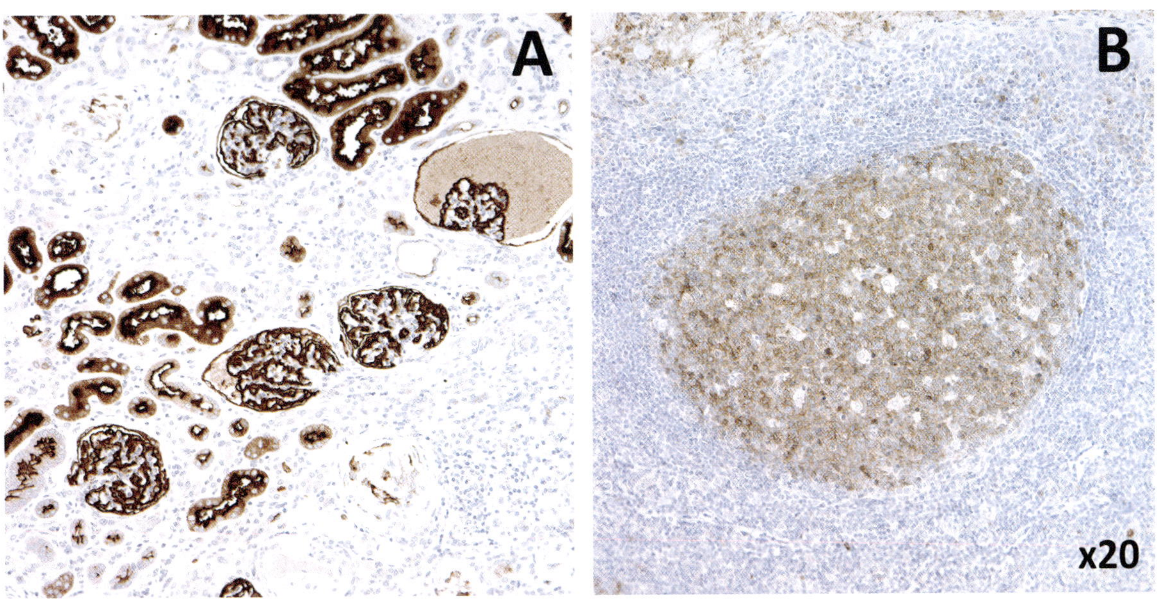

Figure 8.7 CD10 immunohistochemistry staining in renal tissue (A) and lymph node (B)

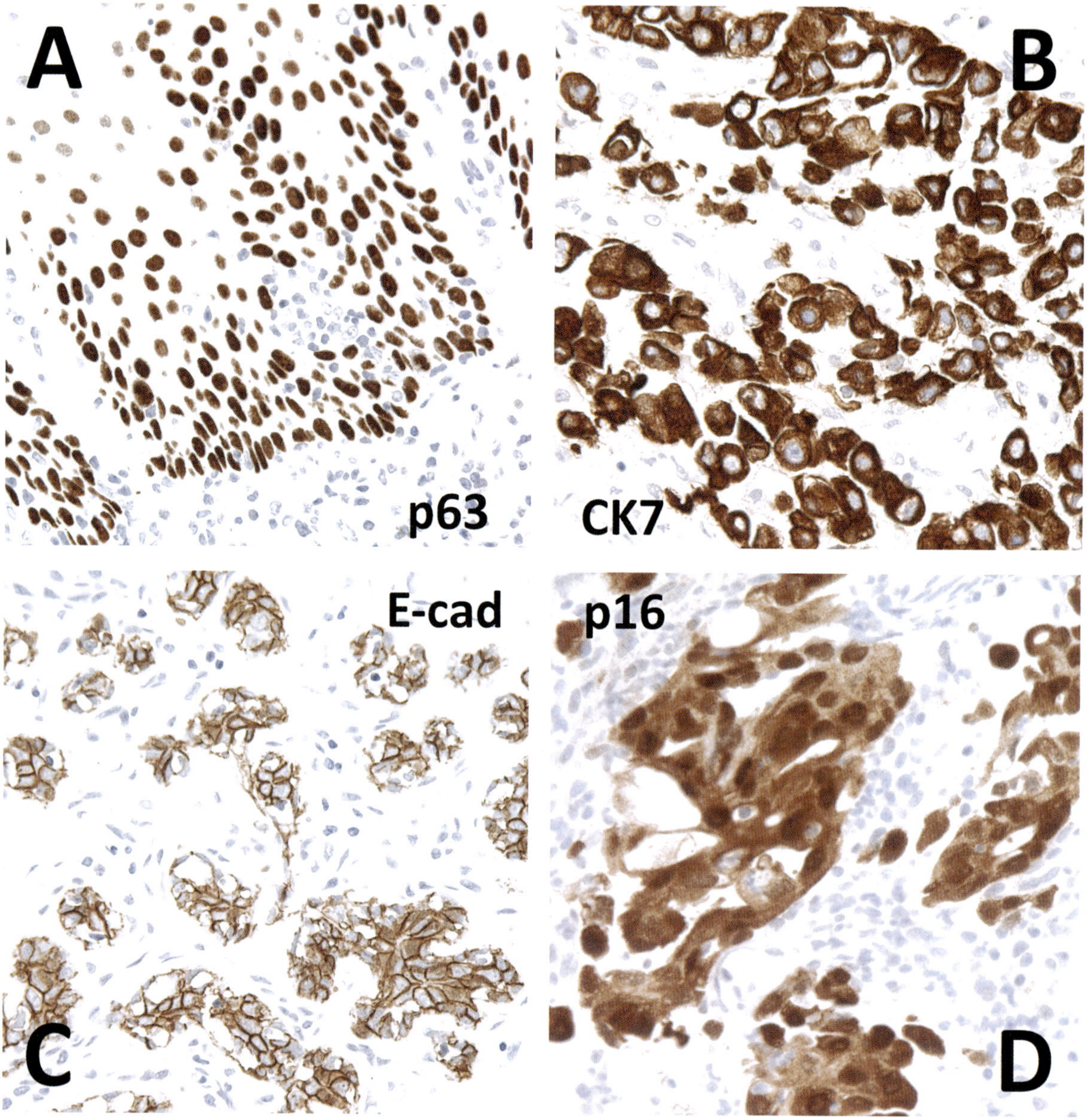

Figure 8.8 The main cellular staining patterns of immunohistochemistry. All images x40

also be monitored over a period of time. Figure 8.10 shows two examples of vimentin IHC staining. Note this V9 vimentin clone does not label skeletal muscle.

Current Status of Antibodies

The main themes when it comes to antibodies are the species of origin, how the antibodies were produced and the forms in which they are available from the market. As stated before, primary antibodies are either mouse or rabbit origin for diagnostic purposes on human tissue. This allows the detection system to be geared for these two species. The choice of clones can be overwhelming. Not all antibodies are created equal. Some are more robust and reliable than others. Resources such as NordiQC can be helpful to a certain extent, but it is ultimately up to the laboratory to find the best clone to suit its requirements. Unfortunately,

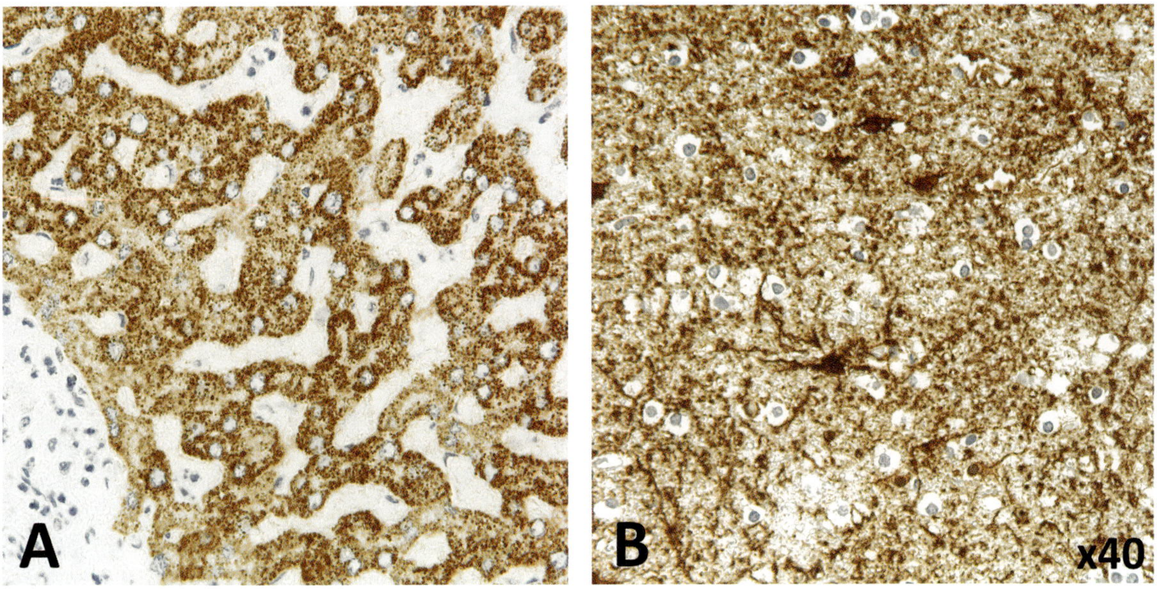

Figure 8.9 A speckled (A) and granular (B) cytoplasmic staining variation

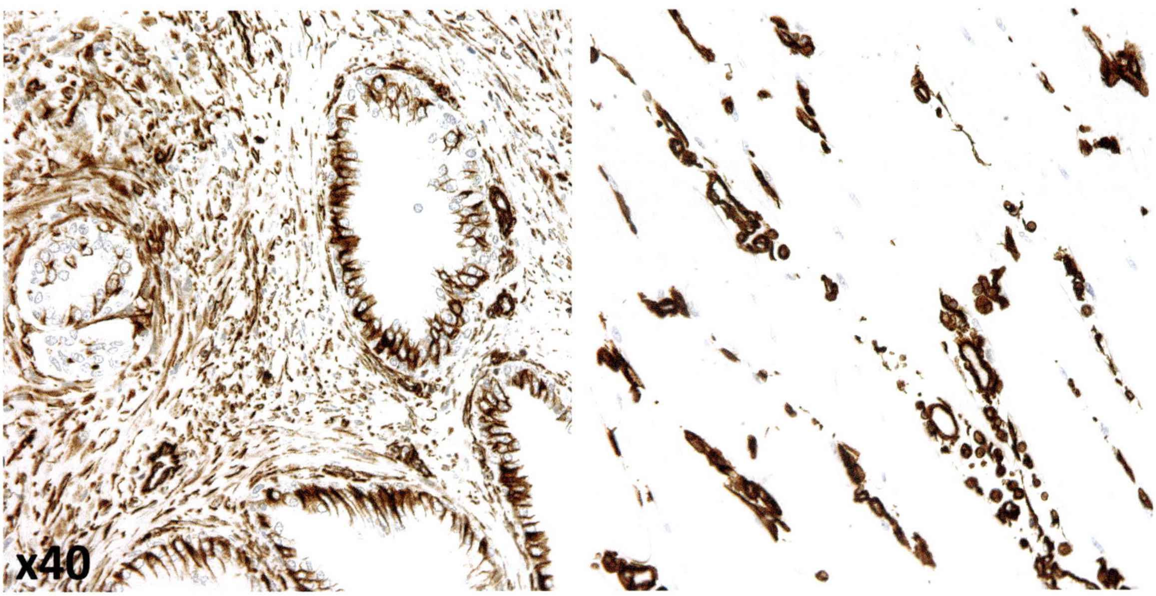

Figure 8.10 Vimentin as a surrogate immunohistochemical assay control

the only way to be successful is by attaining appropriate optimizing and validating protocols.

Concentrate and Ready to Use

Antibody clones are more robust, reliable and easily accessible today than in the past. Vendors are marketing pre-dilute RTU antibodies more aggressively, making them more readily accessible and competitively priced than concentrates. In the early days of IHC, most antibodies were purchased from the manufacturer as concentrates either in liquid form or lyophilized as a powder. Reconstitution with sterile water was required to attain the concentrate antibody. The onus was on the laboratory to optimize and find a suitable working titre, which is dependent on tissue fixation and processing strategy.

The notion of RTUs would not have been readily accepted 20–30 years ago because they would not have been reliable. A big issue that needed to be overcome was the lack of standardization in tissue fixation and processing. It was like the 'Wild West', a state of lawlessness with fixation standards differing between laboratories. Some of us remember using mercury or zinc in fixatives for optimal morphology or perhaps using chloroform for lipid processing. A concerted effort to standardize tissue fixation and processing (to a certain degree) has made RTUs a viable option.

At the present moment, the choice is as wide as ever with both concentrates and RTU antibodies available from many vendors. There is a slight trend in purchasing RTU primary antibodies for routine assays and 'tweaking' retrieval and incubation parameters to personal taste. Some companion diagnostic assays are only available as an RTU and vendors have the ability to 'lock' the assay to an instrument. Roche Ventana's PD-L1 clone SP263 on the BenchMark ULTRA platform for non-small cell lung carcinoma investigations is one example. Regardless, the quality of antibodies becomes a moot point if they are employed in tissue sections with a high degree of necrosis. It is best to always nominate viable tissue for IHC because necrotic debris is notorious for causing increased background staining.

Monoclonal and Polyclonals

Another observed change when compared to 20 years ago is that laboratories are preferring monoclonal antibodies over polyclonals. Some rabbit monoclonals can match the degree of sensitivity offered by polyclonals and, coupled with the traditional superior specificity offered by monoclonals, they have become more popular. The monoclonal antibodies have always had the desired specificity but have now also caught up in the degree of sensitivity. However, polyclonal antibodies are still quite useful. Take for example the S100 protein. This antibody has been around for a long time, mainly used for melanoma and neuronal studies. The correct perspective to adopt is that every antibody must go through a validation process and it is not as simple as picking a monoclonal over a polyclonal antibody by default every time. Remember successful IHC is also based on pre-analytical factors such as tissue fixation.

Take for example, the mismatch repair (MMR) proteins for microsatellite instability. In the past some of these clones were not very robust nor reliable. The MMR proteins are susceptible to suboptimal fixation and processing, especially when applying them to colorectal carcinoma cases. Degradation in IHC staining can easily occur for surgical bowel specimens that are not opened and cleaned as soon as possible after resection and before subjecting them to formalin fixation. Being sensitive to the effects of poor fixation, suboptimal staining was a common occurrence for these MMR proteins.

Whether the current improvement in IHC staining is due to better and more robust primary antibodies or because of a concerted effort to standardize fixation and processing is debatable. Perhaps it is a combination of both. It seems MMR assays are now more reliable and better overall because laboratories have realized fixation and processing of tissue for histology is extremely important. Take endoscopy biopsies of the bowel as evidence. These 2–3 mm biopsies are routinely subjected to formalin fixation as soon as they are sampled, ensuring optimal fixation. Rarely has an MMR IHC panel failed with endoscopic biopsies.

Antibody Cocktails

Antibody cocktails can be most useful in certain scenarios, and there are specific applications when multiple antibodies are utilized in one IHC assay in order to gain more information. Most commonly an antibody cocktail results in a two-colour development. For instance, PIN4 cocktails are used quite often in prostate pathology. This cocktail contains multiple markers for basal cells such as p63, CK5, CK14 or CK34βE12 and AMACR to investigate prostate intraepithelial neoplasia versus invasive carcinoma. As Figure 8.11 shows, it is a dual chromogenic IHC stain with DAB brown chromogen labelling the basal cell markers and Fast Red chromogen for the AMACR marker.

In this double labelling technique, the antibodies are applied to the tissue and the chromogen developed in sequence: DAB brown first, followed by Fast Red. The alternative to the PIN4 cocktail is to stain tissue sections for basal cell markers and AMACR separately on two different slides. Interpretation of whether prostate lesions are benign or malignant may be more difficult if the information required is lost in a subsequent

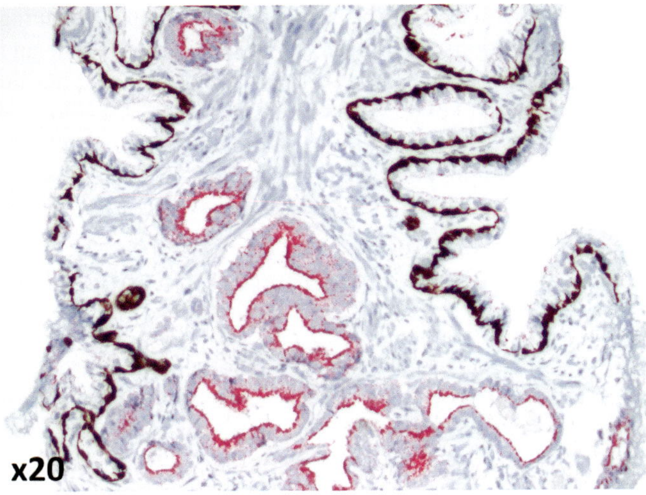

Figure 8.11 PIN4 immunohistochemical staining on prostate core biopsy

section. An obvious advantage of the PIN4 dual stain is that it saves tissue, only requiring one slide, and is therefore particularly useful in prostate transrectal ultrasound (TRUS) needle core biopsies. As a side note, TRUS biopsies are now largely replaced with transperineal biopsies in order to reduce the risk of colon bacteria (some of which are multi-drug resistant) causing infections.

Conversely, double IHC labelling assays take longer to perform and the cost per slide increases. However, the access to IHC automation and the PIN4 antibodies available as a pre-dilute RTU reagent makes the test more achievable. One reason it works so well is that the epitopes do not overlap or co-localize. For example, p63 is a nuclear marker whereas AMACR localizes in the cytoplasm and that in malignant conditions, the basement membranes break apart, resulting in non-staining of cytokeratins. The use of multiple clones and the need for two separate visualization kits means most laboratories run these assays overnight.

Antibody cocktails are also used for one-colour IHC assays. Take for example sentinel lymph node investigations for melanoma. There is a greater chance of highlighting melanoma metastasis if multiple antibodies are deployed in the one assay. Combining Melan A, HMB45 and tyrosinase antibodies into one cocktail and staining the lymph node tissue 'triples' the likelihood of detection, particularly when even one cell is counted as a metastasis. In this situation, there is no need to develop more than one colour IHC. As a screening exercise for the presence of melanoma, pinpointing the exact marker of positivity is not important. Note that the often-used S100 antibody for melanoma has been left out of the cocktail since lymph nodes contain Langerhan's cells, which are also positive for S100 protein.

Cocktails can also be used to differentiate cells within a population. One such example is determining the ratio of B- and T-cells on one tissue section. Complications arise when antigens co-localize to the same area of the cell or the retrieval process of the antibody clones is not compatible. To get around this, investigators have switched to immunofluorescence, using multiple fluorophore channels and then performing image processing. Others have tried various strategies to stain multiple epitopes in one section (Van der Loos 1999). Double and triple staining on FFPE tissue is not impossible but can be quite challenging. Regardless of inherent limitations, with constant discovery of new biomarkers, it is anticipated that there will be more dual staining with antibody cocktails in the future.

Quality Assurance

Quality assurance organizations around the world measure performance characteristics of antibody clones in conjunction with various IHC platforms, including optimal use of tissue controls. NordiQC (www.nordiqc.org) assesses multiple clones of a particular antibody for multiple automation setups and determines the most reliable clone for each scenario. Remember antibodies and in particular their clones are not all created equal. It is therefore up to end users to find the most appropriate clone for their workflow. This task can get very complicated as there is often a mountain load of information to sort through. Choosing a particular antibody clone is only the start. Choice of retrieval method and control tissue are equally important during the validation process of each antibody.

As times progresses, new antibody clones which are proven to be better are replacing clones thought suitable a few years ago. Take for instance the oestrogen receptor antibody. One of the earliest applications of IHC in a diagnostic framework was to assess the oestrogen status of breast cancers. Numerous clones are available and at the present moment, the clones SP1, EP1 and 6 F-11 are widely used. All of these are monoclonal antibodies from either rabbit or mouse, and all have been proven to provide optimal results according to NordiQC (2020). The clone 1D5 in particular has been widely used in the past but seems to have fallen out of favour in routine diagnostic use in Australia. It is interesting to note that the type of automation the laboratory uses does influence the choice of antibody clone. For instance, the SP1 clone has most use on a Roche Ventana Benchmark platform. The EP1 clone is more commonly seen with Agilent Dako machines and the 6 F-11 clone is associated with Leica IHC platforms.

There is nothing to stop the end user from choosing a particular clone for a particular machine. The trend nowadays is to use the clone recommended by the manufacturer of the instrument. Whether this is a good or bad thing is open for debate. Some say the manufacturers now have more control than ever before on how IHC assays are performed. The vendors, on the other hand, highlight the increased regulations and compliance required from organizations such as TGA that leave them with no choice but to 'close' down the platforms in order to achieve IVD status. This is one area that has changed most significantly within the past 30 or so years in diagnostic IHC. The automation is less 'open' than before. Take for example the design of the LabVision Link 48 autostaining system. This machine is totally open and parameters such as incubation times, volume dispense, step progression and reagent use can all be programmed for any protocol desired. In comparison, Dako's Omnis, Leica's Bond III and Ventana's BenchMark ULTRA are all vastly different machines in terms of programmability, especially in the use of third-party reagents. More specifically, certain individual protocols have been locked down, meaning conditions for antigen retrieval, incubation time and temperature parameters cannot be changed. The end user cannot deviate from Roche's PD-L1 protocol when using the clone SP263 for assessing PD-L1 status in non-small cell lung cancers. Not even prolonging incubation times is allowed.

Immunohistochemistry and Molecular Technologies

Molecular analysis of specific tumour-causing or associated mutations has increased within the past few years. Whether this molecular technology will replace IHC entirely is an interesting question. Firstly, to set the context, a little background as to why molecular techniques have been so predominant within histology is offered.

In situ hybridization and sequencing techniques are employed to investigate the DNA or RNA signature of the tumour. The cancer cells' DNA sequence is interrogated to look for changes in the genetic code. In actual effect, these investigations target mutations because it is these mutations that direct a change in the type of proteins the cell produces. Changes in the genetic code may modify the shape and conformity of the synthesized protein, and this alteration in the shape and how the protein folds may render the protein dysfunctional. For example, if a protein acting as an 'on' or 'off' switch for cell replication or synthesis has been modified due to a change in the genetic information, this renders the protein incapable of its proper function. The normal cellular processes stop because the usual checks and balances are ineffective. A failure to regulate cellular signalling pathways in protein production with an out-of-control 'switch' leads to cancer. The 'switch' may be constitutively turned 'on' and as such there is uncontrolled protein synthesis or cellular replication.

The question of where molecular techniques fit in with IHC is being addressed at the present time. The IHC is the detection of cellular proteins which may or may not be present whereas molecular techniques analyse the nucleic acid content of a cell. A change in a gene sequence does not always result in the protein product being altered. There can be 'silent mutations' resulting in a normal protein synthesized by the cell even though there has been a change in the genetic sequence. Another example of a change in DNA when there is no attributable difference in the phenotype is when the genetic sequence is amplified. This amplification would logically result in an increase in protein product, but sometimes this does not occur. Conversely there are times when there is an increase in protein synthesis without gene amplification via ISH studies. In these scenarios other upstream or downstream regulatory factors must be influencing protein synthesis.

Molecular studies do have limitations. For example, they cannot directly measure oestrogen receptor expression. This is important when assessing breast cancer prognosis and treatment options. Another drawback is that the minimum amount of tissue for a reliable molecular result is often greater than that required for histology diagnosis. Conversely, IHC is limited to analysing one or two protein expressions at a time. Testing for epidermal growth factor receptor (EGFR) status is possible with antibodies via IHC, but it is not advised. Many mutational changes may occur within this large domain, and so a better approach is to use next-generation sequencing studies to interrogate the entire EGFR gene. Sequencing the EGFR gene covers many types of possible mutations ranging from a single nucleotide polymorphism (SNPs) to whole areas of deletions. Thus the only way to definitively determine any and every change within this gene's domain is to sequence its DNA and compare it to the wild type sequence.

Similar to IHC and the relationship to conventional special stains, there is also a need for IHC and molecular techniques to coexist. There may be some overlap, but IHC and molecular assays are often complementary. For instance, IHC can be used as a screening test to determine which cases proceed to confirmatory ISH analysis. ALK and ROS1 assays are examples of using IHC to screen only positive cases for further ISH testing.

Figure 8.12 shows additional molecular testing required which clearly highlights the need to perform more analysis on tissue submitted for histology. This prerequisite of doing more and more with less and less material and the flow on effect of a longer turnaround time is a challenge presently faced in every diagnostic histology laboratory. In fact, the most challenging task for any anatomical pathology facility is being given enough tissue to perform all the necessary testing required. Take for example a needle core biopsy that is found to be malignant and has already been subjected to H&E, special and IHC stains. There is the additional molecular component as well as provision of tissue samples for clinical trials. In some cases, the original sample has been exhausted and a repeat biopsy may need to be performed.

Immunohistochemistry can be used as a surrogate for molecular techniques. Nuclear markers such as NKX3.1 are transcription factors derived from the *NKX3.1* gene (Gelmann et al. 2003) regulating cell growth in epithelial prostate tissue. Playing an important role in prostate tissue regulation, NKX3.1 acts as a tumour suppressor due to its ability to restrict uncontrolled growth. Present in both benign and malignant prostates, this antibody is useful in determining prostate metastasis in distant organs (Gurel et al. 2010). By analysing transcription factor expression such as NKX3.1, IHC is moving into areas previously only tested by molecular techniques.

A question often asked about tumour suppressor genes is why positive staining is seen in cancers via IHC, the logic being that staining should be absent because an absence of this tumour suppression would lead to malignancy. This reasoning is true in situations where there is a complete deletion of the *NKX3.1* gene. No gene equates to no protein production, which links to zero tumour suppression. The reason NKX3.1 is also positive in malignant prostate must be related to the degree of mutational change of the gene. This mutated gene is still able to produce the NKX3.1 protein in a form still recognizable by the antibody during IHC staining. A slight change in nucleic acid sequence leading to a minor conformational modified protein, although dysfunctional, is still close enough to the wild type form that the antibody can still bond with it in an IHC stain.

It is the highly specific nature of the protein towards prostate tissue that makes it a useful antibody. Although there is no such thing as an antibody being mutually exclusive to just one specific analyte, IHC is still relied upon because no other technology matches all of the benefits it offers. For instance, NKX3.1 is also found to be positive in some breast lobular carcinomas (Asch-Kendrick et al. 2014). In this instance, there should not be a problem because most breast lobular carcinomas are found in women whilst prostate cancer is exclusive to men.

The knowledge and expertise to successfully use and interpret IHC have always been important and will continually be relied upon moving forward into the future. The mutational analyses of gene sequencing and ISH, in conjunction with IHC, are driving the

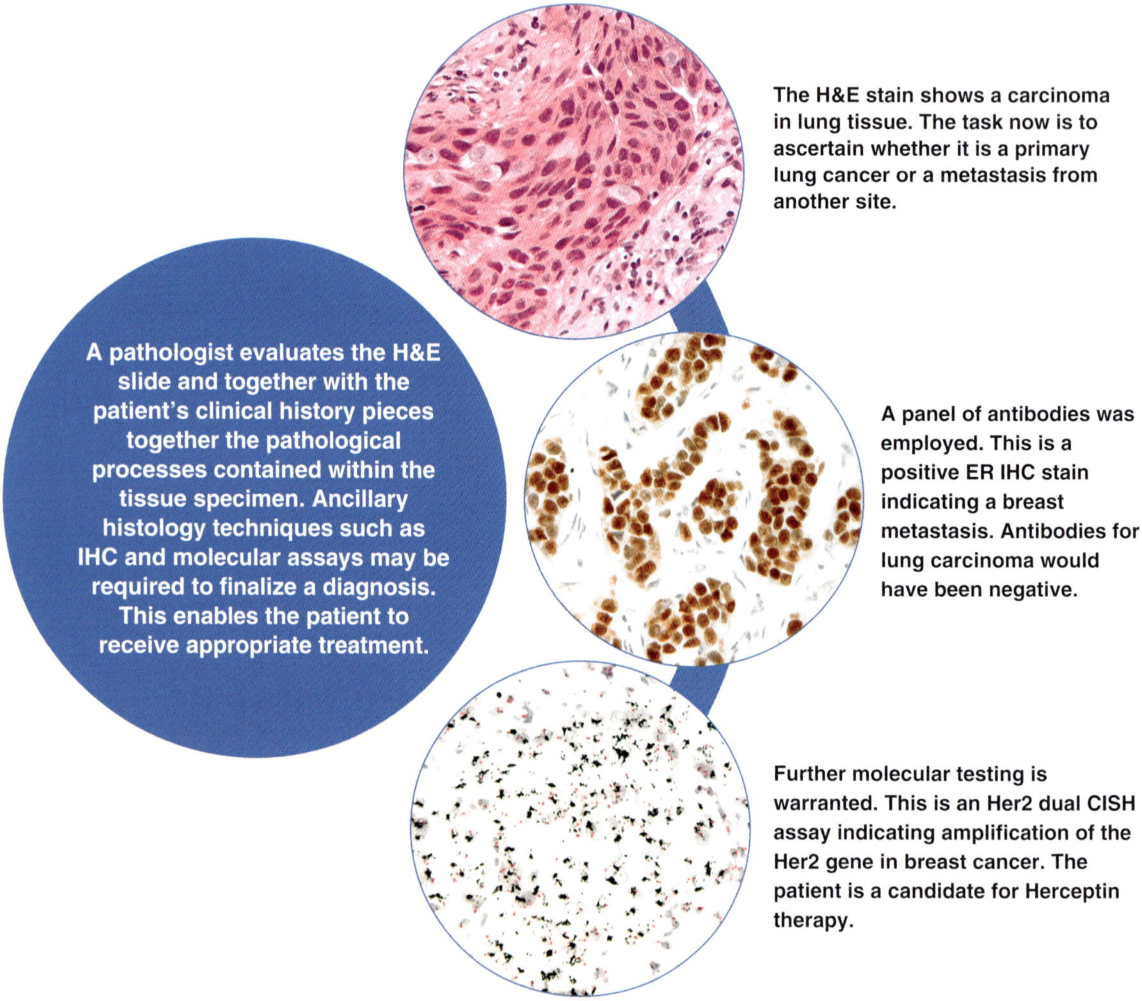

Figure 8.12 Addition of molecular techniques to histological analysis

revolution of personalized medicine and targeted therapy. Specific examples can be found with the diagnostic workup of cancers of the lung, bowel, breast and melanoma.

Lung Pathology

Advances in diagnostics allow tumours to be classified into more and more subtypes. Molecular studies with nucleic acid sequencing have led the charge, but IHC has also been employed with the advantages of being a more rapid and cost-effective assay. Nowhere is this more evident than in lung cancer pathology.

As highlighted in Figure 8.13, malignant lung tumours are classified into two main clinical groups – small cell carcinoma making up 20% and non-small cell carcinoma (NSCLC) making up 80% of all lung cancers (Yu et al. 2009). Within each group, subtypes emerge such as the carcinoids and atypical carcinoids along the neuroendocrine lineage and the squamous cell carcinoma (SCC) and adenocarcinoma within the non-small cell group. All of these subtypes have different therapy regimens and prognosis, stressing the importance for the histology laboratory to provide accurate diagnoses. Lung cancer classification continues to evolve with the discovery of NUT (nuclear protein in testis) carcinoma caused by rearrangement of the *NUT* gene found on 15q14 (Cao et al. 2017) and has shown to be effectively demonstrated with the C52 rabbit monoclonal NUT antibody (Haack et al. 2009). Although NUT examination is not currently in routine clinical use for lung cancer diagnosis, Inamura (2018) has shown NUT carcinoma to be positive for p40, chromogranin A and synaptophysin. A misdiagnosis of SCC or small cell carcinoma is a reality. At this stage, FISH assays for NUT rearrangement are still recommended as the gold standard test (Yatabe et al. 2019).

To highlight the role of IHC, a clinical example is given here using a lesion found within the lung. The abnormal growth must be confirmed as to whether it is a tumour, and if it is, whether it is of primary lung origin or another type of cancer that has metastasized to the lung. Hematoxylin and eosin morphology is employed in order to confirm cytoplasmic mucin and to determine whether the lesion is benign or malignant. If malignant, a typical panel of antibodies consisting of TTF-1 and CK7 is usually requested so as to confirm lung origin. Often TTF-1 IHC is enlisted as the solitary marker for lung adenocarcinoma, especially if the specimen is a needle core biopsy to preserve tissue for further PD-L1 and molecular analyses. If p40, a marker for SCC is also positive, TTF-1 staining trumps p40 indicating adenocarcinoma. Bear in mind that these antibodies are not exclusive to lung lineage, but they are still used with high accuracy in conjunction with the clinical situation and morphology.

When investigating lung lesions, it is common to also include antibodies for mesothelioma. This is a malignant disease of the pleura with strong links to asbestos exposure. A recommended approach to exclude mesothelioma is to include markers for both lung and pleural malignancies, BAP1, calretinin and CK5/6 for mesothelioma, along with the usual TTF-1 and CK7 lung antibodies (Ordonez 2003). Note CK7 may show positivity for both conditions.

Once a cancer of lung origin is established, the next step is classification. For neuroendocrine differentiation, the common markers are synaptophysin, chromogranin and CD56. Recently, a novel marker known as insulinoma-associated protein 1 (INSM1) has been reported to surpass the three in terms of sensitivity and specificity (Rooper et al. 2017).

Non-small cell lung cancers possess a plethora of antibodies to highlight the epithelial nature of the tumour and to subclassify them into squamous cell type or glandular adenocarcinoma distinction. Hematoxylin and eosin morphology can be helpful along with specific markers p40, p63 and CK5/6 for squamous differentiation (Yatabi et al. 2019). Adenocarcinoma markers are typically TTF-1 and Napsin A positive. Lung adenocarcinoma is then

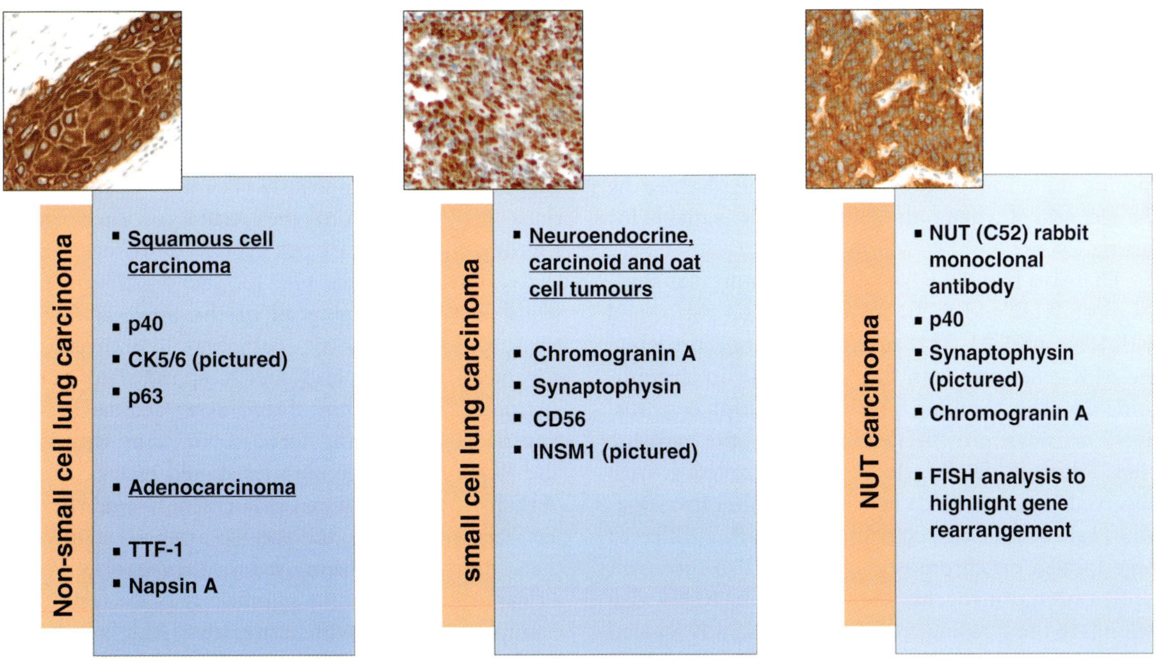

Figure 8.13 Subdivisions of lung cancer

further investigated for EGFR, ALK, ROS1 and PDL1 status.

Next-generation sequencing is the current and preferred mode of molecular testing to determine EGFR status. The EGFR domain on chromosome 7 and the tyrosine kinase signalling pathway have been shown to be a predominant driving force of uncontrolled cellular proliferation. Targeting therapies to these molecular oncogenic sites is the current mainstay of personalized medicine by way of finding mutations which interfere in the normal EGFR pathway (Lynch et al. 2004). Small molecule inhibitors are then deployed to arrest the overexpression of these growth factors, but the key is finding patients who harbour these mutations.

Many types of mutations are attributed to EGFR. These include single nucleotide pleomorphisms, deletions and insertions causing frameshift mutations. The most common are the substitution of amino acid leucine with arginine at position 858 on exon 21 (L858R) and the frameshift deletion on exon 19 of the *EGFR* gene (Zhuo et al. 2017). Next-generation sequencing assays have the ability to search for all mutations. On the other hand, IHC is restricted to the protein products of specific mutations. As such, investigators such as Brevet and colleagues (2010) have used mutation-specific clones 43B2 for the L858R point mutation and 6B6 for the deletion on exon 19 successfully. To prove the continuing evolution of antibodies in IHC, Kim and colleagues (2015) used different clones a few years later to the same effect. Regardless, there is not one clone that will determine all mutations described in the *EGFR* gene to date. Employing specific clones for specific mutations is not feasible, as highlighted by the scenario of when only scant tissue is available for testing.

There is a frontier where IHC and molecular studies meet. ALK and ROS1 analysis can be performed with IHC and ISH. ALK rearrangement occurs when the ALK gene fuses with the *EML4* gene on chromosome 2p. The resulting protein transcript constitutively activates growth factors within the tyrosine kinase domain, leading to the uncontrolled growth observed in cancer (Soda et al. 2007). Other investigators (Takeuchi et al. 2009) found *KIF5B*, a different gene located on chromosome 10, can also fuse with ALK, causing oncogenic overexpression. ROS1 also belongs to the tyrosine receptor kinase family located on chromosome 6. Many gene fusion partners have been identified, but the CD74-ROS1 combination is the most prevalent (Bubendorf et al. 2016). Due to both ALK and ROS1 being oncogenic, specific tyrosine kinase inhibitors are available to 'turn off' the uncontrolled growth switch. This is the rationale for identifying NSCLCs harbouring these gene rearrangements.

The traditional FISH technique of using dual-colour break-apart probes is considered the gold standard, but many laboratories do not have the resources to perform this assay. As a result, reference labs are tasked to do this testing, which increases turnaround times. Immunohistochemical assays are more accessible, which explains why they are being used as a surrogate 'molecular' screening test. Robust and reliable antibody clones are available to identify the protein products of these gene fusions. For their specificity and sensitivity, the D5F3 and 5A4 clones for ALK (Conklin et al. 2013) and the D4D6 and SP384 clones for ROS1 (Conde et al. 2019) are recommended for IHC. Figure 8.14 shows lung adenocarcinoma positive for ROS1 IHC clone SP384 (A) and ALK IHC clone D5F3 (B). As a screening test, only positive ALK and ROS1 IHC are referred for confirmatory FISH assay. Similar to Her2 breast IHC, a negative IHC result for ALK and ROS1 do not require further FISH testing.

These two assays are examples of companion diagnostic tests which have seen a rise within the personalized medicine sphere – that is, a test developed in relation to a therapeutic agent for the specific purpose of identifying patient populations who are the most likely to benefit from the drug. For logistical reasons, NSCLCs are submitted for ALK, ROS1 and EGFR assays simultaneously. Therapy recommendations are taken from the results of each assay. Immunohistochemistry has evolved and continues to evolve into a valuable tool for theranostic purposes whilst also maintaining all of the other traditional roles within diagnostic pathology. However, this advancement must also match appropriate quality assurance, quality control and assay standardization improvements moving forward. In cases with ALK and ROS1 testing, laboratories should include as part of their reporting regimen a statement to confirm IHC has been performed, the specific antibody clone and the automation platform used for the assay, as well as a clear explanation of the significance of the result. For example, NSCLCs with a negative ALK result are unlikely to respond to specific inhibitors to ALK.

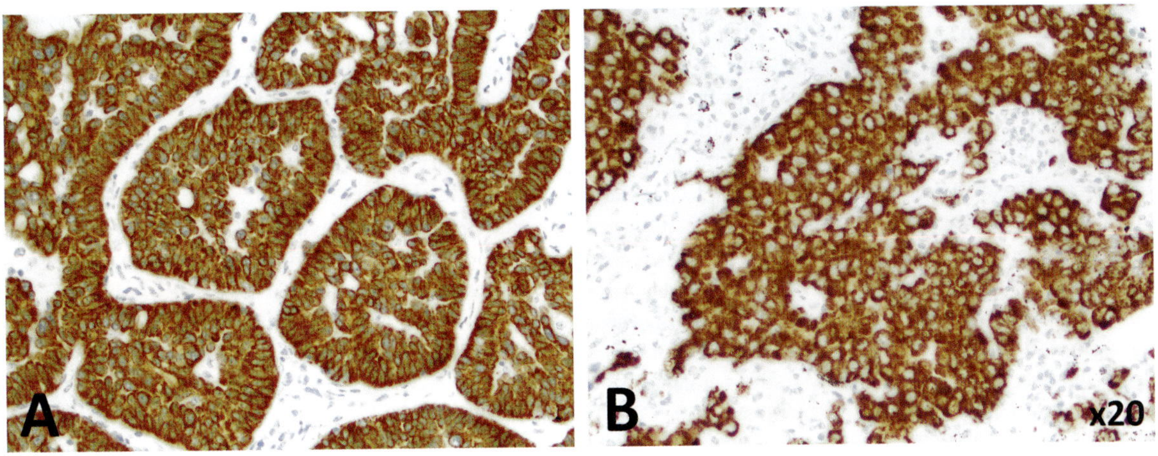

Figure 8.14 Lung adenocarcinoma positive ROS1 (A) and ALK (B) immunohistochemical stains

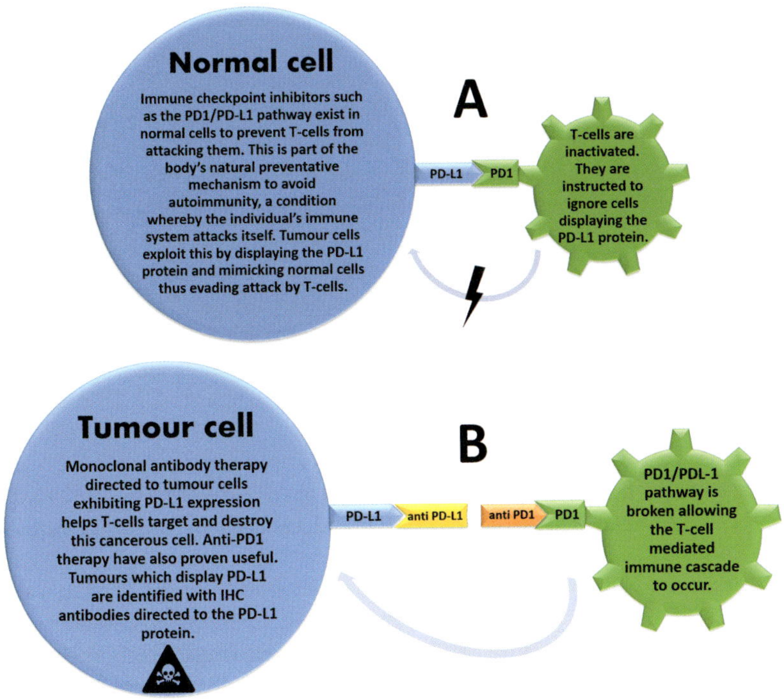

Figure 8.15 The PDL-1 pathway simplified

Note: Simplified representation omitting cascade factors such as T-cell receptor binding required to activate the T-cell response

The latest addition to the NSCLC testing armoury and also in other non-pulmonary cancers is the investigation of checkpoint inhibitors such as programmed cell death-ligand 1 (PD-L1). Figure 8.15 simplifies the rationale for testing PD-L1 status in NSCLC. It highlights how tumour cells evade destruction from immune T-cells by mimicking a normal cell, displaying and binding the PD-L1 to programmed cell death 1 (PD1) protein (Dyck and Mills 2017). T-cells are instructed not to attack cells exhibiting PD-L1 (A). Monoclonal antibody therapy to both PD-L1 and PD1 are available to 'break' this checkpoint so T-cells are activated (B).

Using IHC to identify PD-L1-positive tumours, a scoring algorithm specific to the PD-L1 clone is used to determine whether a tumour is positive or negative by way of cut-off values. The key significance is the exact PD-L1 clone employed for IHC and, to an extent, the type of automation, reagents and incubation parameters used. Several different PD-L1 clones are available from vendors ranging from Roche, Agilent, Spring Bioscience, Abcam and Cell Signalling. Investigators such as Parra and colleagues (2018) have tried to find the most useful clone for the Leica Bond Max IHC platform whilst other workers targeted a specific PD-L1 antibody such as clone 28–8 (Koppel et al. 2018) or clone 22C3 (Ilie et al. 2017) on different automated IHC instruments.

At the moment, end users can purchase any PD-L1 clone to apply to their specific automated or manual IHC platforms. These assays are known as an in house *in vitro* diagnostic assay or a laboratory-developed test. The onus is on the laboratory to carefully verify and validate its use and prove it is fit for purpose with stringent quality assurance measures. Most IHC laboratories find it simpler to use the manufacturer-endorsed clone because of the rigorous product research and development required for regulatory status such as FDA approval in the United States and TGA IVD category in Australia. You might as well use all of the hard work the vendor has done in bringing this product to market. For instance, a laboratory using the Roche Ventana BenchMark ULTRA IHC platform would be directed to use the SP263 clone for NSCLC assays. Due to this assay's IVD status as a companion diagnostic test, Roche has locked the protocol. The laboratory cannot change parameters such as epitope retrieval, incubation times or temperature settings. On the other hand, if a laboratory uses the Dako Omnis IHC platform, the same NSCLC workup uses the 22C3 clone for which the protocol is also locked by the vendor and as such, the PD-L1 IHC assay becomes 'plug and play'. However, the laboratory must still conduct a verification process.

This is a consequence of more and more standardization being applied to the discipline of IHC. Similar to Leica locking down their Oracle HER2 assay for the Bond IHC platform (Nguyen 2011) as more biomarkers are identified by IHC for specific treatment strategies, there is no doubt manufacturers will continue to lock down protocols for their instruments in the future. For this to occur successfully, the emphasis must be made on optimal tissue fixation and processing. This is the denominator and is critical in histology laboratories. There must not be huge variations in tissue-processing protocols between laboratory A and laboratory B, and this is the single biggest challenge facing IHC today. The robustness of clones, the reliability of automation and the availability of appropriate tissue controls are valid issues, but they all pale in significance when the quality of the analyte, being the test tissue submitted for IHC, is suboptimal.

Knowing the specific PD-L1 clone used is important for the oncologist because monoclonal antibody therapy clinical trials are available for specific PD-L1 clones. On assessment, there are clones which score the membrane staining of tumour cells whilst in other situations, evaluation of the immune cell staining within the tumour environment is required. It is important to know the scoring algorithm for specific clones. Figure 8.16 shows NSCLC negative for PD-L1 IHC (A) and a strong positive membranous labelling (B). These images are easy to interpret, but in reality, it can be difficult with tumour heterogeneity and macrophages also staining positive (C), which can mimic cancer cells. The IHC platform and the specific PD-L1 clone influences treatment decisions and therapeutic drugs such as nivolumab (Opdivo) or pembrolizumab (Keytruda) as examples of monoclonal antibody therapies (Silva et al. 2017). Further advancements on PD-L1 status have directives in place to use a specific clone for specific disease states. As stated previously, the PD-L1 clone SP263 RTU has been verified IVD status in Australia and is indicated for use on Roche Ventana BenchMark ULTRA platforms specifically for NSCLC investigations. However, for analysis of triple-negative breast tumours – being oestrogen, progesterone and Her2 negative – Roche mandates the PD-L1 clone to use is SP142.

Tests for EGFR, ALK, ROS1 and PD-L1 status are all examples of companion diagnostic assays. Patients qualify for either small biological inhibitors or humanized monoclonal antibody therapy based on the results of these tests. The increased responsibility of providing an accurate theranostic test via IHC assay is more crucial than ever. Using IHC for this specific arm of personalized medicine will continue to grow in the future as new biomarkers are identified.

Melanoma

Melanoma can be difficult to diagnose as it is a heterogeneous malignancy and many types can be

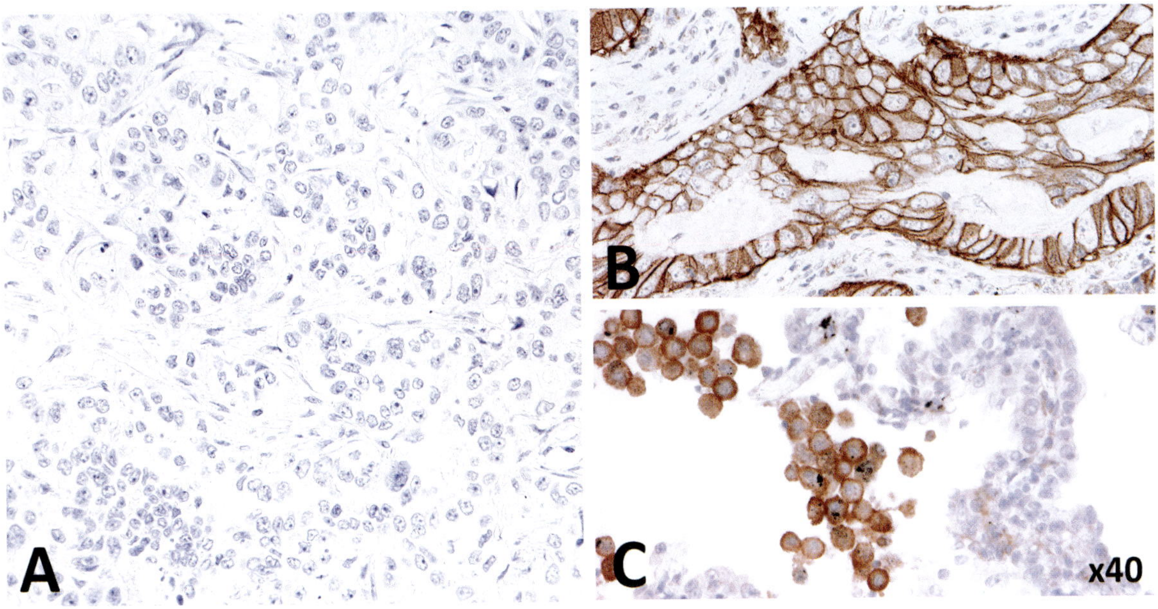

Figure 8.16 NSCLC with PD-L1 IHC

encountered. Several scoring classification systems have been devised, starting with Clark levels from the 1960s and Brestlow's classification introduced in the 1970s to measure depth of tumour invasion in skin. The tumour, node and metastasis (TNM) staging system derived by the American Joint Committee on Cancer (Bartlett and Karakousis 2015) is in current use. Although imaging techniques are available, current best practice is tissue biopsy confirmed by morphology and IHC with subsequent molecular sequencing for activating mutations. Figure 8.17 demonstrates a lesion found in lung tissue with the cut surface of the nodule exposed. The first line of enquiry is to determine whether the tumour is a lung primary or a metastasis from another site. The pigmentation is a clue as to the origin of this cancer.

Many antibodies are available for melanoma IHC workup. Common IHC markers include Melan A, HMB-45, S100 and SOX10. Some markers are more specific whilst others are more sensitive. Historically, the standard antibody for diagnosing melanomas with IHC is the S100 protein. There are, however, melanomas that are S100 negative. Remember tumours do not read textbooks. Since they are 'out of control', they may or may not express certain proteins attributed to melanocytic lineage. The more specific markers for melanocytes are known to be HMB-45, Melan A and MART-1. The more sensitive antibodies are S100 and SOX10, but, unfortunately, these two also recognize other tissue entities. Figure 8.18 shows a melanoma arising in skin H&E stained (A) and corresponding Melan A IHC stain (B).

The list of available antibodies continues to grow in line with the increasing use of IHC in melanoma and sentinel lymph node workup. These include tyrosinase, microphthalmia transcription factor (MITF) and PRAME (Kim and Meehan 2017; Lezcano et al. 2018). PRAME is an abbreviation for preferentially expressed antigen in melanoma and is another IHC marker that shows great promise. The availability of new markers coming on to the market all the time presents a conundrum for laboratories. With so much choice it can be difficult to ascertain the valuable ones for an individual laboratory's needs. The IHC laboratory is therefore tasked and continually faces the challenge to seek out the most robust and reliable antibodies for their needs.

Presently a universal antibody for all melanoma scenarios is not available and usually a panel consisting of a combination of antibody clones is requested to cover both the high sensitivity and high specificity required for an accurate diagnosis. Some laboratories use a combination of antibodies in the 'cocktail' described previously. An added complexity is that all of the antibodies mentioned recognize the full gamut of benign, pre-malignant and malignant conditions.

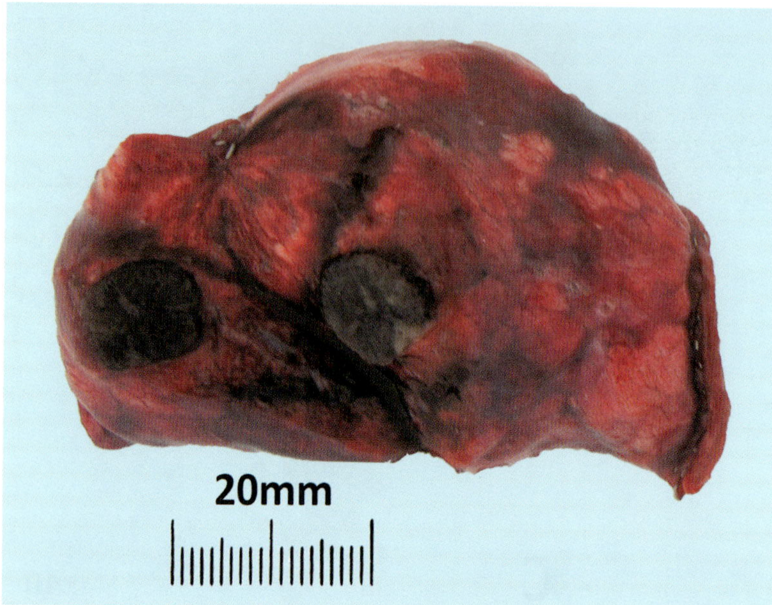

Figure 8.17 Lung nodule for histological analysis

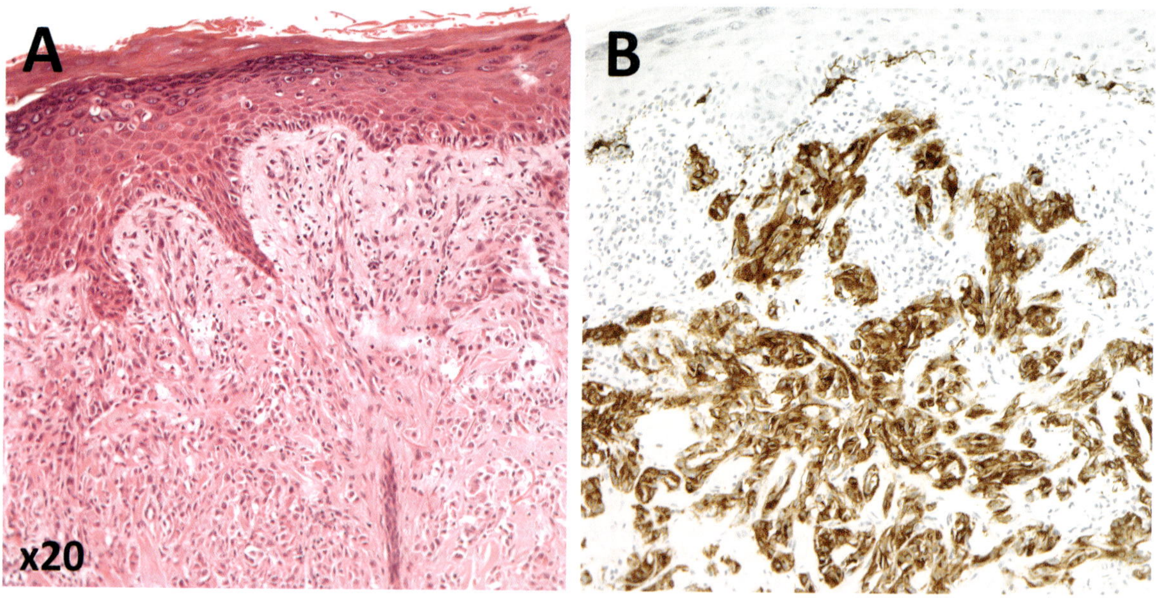

Figure 8.18 Melanoma hematoxylin and eosin stained (A) and corresponding Melan A immunohistochemical stain (B)

The reporting pathologist must be able to confidently identify benign states from malignancy. Often proliferation markers such as Ki-67 are used to measure the cell cycle activity and therefore how aggressive the tumour is. Similar to melanocytic specific antibodies, other proliferation markers are now available in the form of PHH3 (Nielsen et al. 2013), but, once again, it is important for the IHC laboratory to validate the clones to be used routinely. Immunohistochemistry in its present form has proven reliable and necessary in the diagnosis of melanoma (Compton et al. 2015).

Similar to NSCLC, diagnostic emphasis is placed upon molecular characteristics of melanoma. The mutations within the EGFR pathway mentioned previously in NSCLC (Franklin et al. 2002) have also been identified as therapeutic targets for melanoma, especially the BRAF gene. In association with the RAS, MEK and ERK genes, BRAF belongs to a cascading family of genes known as the mitogen activation protein kinase (MAPK) pathway, a cell-signalling and proliferation control area. This can be thought of as a 'switch' for cellular growth and proliferation. Appropriate cellular regulation turns the switch on and off as required. When mutated, it is as if the 'switch' is constantly on. About 70% of melanomas acquire a mutation in this area (Scolyer et al. 2011), leading to loss of regulation and uncontrolled proliferation and growth. Targeted therapy is therefore directed towards these constitutive activation mutational events. About 50% of melanomas harbour a mutation in BRAF and approximately 85% BRAF mutations have the V600E variety (Davis et al. 2019). The nomenclature V600E tells us that the mutation has substituted the amino acid valine (V) for glutamic acid (E) at position codon 600 within the protein chain due to a consequence of the nucleotide base thymine being substituted with adenine at nucleotide 1799. In other words, this single nucleotide polymorphism or 'snip' of a nucleotide base T to A changes the conformational shape of the resulting protein. This slight change in protein shape leaves the switch constantly stuck in the 'on' position.

The BRAF VE1 clone is a specific antibody available for the IHC detection of the BRAF V600E mutation. The limitation, however, is the lack of specificity for other types of BRAF mutations such as V600K, V600R and so on. Similar to EGFR, it is not feasible to have multiple antibody clones to cover all of the specific mutations encountered in melanoma. Molecular techniques such as next-generation sequencing have the ability to scan for all the mutations within this BRAF and other MAPK genes within the one assay by analysing tumour DNA profiles and comparing that to the normal 'wildtype' profile.

Targeted therapy employs inhibitors such as vemurafenib to turn this cascade 'switch' off, thereby downregulating cell proliferation and uncontrolled growth. This therapy often works for a period of time before there is an inherent resistance development by the tumour (Chapman et al. 2011). The next step is understanding the acquired resistance to this line of therapy. Another avenue of targeted therapy is using monoclonal antibodies to help the body's immune system fight the melanoma. Similar to NSCLCs, checkpoint inhibitors have been deployed to aid the T-cells in identifying and destroying the cancer cells. As highlighted previously, the PD1 protein on the immune T-cells recognizes and binds to the PD-L1 protein on healthy cells, which prevents the immune T-cells from attacking and destroying these healthy cells. In essence, this prevents autoimmunity whereby the body attacks itself. Tumour cells have this ability to display the PD-L1 protein as well, thereby mimicking healthy cells and thus avoiding attack from the immune T-cells. Monoclonal antibodies directed towards the PD-L1 protein bind to it and break this combination, thereby allowing the immune cells to attack the tumour cell. There is now a more concerted effort to identify other checkpoint inhibitors as therapeutic targets, and when these biomarkers are identified, IHC will continue to play a role in selecting populations of patients who are most likely to benefit from a particular line of therapy.

Bowel Cancer

Immunohistochemistry is extremely useful in the pathology of bowel cancers. Figure 8.19 shows an adenocarcinoma (arrow) adjacent to normal bowel. The diagnosis of primary bowel cancer is relatively straightforward for this specimen. The H&E morphology alone should be adequate for a confident diagnosis, but if IHC is required, many markers are available to direct lineage to the bowel.

One of the more common scenarios is determining bowel origin in metastatic tumours. After morphological assessment with H&E stain, the pathologist employs a panel of IHC markers specific for the situation in order to elucidate the exact origin of the tumour as outlined previously. If the lesion is in the lungs, for example, antibodies for lung origin such as TTF1 or CK7 are included. If there is clinical suspicion of bowel involvement, then antibodies such as CK20, CDX 2 or SATB2 are employed. The staining result will pinpoint the tumour's colonic origin as indicated in Table 8.1.

Another clinical situation in which IHC is used extensively is when investigating for Lynch syndrome, an autosomal dominant genetic disease commonly associated with increased risk of colorectal, uterine and some other cancers. The term 'Lynch syndrome' is used interchangeably with 'hereditary nonpolyposis colorectal carcinoma' (HNPCC), which can lead to confusion, especially when used to describe non-bowel cancers such as those originating from the endometrium. In addition, HNPCC suggests that these colorectal cancers do not arise from numerous polyps, but in actual fact they do (Grenert 2016). Regardless, within the context of bowel cancer, HNPCC has been given a distinct entity whereby clinically it is typically seen in cohorts younger than 50 years of age, occurring in the proximal bowel. Histologically the adenocarcinoma is often poorly differentiated and contains abundant mucin with signet ring morphology, and lymphocytic aggregation is present at the tumour site (Cai et al. 2003).

There is also a molecular basis to Lynch syndrome, and it is in this area that IHC testing is directed. Mutational events have been found within an area of the genome known as variable nucleotide tandem repeats (VNTR). These are regions of non-coding DNA identified by short repeats of nucleotide bases. For example, the sequence of nucleotide bases 5'GTTAC3' is repeated multiple times within this region of DNA. These repeats are known as microsatellites and they are useful in other applications such as paternity testing and forensic DNA fingerprinting. The histology laboratory can also use microsatellites to match a tissue sample belonging to a specific patient in the event of a mix-up with another patient's tissue specimen during processing. The VNTRs are sometimes referred as short tandem repeats, minisatellites and simple sequence repeats. All of these terms mean the same thing. Due to the nature of these repeating DNA sequences, the enzyme DNA polymerase may make mistakes caused by 'slippages' during DNA replication. It is the function of the mismatch repair (MMR) proteins to repair these errors. If they fail, mutations occur as a result of incorrect base pairing or adenosine pairing with guanine as an example of a point mutation, or there are insertion or deletion loops, resulting in a frameshift mutation. When these errors occur in microsatellite regions, the term 'microsatellite instability' (MSI) is often referenced. The relationship of MSI and dysfunctional MMR proteins is well established in HNPCC (Lynch et al. 1998).

Table 8.1 Typical immunohistochemical panel for bowel cancer

Antibody	Staining pattern	Result
CK7	Cytoplasmic	negative
TTF1	Nuclear	negative
CK20	Cytoplasmic	positive
CDX2	Nuclear	positive
SATB2	Nuclear	positive

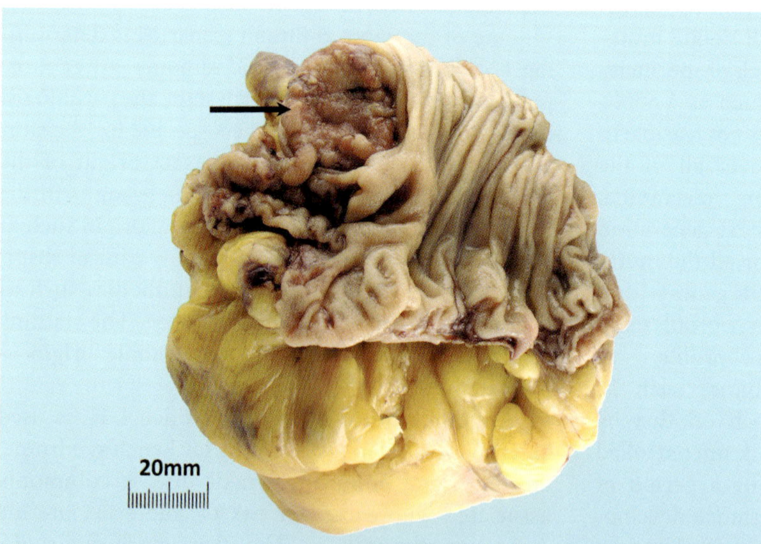

Figure 8.19 Adenocarcinoma of bowel (arrow)

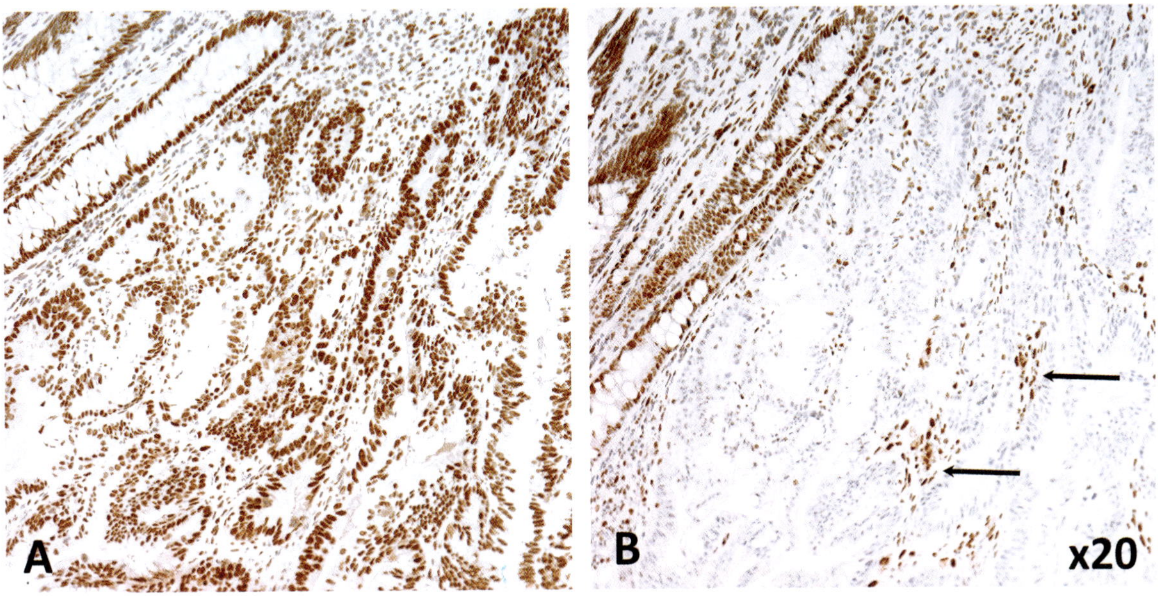

Figure 8.20 Bowel cancer with MMR proteins present for MSH2/MSH6 (A) and absent for MLH1/PMS2 (B)

Although there are many proteins within the MMR family, IHC commonly analyses four. These are the MLH1, PMS2, MSH2 and MSH6 proteins. These MMR proteins exist as complexes; the MSH-2 and MSH-6 act together to search for incorrect base pairing or insertion and deletion loops caused by DNA slippages. MLH-1 and PMS-2 then come along to start the MMR process. In IHC, these proteins are localized within the nuclear region of the cell and are seen in normal and tumour tissue. The IHC interpretation is simple most of the time. Wildtype MMR genes producing normal MMR proteins stain positively for IHC. A mutation to the MMR genes causing MMR dysfunctional proteins show an absence of IHC staining. If MSH2 staining is absent, meaning there is loss of the MMR protein function at the MSH2 gene, then MSH6 should be absent too. This is because MHS2 and MSH6 exist as pairs. Similarly, if MLH1 staining is absent, then PMS2 should correspond to this and be absent too. Figure 8.20 shows the combination of MSH2/MSH6 positive staining (A) and MLH1/PMS2 negative staining (B). Stromal cells and lymphocytes serve as internal control (arrows).

When interpreting IHC staining results, it is sometimes the absence of staining that is critical. In this example of MSI, the absence of IHC staining for MMR proteins means a 'positive result' for the possibility of Lynch syndrome (Shia 2008). This situation is unique to most other IHC settings whereby the presence of staining is the positive result. For instance, a positive S100 IHC is indicative for melanoma or a positive GATA3 IHC is suggestive for breast cancer. With regards to HNPCC, it is important to clearly state the IHC result in a non-ambiguous manner. For instance, best practice would not state whether the IHC stains were 'positive' or 'negative'. A better alternative would include within the report a description of MMR proteins as being 'present' or 'absent'.

However, there are instances where hypermethylation of the MLH1 protein will also render an absence in IHC staining. Processes such as methylation and phosphorylation inducing changes to gene function without generating mutations are known collectively as epigenetic changes. This means that in some cases, the MLH1 IHC staining will be absent but the subsequent PMS2 IHC will show positivity.

Immunohistochemistry is commonly employed as a screening test for Lynch syndrome. Any abnormality seen will be referred to molecular testing via polymerase chain reaction (PCR) and electrophoresis analysis. If Lynch syndrome is confirmed due to defective MMR genes, the immediate and extended family members of the patient will benefit from being subjected to closer surveillance. Another interesting note is that colorectal cancer in the setting of Lynch syndrome seems to have a better prognosis.

Investigators such as Lee and colleagues (2018) are targeting the associated high levels of T-cells found within the tumour microenvironment as a potential line of targeted therapy.

On a technical note, it is important to highlight that optimal fixation of tissue plays a crucial role in the success of MMR proteins. Quite often investigations for MSI are performed on bowel resections. Good laboratory practice for tissue fixation and processing requires the laboratory to open the bowel specimen and clean out the contents after surgical removal without delay. This allows the fixative to penetrate the mucosal lining for optimal fixation. Any hindrance to this operation results in suboptimal MMR IHC because the panel of four MMR antibodies are susceptible to deficiencies in tissue fixation and processing. They are not as forgiving as some other more robust antibodies.

Poor fixation and processing often manifest as heterogeneous, patchy and non-uniform staining of the tumour. Compare this to MSI IHC investigations performed on colorectal endoscopic biopsies whereby a high-quality IHC stain is consistently achieved because these biopsies are on average 3 mm in size and placed into fixative immediately after sampling from the patient. The pre-analytic factors of small endoscopy biopsies are easier to control and optimize when compared to a large bowel resection. Conversely, it is preferable to perform analysis for Lynch syndrome on large bowel resections to overcome possible areas of true tumour heterogeneity. Sampling the entire tumour would allow a more representative account of the cancer. Knowing MMR proteins exist in normal cells, an assessment of internal tissue controls is straightforward and should consist of stromal elements and the surrounding lymphocytes (Ruszkiewicz et al. 2002). Similar to NSCLC and melanoma, molecular sequencing within the EGFR and MAPK pathway is also utilized for bowel cancer.

Breast Pathology

The use of IHC in breast pathology has been around for a very long time. One of the first original predictive and prognostic markers utilized were the ER and PR antibody assays to ascertain hormone receptor status of the tumour. Breast cancers that are ER positive may benefit from anti-oestrogen therapy agents such as Tamoxifen (Mies 2016). Patients with breast tumours that are ER negative would not respond to anti-oestrogen therapy – another example of personalized medicine in selecting the candidates who are most likely able to respond to a certain line of therapy. In addition to ER and PR status, another marker was subsequently identified to add to the targeted therapy regime in the form of Her2 receptor status. Her2 belongs to the epidermal growth factor receptor family. Breast cancers exhibiting Her2 gene amplification are likely to increase Her2 protein synthesis, leading to one of the hallmarks of cancer, uncontrolled cellular growth. Patients with Her2 overexpression have been shown to respond well to monoclonal antibody immunotherapy agents such as Herceptin (Moelans et al. 2010).

The three markers of ER, PR and Her2 form the trinity of the current breast IHC diagnostic panel. Some laboratories go one step further and routinely include a proliferation marker such as Ki67 to gauge how mitotically 'active' the tumour is. All of these IHC assays are routinely performed on FFPE tissue. Hence a routine breast IHC panel consisting of ER, PR, Her2 and Ki67 is quite commonplace. Other antibodies worthy of note are E-Cadherin to differentiate ductal differentiation from that of lobular and CK7 and GATA3 to help identify distant metastases of breast origin. As is often the case, antibodies such as CK7 and GATA3 are expressed in other cell types and tissue locations, so it is important to remember this and interpret IHC antibodies within the context of a given clinical situation.

Not only has breast cancer pathology been used by IHC as one of the pioneers of targeted therapy, it is also one of the first instances where pathologists have been asked to perform a quantitative type of analysis using IHC. Traditional IHC assays seek the presence or absence of a protein. If the protein of interest is present, it is designated by a colour reaction and if it is absent, no colour formation is observed. In simple terms, there are two possible results: either the protein is present and observable, or it is not. The use of IHC in breast pathology changes this paradigm. Now the answers sought include whether a protein is present, and if so, how much of it is present. A grading system counts the number of positive tumour cells within the entire population of cancer cells present. The requirement to provide such an answer in terms of quantity brings several challenges. Some of these pivots around accuracy, precision, reproducibility and objectivity themes. For ER and PR status, it has been decided that a positive result is one that contains more than or

Table 8.2 Summary of Her2 IHC staging (Wolff et al. 2018)

IHC staining pattern	HER2 score	Her2 status
Cancer cells show intense complete membrane staining in > 10% of the invasive tumour population.	3+	Positive
Cancer cells show weak to moderate complete membrane staining in > 10% of the invasive tumour population.	2+	Equivocal
Cancer cells show weak/faint incomplete membrane staining in > 10% of the invasive tumour population.	1+	Negative
Cancer cells show weak/faint incomplete membrane staining in ≤ 10% of the invasive tumour population or when no staining is observed.	0	Negative

equal to 1% positively stained tumour cells within the entire population of cancer cells present (Hammond et al. 2010). Interpreting and deciding a Her2 status requires more effort because the score is divided into four categories with three groups as highlighted in Table 8.2.

Note that only the invasive breast carcinoma portion is subjected to HER2 scoring. Accompanying *in situ* carcinoma that may be present is not to be considered when assessing for Her2 status. In the not so distant past, every breast cancer underwent Her2 ISH even if the Her2 IHC was negative (National Breast and Ovarian Cancer Centre and Australian Cancer Network 2008). Nowadays, this has changed due to the good concordance achieved between Her2 IHC and ISH and the high confidence placed on IHC as a stand-alone test. Negative Her2 IHC (score 1+ and 0) do not require ISH studies. Breast cancers that are judged to be positive (score 3+) or equivocal (score 2+) by IHC are further referred for HER2 ISH. Figure 8.21 demonstrates an invasive breast cancer H&E stained (A) with corresponding Her2 IHC (B) and Her2 ISH (C). Single-probe or dual-probe ISH assays are available for the specific purpose of testing for HER2 gene amplification located on chromosome 17. As such, there are now two methods to assess HER2 status. Access to Herceptin therapy can be decided by IHC to determine whether HER2 protein is overexpressed or by ISH to ascertain amplification of the HER2 gene. Knowing HER2 gene amplification invariably leads to HER2 protein overexpression, the gold standard assay for HER2 status therefore is with the ISH evaluation; IHC, however, has proven a reliable surrogate for this form of molecular test and is often used as the lone indicator when the IHC result is negative in deciding Her2 status.

In addition to using IHC as a companion diagnostic test for breast cancers, it has also been successfully employed for determining lymph node status of a breast cancer patient. The presence of cancer cells within regional lymph node tissue provides clear evidence of active spread from the primary tumour site. The lymphoid tissue of greater emphasis are the sentinel lymph nodes and epithelial markers such as pan cytokeratin AE1/3 clones or Cam 5.2 are routinely deployed to visualize breast micro and macro metastases at these sites. The resulting presence or absence of cancer cells as indicated via IHC have treatment and prognosis implications. Breast cancer treatments are continually evolving. Laboratories are now currently performing IHC on breast sentinel nodes for the presence of isolated tumour cells up to 20 µm or micro metastases of less than 2 mm because there is no automatic requirement of axillary dissection at these sizes. Patients can be monitored more closely or given axillary radiotherapy for the remaining nodes in lieu of surgery. This area of assessing axillary treatment decisions, however, is rapidly changing.

On a technical note, the laboratory receives breast needle cores as well as mastectomy for investigation. Quite often a breast needle core is performed when there is clinical suspicion of breast cancer. This procedure is favoured because it is minimally invasive and the patient recovers with less morbidity. Upon viewing the H&E slide the pathologist will order the breast IHC panel if it is malignant. A breast core biopsy found to contain malignant cells is commonly followed by a wide local excision or total mastectomy. It is important to note that even when IHC was performed on the previous needle core biopsy, a repeat IHC breast panel is performed on the subsequent 'big' specimen. The reasons are many.

Breast cancers can be heterogeneous in nature and the lesion may exhibit more than one phenotype. Some areas of the tumour can be ER negative but within other areas of the same specimen the cancer cells are ER positive. Depending on the exact area where the

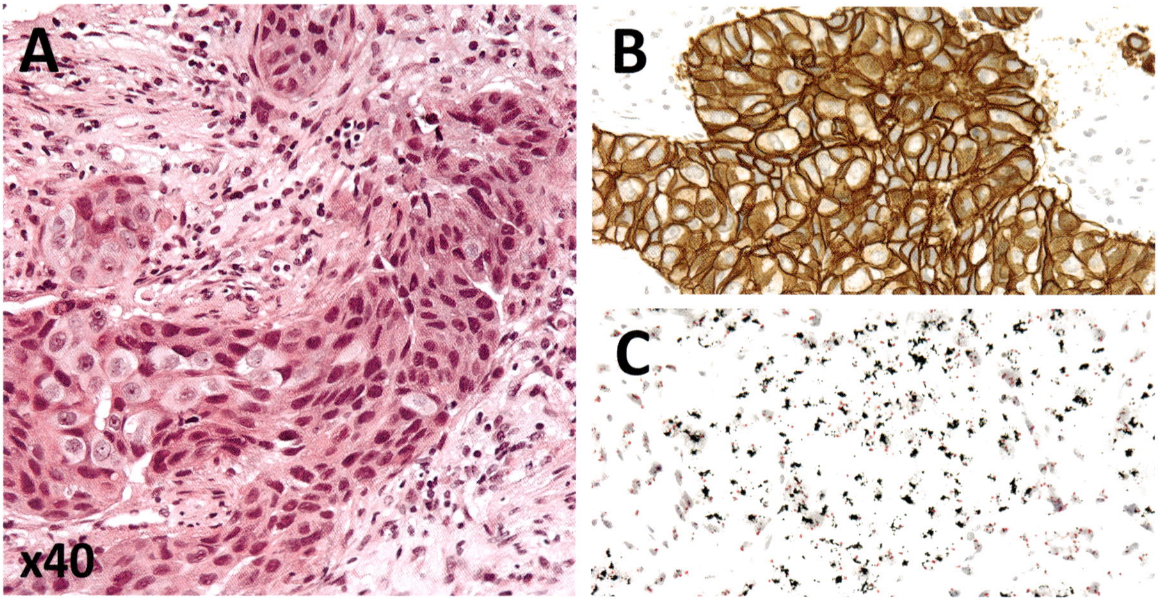

Figure 8.21 Hematoxylin and eosin stain of invasive breast cancer (A) with Her2 immunohistochemistry staining (B) and corresponding HER 2 *in situ* hybridization (C)

needle has sampled for core biopsy, the basis of the pathology report is generated for the needle core sample. When the time comes to examine the larger mastectomy or wide local excision, the IHC is repeated on a representative tumour block that is more likely to contain the entire lesion whereby it is possible for the pathologist to observe the degree of heterogeneity.

Other reasons for performing hormone receptors initially on core biopsy and to repeat them on subsequent excision are based on a technical and clinical perspective. For instance, tissue fixation and processing are vastly superior for core biopsies, which follows that IHC should be optimal for an accurate result. In addition, the patient may undergo neoadjuvant therapy prior to wide local excision therefore requiring hormone status via IHC. Or perhaps the tumour phenotype has changed due to some other basis. It is current best practice to determine ER, PR and Her2 status on the 'big' excision biopsy even though it was previously performed on the patient.

Breast IHC is served by many different antibody clones, and it is incumbent on the laboratory to choose the best one for their breast cancer service. Take ER, for example; throughout the years many clones have come and gone, some good and some bad, and choosing the right clone requires careful consideration of a number of factors. Obviously, the clone picked to be the routine marker for ER status would need to be highly sensitive and specific as well as reliable and robust. Quite often the type of automation and instrumentation supplied by a specific vendor influences the choice of clone. The latest addition to the breast cancer workup is testing for PD-L1 status using the clone SP142 for ER, PR and Her2 IHC (triple) negative breast cancers. Figure 8.22 shows an H&E of a breast cancer (A). Subsequent hormone receptors and Her2 IHC were all negative, but the tumour was shown to be PD-L1 positive with clone SP142 (B). This patient is a candidate for checkpoint inhibitor immunotherapy.

Conclusion

The anatomical pathology laboratory is entrusted to investigate many diseases, most of which comprise tumour diagnoses and prognoses. To this end, it has a crucial role to play in the management of cancer. Not only does tissue diagnosis confirm the presence of cancer, but it can also subtype tumours and in some situations, adds further prognostic information or dictates treatment options. Immunohistochemistry is a critical component of this mandate with the majority of assays being performed on FFPE tissue. Traditional H&E morphology and special stains can only provide a finite resource when it comes to

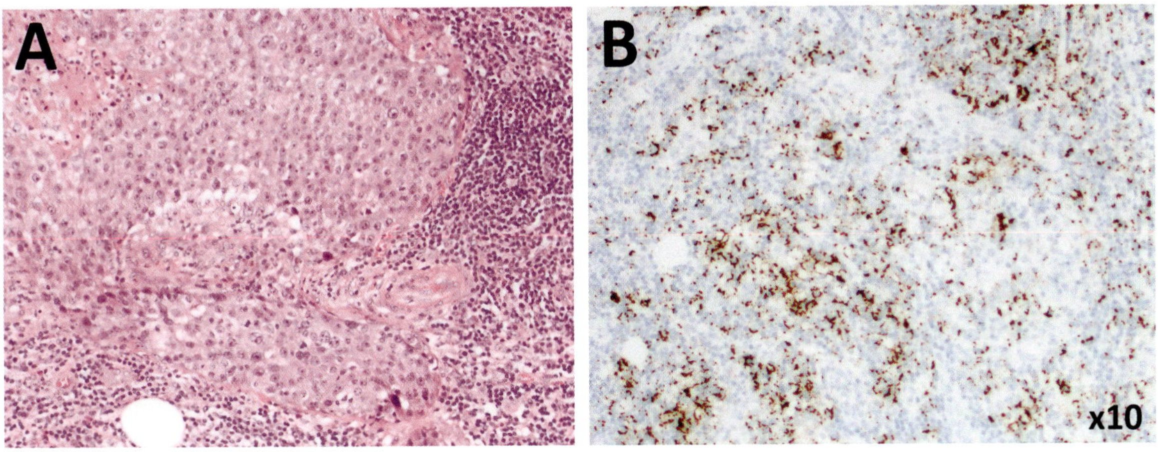

Figure 8.22 Triple-negative breast cancer hematoxylin and eosin (A) showing PDL1 positivity with clone SP142 (B)

subtyping tumours to find treatment for specific cancers. Immunohistochemistry offers an additional layer for these investigations by complementing traditional histology techniques. Some argue it is another 'special stain' while others view IHC as a bridge between traditional morphology and the frontier of molecular testing. Regardless of personal viewpoints, IHC is an effective analytical tool that fits with H&E, special stains and molecular assays.

There are common themes within IHC. The issue of standardization remains a challenge, particularly in the pre-analytical domain of tissue fixation and processing. If a high level of consistency is achieved to a set 'standard' in this regard, RTU antibodies can be employed routinely with readily available detection kits. The progress of robotics to attain a level of automation that is 'load and walk away' has contributed to the wide acceptance of this technology for both diagnostic applications and research projects. However, an optimized and calibrated IHC assay still requires the expertise of technical laboratory personnel. Each antibody must be validated to ascertain it is fit for purpose, and standard practice is to use suitable control tissue.

The requirements from the laboratory for offering IHC in terms of facility and consumables are not onerous. In fact, the technology is so widely available that IHC has become firmly entrenched in both large and small institutions. It is a necessary tool in histology, employed in both qualitative and quantitative analyses because of its versatility. An additional dimension to IHC is the area of companion diagnostics for personalized medicine. New biomarkers for treatment modalities are continually being sought, but there is still a high demand for the 'common' variety of antibodies. Markers to differentiate epithelial lesions from melanoma or sarcoma are still required for accurate diagnoses, and IHC assays of this nature will be performed for the foreseeable future.

Current staining protocols and antibodies have evolved to be more streamlined. The concept of standardization has reduced the many variables attributed to the IHC assay to just two. In most cases, these considerations are the type of epitope retrieval (if required) and the working antibody titre. The use of RTU antibodies reduces the assay down to the one parameter of antigen retrieval. Clinical examples taken from cancers of the lung, breast, bowel and melanoma have shown the importance of IHC in diagnostic histopathology. The new frontier of molecular testing for tumour mutations will evidently increase IHC assays as companion diagnostic devices. Complementing molecular technologies, differentiating tumour origins and selecting patients for personalized treatments are the main roles of IHC in its current status.

References

Asch-Kendrick RJ, Samols MA, Lilo MT, Subhawong AP, Sharma R, Illei PB, Argani P, Cimino-Mathews A 2014. NKX3.1 is expressed in ER-positive and AR-positive primary breast carcinomas. *J Clin Pathol* **67**(9):768–71.

Bartlett EK, Karakousis GC 2015. Current staging and prognostic factors in melanoma. *Surg Oncol Clin N Am* **24** (2):215–27.

Brevet M, Arcila M, Ladanyi M 2010. Assessment of EGFR mutation status in lung adenocarcinoma by immunohistochemistry using antibodies specific to the two major forms of mutant EGFR. *J Mol Diagn* **12**(2):169–76.

Browne MA, Howard CV, Jolleys GD 1995. Principles of stereology. In Wootton R, Springall DR, Polak JM, eds. *Image analysis in histology: Conventional and confocal microscopy*. Cambridge University Press; 96–120.

Bubendorf L, Büttner R, Al-Dayel F, Dietel M, Elmberger G, Kerr K, López-Ríos F, Marchetti A, Öz B, Pauwels P, Penault-Llorca F, Rossi G, Ryška A, Thunnissen E 2016. Testing for ROS1 in non-small cell lung cancer: A review with recommendations. *Virchows Arch* **469** (5):489–503.

Cai SJ, Xu Y, Cai GX, Lian P, Guan ZQ, Mo SJ, Sun MH, Cai Q, Shi DR 2003. Clinical characteristics and diagnosis of patients with hereditary nonpolyposis colorectal cancer. *World J Gastroenterol* **9**(2):284–7.

Cao J, Chen D, Yang F, Yao J, Zhu W, Zhao C 2017. NUT midline carcinoma as a primary lung tumor: A case report. *J Thorac Dis* **9**(12):e1045–9.

Chapman PB, Hauschild A, Robert C, Haanen JB, Ascierto P, Larkin J, Dummer R, Garbe C, Testori A, Maio M, Hogg D, Lorigan P, Lebbe C, Jouary T, Schadendorf D, Ribas A, O'Day SJ, Sosman JA, Kirkwood JM, Eggermont AMM, Dreno B, Nolop K, Li J, Nelson B, Hou J, Lee RJ, Flaherty KT, McArthur GA 2011. Improved survival with vemurafenib in melanoma with BRAF V600E mutation. *N Engl J Med* **26**(364): 2507–16.

Compton LA, Murphy GF, Lian CG 2015. Diagnostic immunohistochemistry in cutaneous neoplasia: An update. *Dermatopathology (Basel)* **2**(1):15–42.

Conde E, Hernandez S, Martinez R, Angulo B, De Castro J, Collazo-Lorduy A, Jimenez B, Muriel A, Mate JL, Moran T, Aranda I, Massuti B, Rojo F, Domine M, Sansano I, Garcia F, Felip E, Mancheño N, Juan O, Sanz J, Gonzalez-Larriba JL, Atienza-Cuevas L, Arriola-Arellano E, Abdulkader I, Garcia-Gonzalez J, Camacho C, Rodriguez-Abreu D, Teixido C, Reguart N, Gonzalez-Piñeiro A, Lazaro-Quintela M, Lozano MD, Gurpide A, Gomez-Roman J, Lopez-Brea M, Pijuan L, Salido M, Arriola E, Company A, Insa A, Esteban-Rodriguez I, Saiz M, Azkona E, Alvarez R, Artal A, Luz Plaza M, Aguiar D, Enguita AB, Benito A, Paz-Ares L, Garrido P, Lopez-Rios F 2019. Assessment of a new ROS1 immunohistochemistry clone (SP384) for the identification of ROS1 rearrangements in patients with non–small cell lung carcinoma: The ROSING Study. *J Thorac Onco* **14**(12):2120–32.

Conklin CMJ, Craddock KJ, Have C, Laskin J, Couture C, Ionescu DN 2013. Immunohistochemistry is a reliable screening tool for identification of ALK rearrangement in non-small cell lung carcinoma and is antibody dependent. *J Thorac Oncol* **8**(1):45–51.

Dako 2020. Omnis EnVision Flex, High pH GV800 Instructions for use. Agilent Technologies (online). Available at www.agilent.com/cs/library/packageinsert/public/PD04120EFG_02.pdf (Accessed 16 June 2021).

Davis LE, Shalin SC, Tackett AJ 2019. Current state of melanoma diagnosis and treatment. *Cancer Biol Ther* **20** (11):1366–79.

Dyck L, Mills KHG 2017. Immune checkpoints and their inhibition in cancer and infectious diseases. *Eur J Immunol* **47**(5):765–79.

Engel P, Boumsell L, Balderas R, Bensussan A, Gattei V, Horejsi V, Jin BQ, Malavasi F, Mortari F, Schwartz-Albiez R, Stockinger H, Van Zelm MC, Zola H, Clark G 2015. CD nomenclature 2015: Human leukocyte differentiation antigen workshops as a driving force in immunology. *J Immunol* **195**(10):4555–63.

Franklin WA, Veve R, Hirsch FR, Helfrich BA, Bunn PA Jr 2002. Epidermal growth factor receptor family in lung cancer and premalignancy. *Semin Oncol* **29**(1 Suppl 4):3–14.

Galimberti V, Cole BF, Zurrida S, Viale G, Luini A, Veronesi P, Baratella P, Chifu C, Sargenti M, Intra M, Gentilini O, Mastropasqua MG, Mazzarol G, Massarut S, Garbay JR, Zgajnar J, Galatius H, Recalcati A, Littlejohn D, Bamert M, Colleoni M, Price KN, Regan MM, Goldhirsch A, Coates AS, Gelber RD, Veronesi U 2013. International Breast Cancer Study Group Trial 23–01 investigators. Axillary dissection versus no axillary dissection in patients with sentinel-node micrometastases (IBCSG 23–01): A phase 3 randomised controlled trial. *Lancet Oncol* **14** (4):297–305.

Gelmann EP, Bowen C, Bubendorf L 2003. Expression of NKX3.1 in normal and malignant tissues. *Prostate* **55**:111–17.

Grenert, JP 2016. Hereditary nonpolyposis colorectal cancer and Lynch syndrome. In Leonard DGB, ed. *Molecular pathology in clinical practice*. Springer; 339–50.

Gurel B, Ali TZ, Montgomery EA, Begum S, Hicks J, Goggins M, Eberhart CG, Clark DP, Bieberich CJ, Epstein JI, De Marzo AM 2010. NKX3.1 as a marker of prostatic origin in metastatic tumors. *Am J Surg Pathol* **34** (8):1097–105.

Haack H, Johnson LA, Fry CJ, Crosby K, Polakiewicz RD, Stelow EB, Hong SM, Schwartz BE, Cameron MJ, Rubin MA, Chang MC, Aster JC, French CA 2009. Diagnosis of NUT midline carcinoma using a NUT-specific monoclonal antibody. *Am J Surg Pathol* **33**(7):984–91.

Hammond ME, Hayes DF, Dowsett M, Allred DC, Hagerty KL, Badve S, Fitzgibbons PL, Francis G, GoldsteinNS, Hayes M, Hicks DG, Lester S, Love R, Mangu PB, McShane L, Miller K, Osborne CK, Paik S, Perlmutter J, Rhodes A, Sasano H, Schwartz JN, Sweep FC, Taube S, Torlakovic EE, Valenstein P, Viale G, Visscher D, Wheeler T, Williams RB, Wittliff JL, Wolff AC, American

Society of Clinical Oncology, College of American Pathologists 2010. American Society of Clinical Oncology/ College of American Pathologists guideline recommendations for immunohistochemical testing of estrogen and progesterone receptors in breast cancer. *Arch Pathol Lab Med* **134**(6):907–22.

Ilie M, Khambata-Ford S, Copie-Bergman C, Huang L, Juco J, Hofman V, Hofman P 2017. Use of the 22C3 anti-PD-L1 antibody to determine PD-L1 expression in multiple automated immunohistochemistry platforms. *PLoS One* **12** (8):e0183023.

Inamura K 2018. Update on immunohistochemistry for the diagnosis of lung cancer. *Cancers* **10**(3):72.

Kim CH, Kim SH, Park SY, Yoo J, Kim SK, Kim HK 2015. Identification of EGFR mutations by immunohistochemistry with EGFR mutation-specific antibodies in biopsy and resection specimens from pulmonary adenocarcinoma. *Cancer Res Treat* **47**(4): 653–60.

Kim RH, Meehan SA 2017. Immunostain use in the diagnosis of melanomas referred to a tertiary medical center: A 15-year retrospective review (2001–2015). *J Cutan Pathol* **44**: 221–7.

Koppel C, Schwellenbach H, Zielinski D, Eckstein S, Martin-Ortega M, D'Arrigo C, Schildhaus HU, Rüschoff J, Jasani B 2018. Optimization and validation of PD-L1 immunohistochemistry staining protocols using the antibody clone 28-8 on different staining platforms. *Mod Pathol* **31**(11):1630–44.

Koulis C, Yap R, Engel R, Jardé T, Wilkins S, Solon G, Shapiro JD, Abud H, McMurrick P 2020. Personalized medicine: Current and emerging predictive and prognostic biomarkers in colorectal cancer. *Cancers (Basel)* **12**(4):812.

Kővári B, Turkevi-Nagy S, Báthori Á, Fekete Z, Krenács L 2020. Syntaxin 1: A novel robust immunophenotypic marker of neuroendocrine tumors. *Int J Mol Sci* **21**(4):1213.

Lee SJ, Jun SY, Lee IH, Kang BW, Park SY, Kim HJ, Park JS, Choi GS, Yoon G, Kim JG 2018. CD274, LAG3, andIDO1 expressions in tumor-infiltrating immune cells as prognostic biomarker for patients with MSI-high colon cancer. *J Cancer Res Clin Oncol* **144**(6):1005–14.

Leica 2019. Refine detection kit Cat#DS9800 Instructions for use. Leica Biosystems Newcastle Ltd.

Lezcano C, Jungbluth AA, Nehal KS, Hollmann TJ, Busam KJ 2018. PRAME expression in melanocytic tumors. *Am J Surg Pathol* **42**(11):1456–65.

Lynch HT, Smyrk T, Lynch JF 1998. Molecular genetics and clinical-pathology features of hereditary nonpolyposis colorectal carcinoma (Lynch syndrome): Historical journey from pedigree anecdote to molecular genetic confirmation. *Oncology* **55**(2):103–8.

Lynch TJ, Bell DW, Sordella R, Gurubhagavatula S, Okimoto RA, Brannigan BW, Harris PL, Haserlat SM, Supko JG, Haluska FG, Louis DN, Christiani DC, Settleman J, Haber DA 2004. Activating mutations in the epidermal growth factor receptor underlying responsiveness of non-small-cell lung cancer to gefitinib. *N Engl J Med* **350**(21):2129–39.

Mies, C 2016. Breast cancer. In: Leonard DGB, ed. *Molecular pathology in clinical practice*. Springer; 433–46.

Moelans CB, Kibbelaar RE, Van den Heuvel MC, Castigliego D, De Weger RA, Van Diest PJ 2010. Validation of a fully automated HER2 staining kit in breast cancer. *Cell Oncol* **32**(1–2):149–55.

Moll R, Franke WW, Schiller DL, Geiger B, Krepler R 1982. The catalog of human cytokeratins: Patterns of expression in normal epithelia, tumors and cultured cells. *Cell* **31**(1):11–24.

National Breast and Ovarian Cancer Centre and Australian Cancer Network 2008. *The pathology reporting of breast cancer. A guide for pathologists, surgeons, radiologists and oncologists (3rd edition)*. National Breast and Ovarian Cancer Centre.

Nguyen T 2011. Oracle HER2 Bond immunohistochemistry system validation. *Journal of Histotechnology***34**(2):79–87.

Nielsen PS, Riber-Hansen R, Jensen TO, Schmidt H, Steiniche T 2013. Proliferation indices of phosphohistoneH3 and Ki67: Strong prognostic markers in a consecutive cohort with stage I/II melanoma. *Mod Pathol* **26**(3):404–13.

NordiQC 2020. Assessment run B29. NordiQC (online). Available at www.nordiqc.org/downloads/assessments/132_2.pdf (Accessed 1 July 2021).

Ordonez NG 2003. The immunohistochemical diagnosis of mesothelioma: A comparative study of epithelioid mesothelioma and lung adenocarcinoma. *Am J Surg Pathol* **27**(8):1031–51.

Paez JG, Jänne PA, Lee JC, Tracy S, Greulich H, Gabriel S, Herman P, Kaye FJ, Lindeman N, Boggon TJ, Naoki K, Sasaki H, Fujii Y, Eck MJ, Sellers WR, Johnson BE, Meyerson M 2004. EGFR mutations in lung cancer: Correlation with clinical response to gefitinib therapy. *Science* **304**(5676):1497–500.

Parra ER, Villalobos P, Mino B, Rodriguez-Canales J 2018. Comparison of different antibody clones for immunohistochemistry detection of programmed cell death ligand 1 (PD-L1) on non-small cell lung carcinoma. *Appl Immunohistochem Mol Morphol* **26**(2):83–93.

Ruszkiewicz A, Bennett G, Moore J, Manavis J, Rudzki B, Shen L, Suthers G 2002. Correlation of mismatch repair genes immunohistochemistry and microsatellite instability status in HNPCC-associated tumours. *Pathology* **34**(6):541–7.

Roach C, Zhang N, Corigliano E, Jansson M, Toland G, Ponto G, Dolled-Filhart M, Emancipator K, Stanforth D, Kulangara K 2016. Development of a companion diagnostic

PD-L1 immunohistochemistry assay for pembrolizumab therapy in non-small-cell lung cancer. *Appl Immunohistochem Mol Morphol.* **24**(6):392–7.

Rolls G 2021. Fixation and fixatives (2): Factors influencing chemical fixation, formaldehyde and glutaraldehyde. Leica Biosystems (online). Available at www.leicabiosystems.com/knowledge-pathway/fixation-and-fixatives-2-factors-influencing-chemical-fixation-formaldehyde-and-glutaraldehyde (Accessed 29 July 2021).

Rooper LM, Sharma R, Li QK, Illei PB, Westra WH 2017. INSM1 demonstrates superior performance to the individual and combined use of synaptophysin, chromogranin and CD56 for diagnosing neuroendocrine tumors of the thoracic cavity. *Am J Surg Pathol* **41** (11):1561–9.

Schweizer J, Bowden PE, Coulombe PA, Langbein L, Lane EB, Magin TM, Maltais L, Omary MB, Parry DA, Rogers MA, Wright MW 2006. New consensus nomenclature for mammalian keratins. *J Cell Biol* **174** (2):169–74.

Scolyer RA, Long GV, Thompson JF 2011. Evolving concepts in melanoma classification and their relevance to multidisciplinary melanoma patient care. *Mol Oncol* **5** (2):124–36.

Shia J 2008. Immunohistochemistry versus microsatellite instability testing for screening colorectal cancer patients at risk for hereditary nonpolyposis colorectal cancer syndrome. Part I. The utility of immunohistochemistry. *J Mol Diagn* **10**(4):293–300.

Silva AP, Coelho PV, Anazetti M, Simioni PU 2017. Targeted therapies for the treatment of non-small-cell lung cancer: Monoclonal antibodies and biological inhibitors. *Hum Vaccin Immunother* **13**(4):843–53.

Soda, M, Lim Choi Y, Enomoto M, Takada S, Yamashita Y, Ishikawa S, Fujiwara SI, Watanabe H, Kurashina K, Hatanaka H, Bando M, Ohno S, Ishikawa Y, Aburatani H, Niki T, Sohara Y, Sugiyama Y, Mano H 2007. Identification of the transforming EML4–ALK fusion gene in non-small cell lung cancer. *Nature* **448** (7153):561–6.

Takeuchi K, Choi YL, Togashi Y, Soda M, Hatano S, Inamura K, Takada S, Ueno T, Yamashita Y, Satoh Y, Okumura S, Nakagawa K, Ishikawa Y, Mano H 2009. KIF5B-ALK, a novel fusion oncokinase identified by an immunohistochemistry-based diagnostic system for ALK-positive lung cancer. *Clin Cancer Res* **15**(9):3143–9.

Terata K, Saito H, Nanjo H, Hiroshima Y, Ito S, Narita K, Akagami Y, Nakamura R, Konno H, Ito A, Motoyama S, Minamiya Y 2017. Novel rapid-immunohistochemistry using an alternating current electric field for intraoperative diagnosis of sentinel lymph nodes in breast cancer. *Sci Rep* 7:2810.

Van der Loos CM 1999. *Immunoenzyme multiple staining methods*. First edition. Garland Science.

Vartanian RK, Leung JK, Davis JE, Kim YB, Owen DA 1998. A novel Alcian yellow-toluidine blue (Leung) stain for Helicobacter species: Comparison with standard stains, a cost-effectiveness analysis, and supplemental utilities. *Mod Pathol* **11**(1):72–8.

Wolff AC, Hammond MEH, Allison KH, Harvey BE, Mangu PB, Bartlett JMS, Bilous M, Ellis IO, Fitzgibbons P, Hanna W, Jenkins RB, Press MF, Spears PA, Vance GH, Viale G, McShane LM, Dowsett M 2018. Human epidermal growth factor receptor 2 testing in breast cancer: American Society of Clinical Oncology/College of American Pathologists Clinical Practice Guideline Focused Update. *J Clin Oncol* **36**(20):2105–22.

Wolff AC, Hammond ME, Schwartz JN, Hagerty KL, Allred DC, Cote RJ, Dowsett M, Fitzgibbons PL, Hanna WM, Langer A, McShane LM, Paik S, Pegram MD, Perez EA, Press MF, Rhodes A, Sturgeon C, Taube SE, Tubbs R, Vance GH, van de Vijver M, Wheeler TM, Hayes DF 2007. American Society of Clinical Oncology/College of American Pathologists guideline recommendations for human epidermal growth factor receptor 2 testing in breast cancer. *J Clin Oncol* **25**(1):118–45.

Yatabe Y, Dacic S, Borczuk AC, Warth A, Russell PA, Lantuejoul S, Beasley MB, Thunnissen E, Pelosi G, Rekhtman N, Bubendorf L, Mino-Kenudson M, Yoshida A, Geisinger KR, Noguchi M, Chirieac LR, Bolting J, Chung JH, Chou TY, Chen G, Poleri C, Lopez-Rios F, Papotti M, Sholl LM, Roden AC, Travis WD, Hirsch FR, Kerr KM, Tsao MS, Nicholson AG, Wistuba I, Moreira AL 2019. Best practices recommendations for diagnostic immunohistochemistry in lung cancer. *J Thorac Onco* **14**(3):377–407.

Yu J, Kane S, Wu J, Benedettini E, Li D, Reeves C, Innocenti G, Wetzel R, Crosby K, Becker A, Ferrante M, Cheung WC, Hong X, Chirieac LR, Sholl LM, Haack H, Smith BL, Polakiewicz RD, Tan Y, Gu TL, Loda M, Zhou X, Comb MJ 2009. Mutation-specific antibodies for the detection of EGFR mutations in non-small-cell lung cancer. *Clin Cancer Res* **15**(9):3023–8.

Zhuo M, Zheng Q, Zhao J, Wu M, An T, Wang Y, Li J, Wang S, Zhong J, Yang X, Chen H, Jia B, Dong Z, Gao E, Wang J, Wang Z 2017. Survival difference between EGFR Del19 and L858 R mutant advanced non-small cell lung cancer patients receiving gefitinib: A propensity score matching analysis. *Chin J Cancer Res* **29**(6):553–60.

Chapter 9

Immunohistochemistry for Future Applications

Candice J. Clarke

Overview

Immunohistochemistry (IHC) techniques have been utilized in research and diagnostic pathology since Coon's early work in the 1940s (Dixon et al. 2015). Diagnostic pathology laboratories routinely perform IHC primarily on formalin-fixed paraffin-embedded (FFPE) tissue sections, frozen tissue sections and cytological specimens. Advances in IHC techniques have generally evolved from research and then those which prove to be most cost-effective and adaptable tend to be taken up by diagnostic laboratories. With recent advances in molecular biology techniques to aid in the diagnosis and prognosis of routine pathology specimens there has been a greater requirement for the use of anatomical pathology specimens. The requirements to get a diagnosis from a tissue biopsy can be extensive, with surgeons taking smaller tissue biopsies so as to avoid invasive procedures for the patient. Therefore it is vital to maximize the use of each tissue sample in order to get the most benefit for the patient.

This review covers techniques currently being used and developed in a research setting which may be introduced into a routine diagnostic laboratory soon. There are many forms of multiplex staining techniques, all promoting the discovery of complex biological processes using different types of antibody tagging. Then there are 'next-generation' IHC techniques based on the principles of mass spectrometry. These new techniques allow us to extract even more information from a single tissue section, with both quantitative data and the spatial location of proteins in the tissue. The use of digital pathology and digital image analysis with the assistance of artificial intelligence is becoming a reality. Likewise, the use of tissue microarrays to get the most out of a patient's tissue sample may gain in popularity. By chapter's end, it is hoped, an appreciation will be gained of the technology available now, albeit in a research setting, which may soon find applications in the diagnostic sphere.

The continued advancement of IHC is dynamic, based on clinical need, cost per test and reproducibility. It is a worthwhile exercise to glimpse into the future and be aware of the developing IHC landscape.

Multiplex Staining

Traditional IHC is performed on a single tissue section with one primary antibody. To visualize multiple proteins in the tissue, serial sections are cut and an individual antibody is tested on each tissue section. Multiplex staining allows multiple markers to be visualized on the same tissue section (Fassler et al. 2020). Multiplex staining can be performed either sequentially, with multiple antibodies labelled one after the other, or simultaneously, all labelled at the same time (Dixon et al. 2015). Multiplex staining can be performed on cell preparations, fresh frozen tissue and FFPE with either chromogenic or fluorescent labels to visualize the antibodies of interest (Tan et al. 2020).

Simple multiplex techniques have been well established and are routinely used in diagnostic pathology laboratories. At the moment, they are generally limited to two or three antibody markers on a single tissue section (Carvajal-Hausdorf et al. 2015). The future of multiplex IHC staining lies in the development of up to 50 antibodies within a tissue section. Advanced multiplex techniques of this nature have been developed to be highly accurate, enabling many localization markers in a single cell (Taube et al. 2020).

Planning and validation are two of the key steps to successful multiplex staining techniques, and one of the most important is the selection of the primary antibodies. It is preferred that monoclonal antibodies are used as they provide higher sensitivity and reproducibility (Taube et al. 2020). Before any multiplex method is performed each antibody should be tested and optimized as a single stain with an appropriate control tissue to determine the suitability of the antibody to be used as a marker in the multiplex assay (Taube et al. 2020). There are also two methods to labelling the antibody for visualization; either directly or indirectly (Dixon et al. 2015). A directly labelled antibody has a reporter tag conjugated to the antibody; these may consist of chromogens, fluorophores or metal tags. The indirect method is a two-step process. There are many advantages of multiplex staining, including that multiple antibodies are visualized on the one tissue section to study complex biological interactions (Parra et al. 2020). The most common label used for multiplexing is chromogenic and fluorescent assays.

Chromogenic Multiplex Staining

The most commonly used chromogen to visualize the antibody markers in diagnostic pathology is 3,3'-diaminobenzidine (DAB). Generally, the maximum antibodies which can be visualized with chromogenic detection are two to three depending on the cellular localization of the proteins (Dixon et al. 2015). One of the biggest advantages of chromogenic multiplex staining is that it does not require any specialized microscope equipment and can be performed in a routine diagnostic laboratory either manually or on an automated staining platform (Carvajal-Hausdorf et al. 2015). It is a quick and robust technique which can be visualized using a routine optical microscope found in any pathology laboratory (Taube et al. 2020). No special software is needed to analyse the slides, and they can be sent and analysed for diagnosis in any laboratory (Tan et al. 2020). The downside to chromogenic multiplex staining is that it is not a quantitative method; at best in some situations it can semi-quantitative (Taube et al. 2020). As the interpretation is subjective to the individual pathologist, there can be inter-observer variability (Tan et al. 2020).

Fluorescence Multiplex Staining

Fluorescence multiplex staining has been a popular technique for researchers to answer many biological questions. Basic fluorescence multiplex staining consists generally of three colours – two coloured fluorophores for the antibodies of interest and a stain for the cell nucleus (Hoffmann et al. 2019). In a routine pathology laboratory, immunofluorescence is generally single plex and commonly used in renal and dermatopathology (Carvajal-Hausdorf et al. 2015).

Basic fluorescence multiplex techniques require a simple fluorescence microscope, which can be found in diagnostic pathology facilities with no further purchase of equipment necessary as the technique can be performed manually or on an automated IHC platform. The basic two- and three-colour fluorescence multiplex techniques are easily interpreted by a diagnostic pathologist without the need for imaging software (Hoffmann et al. 2019). The main problem with fluorescence staining is the background autofluorescence and the potential for fluorescence overlap depending on the localization of the markers of interest (Levenson et al. 2015; Parra et al. 2019).

Many novel fluorescence multiplex staining techniques are currently being used for research. A simple search of the published literature will reveal techniques which have been used frequently while others are still under development. Two examples of commercially available kits include Opal (Akoya BioSciences) and Cell DIVE (Leica Microsystems). This area is developing continually as new biological questions need to be answered and the techniques are refined as the technology advances. The methods described next include new and interesting assays which may be adopted into routine diagnostic laboratories in the future. Some are available as commercialized kits whilst others offer real potential for widespread use. These include tyramide signal amplification (TSA), CO detection by indEXing (CODEX) and quantum dot (QD) technology.

Tyramide Signal Amplification

Tyramide signal amplification (TSA) is an IHC multiplex staining technique using fluorescence to visualize protein expression in a single tissue section (Zhang et al. 2017). This multiplex technique is a form of enzymatic amplification with fluorophores conjugated to tyramide molecules (Parra et al. 2020; Viratham Pulsawatdi et al. 2020). Tyramide signal amplification can be used on FFPE tissue comparable to traditional IHC to visualise the co-localization of proteins on a single section (Parra et al. 2020).

Research has shown that up to nine markers can be used to detect proteins in a single tissue section, but most studies use a five or seven multiplex system (Parra et al. 2020). The TSA methods are more sensitive than traditional IHC techniques and can be used to detect low levels of protein in the tissue while using less of the antibodies (Gorris et al. 2018). Tyramide signal amplification works by binding one antibody with the tyramide-bound fluorophore at a time to the epitope of interest followed by a cycle of stripping unbound antibody before the next one is applied in order to avoid non-specific binding (Hofman et al. 2019; Tan et al. 2020; Taube et al. 2020). This sequential cycling starts with the tyramide fluorophore of the first antibody being covalently bound to the tyrosine residues associated with the epitope of interest catalysed by the enzymatic action of horse radish peroxidase (HRP) (Lee et al. 2020; Parra et al. 2019). After the binding of each antibody, the tissue is subjected to 'stripping' in the microwave so as to remove unbound primary and secondary antibodies before the process is repeated for the next antibody (Parra et al. 2017; Hofman et al. 2019; Tan et al. 2020). The unbound antibodies are removed, but due to the covalent bonding, the fluorophore remains (Lee et al. 2020). The tyramide molecules bound to the antibodies generate enzymatic amplification, increasing the sensitivity (Viratham Pulsawatdi et al. 2020).

This sequential cycling process when performed manually can take up to a week, which leaves a large margin for human error and can adversely affect reproducibility. In this context it is not a viable option for a clinical diagnostic laboratory. In recent years, there has been some automation of TSA techniques on existing IHC platforms, allowing for a more rapid result to be obtained (Zhang et al. 2017; Sun et al. 2021). An automated system can perform the same staining processes within a day whilst providing a more uniform and reproducible approach (Tan et al. 2020). There are also commercially available TSA staining kits ranging from three plex to seven plex, depending on the number of antibodies required to be detected in a tissue section. The commercial kits cater for both manual and automated staining using the TSA method (Parra et al. 2019). A big advantage of combining the commercially available kits with an automated system is the level of reproducibility and reliability achieved for clinical diagnostics. For example, Akoya Biosciences have produced a detection kit from their Opal range optimized for use on the Leica Biosystems BOND RX platform (Parra et al. 2019; Viratham Pulsawatdi et al. 2020).

Due to the fluorescent nature of the method, the slide requires an imaging system capable of detecting the multispectral range of the fluorophores (Parra et al. 2020; Shakya et al. 2020). Whole slide imaging (WSI) can be performed, or a region of interest (ROI) selected by a pathologist is scanned (Viratham Pulsawatdi et al. 2020). In comparison, WSI requires more scanning time and results in a larger amount of data then zoning into a ROI. In addition, the data need to be analysed and interpreted correctly, which may require the expertise of an experienced statistician as well as the critical input of a pathologist (Parra et al. 2020; Shakya et al. 2020). These data need to be securely stored. The current trend is that with increasing technology developments and improvement of image resolutions, the data storage requirements inevitably increase (Parra et al. 2020).

Multiplex IHC using TSA is a complex technique which requires careful planning and optimization for a successful outcome. Suitable control tissues are required for extensive optimization with each antibody and include parameters such as optimal antibody dilutions, incubation times, fluorophore intensity and sufficient blocking to ensure the optimal results. When selecting antibody–fluorophore pairings, the protein abundance should be considered. The antibody which is expected to be the most abundantly expressed should be paired with the fluorophore with the weakest intensity and the lowest-expressed antibody should be paired with the fluorophore with the strongest intensity (Lee et al. 2020). The theory and process of performing TSA is the same whether it is performed manually using a microwave for the stripping and retrieval steps or whether it is automated on an IHC staining platform. The planning and optimization steps before commencing the TSA assay are also the same and are highlighted in Figure 9.1 (Parra et al. 2020; Tan et al. 2020).

These steps are important to follow because they produce and maintain a robust and replicable method. Where possible, it is best to use monoclonal antibodies as they have a higher specificity and lower background staining compared with polyclonal antibodies (Parra et al. 2020). The TSA methods also allow the use of antibodies from the same species due to the sequential stripping of the primary and secondary antibodies before the next antibody is applied. This act removes the associated immunoglobulins which may cause unwanted binding in subsequent steps. An unintentional consequence is the potential for steric hindrance when an antibody binds to a site and blocks the binding of further antibodies (Taube et al. 2020). To combat this phenomenon, either reduce the concentration of the conjugated tyramide fluorophore or increase the antibody dilution (Viratham Pulsawatdi et al. 2020). Even if all of these steps are followed, a result may still not be obtained if the tissue is of poor quality at the start. Hence, it is important to maintain good pre-analytical steps because the quality of staining is affected by poor tissue quality. Similar to routine one-colour IHC, there is no substitute for optimal tissue quality. This method cannot correct poorly fixed and processed tissue, and so it is important that routine histology processes are performed to a high standard, including section thickness and appropriate glass slide choice (Parra et al. 2020). Table 9.1 lists the advantages and disadvantages of TSA IHC.

CO Detection by IndEXing (CODEX)

CO detection by indEXing (CODEX) is a fluorescence-based DNA bar coding multiplex imaging platform commercialized by Akoya Biosciences (Parra et al. 2019; Phillips et al. 2021). This platform can be used on cell preparations, fresh frozen and FFPE tissue to detect greater than 50 antibodies at the same time. CODEX is a high throughput technique which can be used to obtain information about the relative abundance and expression of the biomarkers of interest within a spatial context (Goltsev et al. 2018). This is an advantage over other fluorescence multiplex techniques which provide information about the proteins without spatial context. CODEX gives similar spatial information about the antibodies when compared to the more complex mass spectrometry techniques of multiplex ion beam imaging (MIBI) or scanning mass cytometry

Table 9.1 Weighing up the pros and cons of tyramide signal amplification immunohistochemical staining

Advantages	Disadvantages
TSA multiplex staining can be measured semi-quantitatively while still showing spatially the location of the antibody (Tan et al. 2020).	Specialized microscopy/scanning is needed to analyse the slide due to the fluorescent nature of TSA.
It is a sensitive assay which can detect low levels of protein in the tissue as well as potentially useless antibody due to the sensitivity (Parra et al. 2020).	There is the potential for spectral overlap of fluorophores.
Visualise co-localization of proteins, analyse complex biological interactions in a single tissue section (Willemsen et al. 2021).	Requires extensive optimization and expertise.
Can use same species antibodies as the stripping steps performed (Dixon et al. 2015; Lee et al. 2020).	Tissue can be heat sensitive, delicate tissue samples.

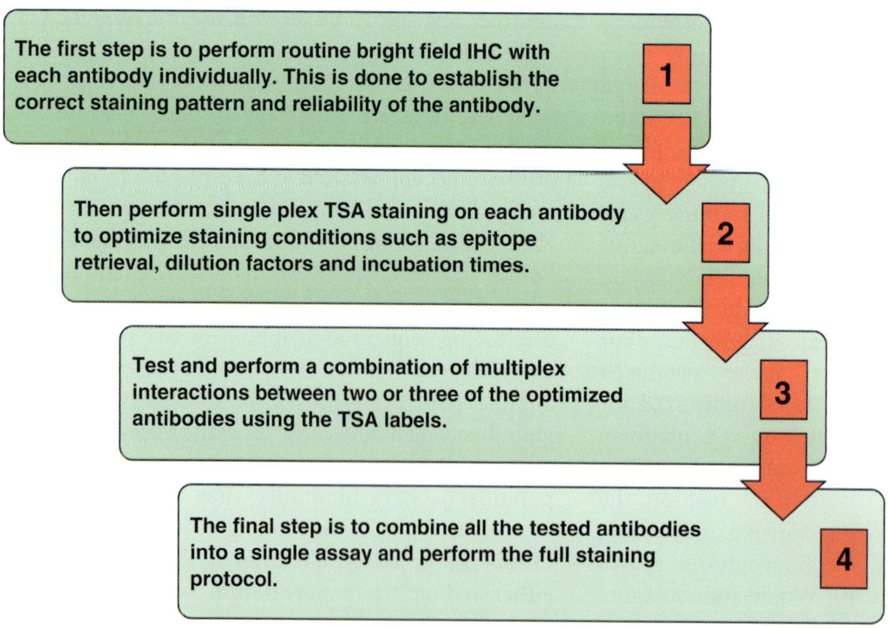

Figure 9.1 Planning a tyramide signal amplification immunohistochemical assay

(SMC) without the expensive equipment. This is its biggest advantage: the CODEX platform does not require expensive imaging equipment and is compatible with a routine three-colour fluorescence microscope set-up (Goltsev et al. 2018, Tan et al. 2020).

To perform the CODEX assay all of the antibodies are conjugated to unique oligonucleotide duplex sequences with 5' overhangs (Parra et al. 2019). All tagged antibodies are applied and incubated on the tissue at the same time. A mixture of the nucleotide bases adenine, guanine, uracil and cytosine is used to create the sequences (Parra et al. 2019). The antibodies are visualized in pairs through a series of labelling cycles; each cycle contains a nucleotide mix of a non-fluorescent 'index' nucleotide and two fluorescently labelled nucleotides (Goltsev et al. 2018). The 'index' nucleotides match to the first positions bound to all antibodies and then each of the two fluorescent bound nucleotides has only one match to bind to according to their unique nucleotide sequence. The pair of antibodies is then imaged using the fluorescence microscope before the fluorescence tags are cleaved and rinsed, and the next cycle is performed (Goltsev et al. 2018). This cycling process is repeated until all of the pairs have been visualized. The order of visualization is antibodies with the shorter 5' overhang first, followed by those with the longest 5' overhang last (Parra et al. 2019).

Due to CODEX not requiring specialized equipment there is no initial purchase of expensive equipment, but the repeat label cycling and imaging uses a considerable amount of time. It is the nature of a time-consuming assay that the longer the procedure is, the higher the chance of errors. It is therefore important to validate and assess the suitability of each antibody with careful planning and selection. The larger the antibody range, the more complex planning is involved. To assist and make the protocol somewhat more manageable, vendors of this technology have made it commercially available in order to alleviate some of the laborious tasks.

Nanocrystal Quantum Dots

Nanocrystal quantum dots (QD) are conjugated to antibodies as fluorescence tags and used as an alternative to chromogen and traditional fluorophores such as FITC and the Alexa Fluor compounds. Visualization is via multispectral imaging technology (Matea et al. 2017). Quantum dots are specially coated nanocrystals which have excellent photostability and can be excited by any wavelength of light. They possess narrow bands of fluorescence emission (Zrazhevskiy and Gao 2013; Parra et al. 2019). Quantum dots do not show endogenous autofluorescence because they have high sensitivity and specificity (Parra et al. 2019). This technology has potential for widespread use, but more research needs to be performed if it is to be used in a clinical setting. The use of QDs for routine immunofluorescence techniques is feasible due to the basic requirement of a fluorescence microscope with appropriate narrow band pass filters for visualization of the tissue.

Next-Generation Immunohistochemistry

Current diagnostic IHC techniques have been around for decades using either chromogen or fluorophore tags to visualize protein expression in tissue sections (Angelo et al. 2014). The next generation of IHC techniques in the research field are being developed because more complex biological questions are being asked. One such method being explored is combining mass spectrometry with IHC in order to study the protein expression of biomarkers in tissue sections (Angelo et al. 2014; Levenson et al. 2015; Rost et al. 2017; Ahmed et al. 2020; Tan et al. 2020).

These techniques are built around a similar technique known as mass cytometry, a system previously used to build tumour profiles and to quantify proteins expressed in single cells but does not show these proteins within a spatial context. Their location within the cell cannot be defined (Bendall et al. 2012). Mass cytometry has been developed by using flow cytometry concepts coupled with mass spectrometry (MS) techniques to measure the protein abundance via antibodies individually tagged with unique metal isotopes (Spitzer and Nolan 2016). This approach was developed and based on the same principles as flow cytometry, a technology to analyse single cells in a cell suspension by using antibodies tagged with fluorophores. A limitation, however, is that flow cytometry can only analyse a certain number of antibodies simultaneously before encountering spectral overlap of the fluorophores (Bendall et al. 2012; Spitzer and Nolan 2016). Mass cytometry, on the other hand, uses metal isotopes as antibody tags and these create a unique peak according to molecular weight. There are no spectral overlap concerns, which allows an increased number of antibodies to be analysed simultaneously for the accurate collection of quantitative data (Bendall et al. 2012; Levenson et al. 2015; Spitzer and Nolan 2016).

Mass cytometry requires specialized equipment and the cells are subject to a series of complex processes to obtain the required data. Techniques may vary with the equipment employed, but the basic concept is explained in Figure 9.2.

The 'mass-to-charge ratio' enables each metal present to be quantitatively measured. As each metal represents an individual antibody, the antibodies present can be quantitatively measured (Bendall et al. 2012; Spitzer and Nolan 2016). Remember, although mass cytometry offers valuable quantitative data of protein expression, it does not provide spatial information of where the proteins are expressed in the tissue (Angelo et al. 2014; Levenson et al. 2015; Parra et al 2019). Traditional IHC-stained sections, on the other hand, are used to visualize the expression of proteins in a tissue of interest whilst also providing important spatial information. These sections are analysed by trained pathologists, but there is the potential for inter-observer variability and they only have the potential to provide semi-quantitative data (Rost et al. 2017; Aljakna et al. 2018). To find the answers to complex biological interactions, there is a need for techniques that can provide spatial visualization of proteins as well as quantification. These requirements have driven researchers to investigate the 'next generation' of IHC techniques known as mass spectrometry IHC (Parra et al. 2019).

Mass Spectrometry Immunohistochemistry

Mass spectrometry immunohistochemistry (MSIHC) is an emerging technique developed to perform IHC on a single tissue section for the purposes of visualization and quantification of multiple proteins. Marrying the two technologies of mass spectrometry and IHC not only allows proteins be localized within tissue sections; MSIHC also enables them to be quantitatively analysed (Aljakna et al. 2018; Parra et al. 2019; Tan et al. 2020). The difference, however, is that antibodies are labelled with metal isotopes instead of enzyme developed chromogen or fluorophores. This is a form of tag mass imaging mass spectrometry (MS), which uses traditional MS techniques to allow the visualization of antibodies or oligonucleotides in a specific region of the tissue on either FFPE or fresh frozen tissue sections (Dixon et al. 2015).

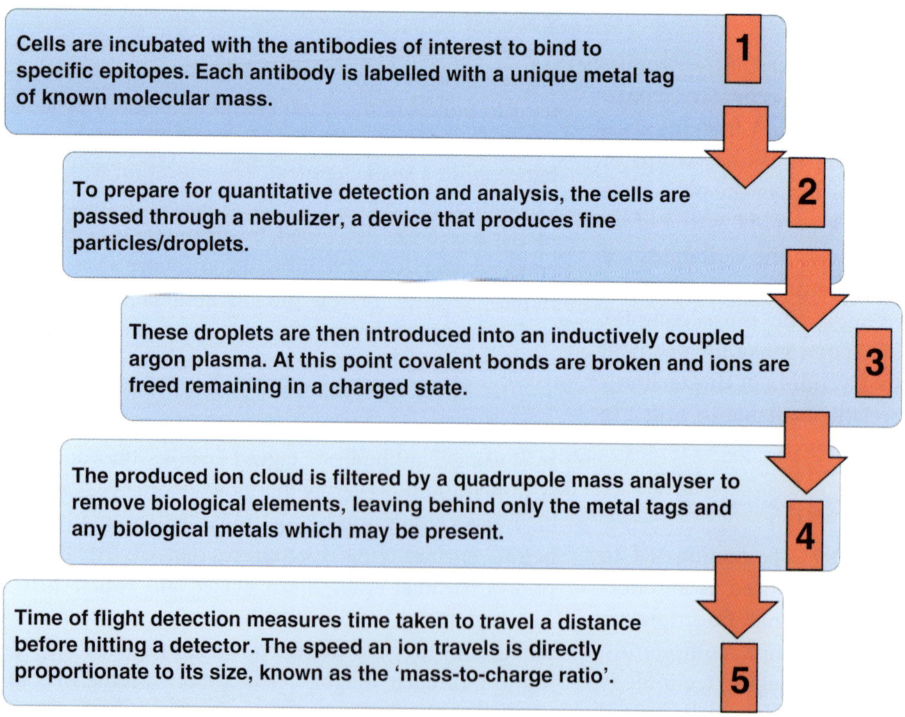

Figure 9.2 Mass cytometry basic concepts

As previously stated, before MSIHC can be performed on FFPE tissue an extensive amount of preparation and optimization is needed (Taube et al. 2020). Performing MSIHC on FFPE tissue sections starts with traditional IHC methods of tissue preparation which include deparaffinising the section, performing appropriate antigen retrieval and executing a blocking step for endogenous enzyme activity (Aljakna et al. 2018). Primary antibodies are labelled individually with a unique isotopically pure metal tag with a known molecular mass (Levenson et al. 2015). All of the primary antibodies are mixed together and incubated on a single tissue section in one incubation step. Mass spectrometry IHC does not require signal amplification to be performed as this is a very sensitive technique (Parra et al. 2019).

As with traditional IHC methods performed on FFPE tissue sections, MSIHC is also impacted by suboptimal pre-analytical events. Poor tissue fixation and processing coupled with inappropriate storage conditions will have a negative impact on results (Rost et al. 2017). It is therefore important to follow standard practices in handling FFPE tissues because there are no workarounds as MSIHC cannot remedy these issues. The antibodies selected should be optimized and tested on tissue prior to MSIHC being performed to ensure they are reliable and exhibit the appropriate staining pattern.

Secondary ion mass spectrometry (SIMS) and laser ablation are two tag mass methods which have been described in reference to imaging mass spectrometry (Levenson et al. 2015; Parra et al. 2019). The major difference between these two techniques is the method in which they are used to liberate, ionize and detect the metal tags from the ROI in the tissue section. The two techniques which have been described for use in MSIHC are multiplex ion beam imaging (MIBI) based on SIMS and scanning mass cytometry (SMC) using laser ablation (Levenson et al. 2015; Parra et al. 2019).

The ROI of the tissue section is rastered using ion beam or laser in a grid-like arrangement to acquire relevant data (Aljakna et al. 2018). The data acquired can then be analysed and an image reconstructed. These images are then pseudo-coloured to represent traditional IHC or immunofluorescence (Angelo et al. 2014). The images can be coloured to mimic a traditional IHC stained section with the counterstaining blue in replacement of the haematoxylin and the antibodies brown to reflect the 3,3'-diaminobenzidine (DAB) chromogen (Rost et al. 2017). This imaging allows visualization of the site of proteins within tissue as well as co-localized proteins for answers to more complex biological questions (Tan et al. 2020).

Multiplex Ion Beam Imaging

This technology uses an ion beam to liberate ions from the tissue surface (Levenson et al. 2015; Parra et al. 2019). The detection system can be either a coupled magnetic detector or time of flight (TOF) mass spectrometer. Both have the ability to detect ions and allow quantitative data collection of each individual antibody. The ion beam scans the surface of the ROI and only removes a depth of 5–10 nm from the superficial layer (Levenson et al. 2015). By removing just this shallow layer, the sample can be rescanned for further tissue analysis. Replication of the experiment can be performed, akin to cutting another FFPE section for a repeat IHC stain. The ability to rescan a ROI area allows an overview scan of the tissue at low resolution to look for more specific ROIs for high-resolution analyses. (Baharlou et al. 2019).

Isotopically pure lanthanides are typically used as the metal tag conjugated to the antibodies (Ahmed et al. 2020). They are ideal labels because lanthanides are rare earth metals and are not generally present in biological samples (Han et al. 2018). In addition, these metal tags do not degrade and are enriched to a single isotope with no cause for overlap or interfering background signals. The potential to tag more than 50 antibodies at once at a resolution of 200 nm renders MIBI a technology that is worth considering for routine diagnostic pathology (Parra et al. 2019).

Scanning Mass Cytometry

This imaging technique employs a laser to ablate and liberate ions for detection (Giesen et al. 2014). Scanning mass cytometry also uses metal isotopes as tags for the antibodies and applies the same basic principles as mass cytometry (Levenson et al. 2015). A laser ablates the ROI, which then passes through a nebulizer and is introduced into inductively coupled plasma before the data is acquired by a TOF detector (Baharlou et al. 2019). Unlike MIBI, this technique removes the entire thickness of the sample, thereby destroying it and forgoing the chance for assay replication or the ability to perform a low-resolution initial scan (Levenson et al. 2015).

Table 9.2 Weighing the pros and cons of mass spectrometry immunohistochemistry

Advantages	Disadvantages
The ability to obtain a considerable amount of information from a single tissue section.	Requires specialized equipment which is generally not found in routine diagnostic pathology laboratories.
Achieving quantitative data whilst visualizing and locating proteins in the tissue section.	Complex techniques require expertise. Extensive optimization and planning of the assay are required.
Efficient use of tissue allows more information to be gained from small and rare tissue samples such as needle core biopsies.	The equipment and the cost of the reagents required are expensive. There is a high capital investment at start-up.
There are no background or crossover of signals. Each metal peak is based on molecular mass of uniquely tagged antibody allowing spectral separation.	Quite laborious. Image acquisition and then data analysis require heavy investment of time and laboratory resources.
This technology is advancing all the time, which should decrease the cost and make the equipment required available to diagnostic pathology laboratories.	Time-consuming, especially if higher image resolutions are required. This means longer scanning times with current technology.

Up to 50 antibodies can be detected in a single tissue section with a resolution between 1 µm and 500 nm (Levenson et al. 2015). The acquisition of images is slow with current technologies taking about one hour to scan a mm^2 of tissue area. This bottleneck will undoubtedly decrease as the technology matures. Table 9.2 summarizes the main advantages and disadvantages of this next-generation IHC system.

Digital Pathology

The need for digital pathology and the ability to work remotely has increased in recent times, particularly with the global COVID-19 pandemic (Hanna et al. 2020). Automated scanning and analysis are also important in remote areas for consultation on difficult or interesting cases, for education and archiving of rare specimens (Wilbur et al. 2015; Borowsky et al. 2020). New technologies such as MSIHC discussed previously will tether on to these digital platforms and as this technology develops, more slide scanning systems are becoming available on the market (Qaiser et al. 2018; Hanna et al. 2019). With the increase in availability and competition they have also become more affordable, making digital slide scanning systems a viable option for many diagnostic laboratories to introduce into their routine workflow. Slide scanners can now perform WSI to allow a pathologist to diagnose from the digital images. Studies have shown that high-quality digital images compare favourably to traditional glass slides and there is good concordance between the two (Wilbur et al. 2015; Hanna et al. 2020). Whole slide imaging can be used diagnostically for not only H&E slides, but also for special stains, frozen sections and IHC.

Many challenges are faced when introducing image analysis from WSI into a diagnostic pathology laboratory, and it is vital to perform solid validation studies. The ability to diagnose from the scanned images is only part of the challenge; there are also many technical difficulties to overcome. One of the most important factors in producing a diagnosable WSI is the quality of the original slides produced for scanning (Hanna et al. 2020). It is important that the slides and coverslips are not cracked or broken and there are no artefacts or bubbles on the slide surface beneath the coverslip (Dimitriou et al. 2019; Hanna et al. 2020). Coverslips also need to be carefully positioned and slides must be clean and free of markings. These quality control processes are important to obtain an image suitable for diagnostic purposes. A technical limitation includes the inability to use polarization in cases for amyloid (Borowsky et al. 2020; Hanna et al. 2020). There can also be an issue with histochemical and IHC slides, especially when investigating for microorganisms such as *Helicobacter pylori*. Their small size renders a degree of difficulty for accurate diagnoses (Hanna et al. 2020).

The scanning of the slides and creating the WSI is only part of the process in being able to diagnose from the digital images. It is also important to have quality images readily accessible. If the pathologist does not have reliable internet and/or network connections, the images may load very slowly or with poor resolution. One of the biggest issues and costs associated with digital pathology are the large amounts of data produced and the need to store these data (Dimitriou et al. 2019; Fassler et al. 2020). Other equipment needed includes a computer capable of handling the large image files and a quality screen to display the images. (Wilbur et al. 2015). The ability to display more than image at a time is also important as pathologists often compare more than one slide at once, particularly with IHC slides where they may be comparing two different cell populations (Davidson et al. 2019).

Digital Image Analysis Using Artificial Intelligence

Parallel with advances in slide scanners and diagnostics for WSI, there have also been improvements in digital image analysis (DIA) methods with computer-assisted diagnostic techniques (Fassler et al. 2020). Interpretation of IHC slides by pathologists is subjective, and the interpreted result can be subject to intra- and inter-observer variability (Hall et al. 2008; Wilbur et al. 2015; Koopman et al. 2018). With the assistance of artificial intelligence (AI) and machine-based learning, DIA platforms can aid in the provision of more objective diagnostic outcomes (Koopman et al. 2019). There have been many studies dedicated to DIA of Her2 IHC in breast and gastro-oesophageal cancer (Hall et al. 2008; Qaiser et al. 2018; Shamai et al. 2019). The Her2 status of a patient is obtained by using a combination of IHC and *in situ* hybridization (ISH). A negative case is 0 or 1+, equivocal 2+ and positive is score3+ for IHC. *In situ* hybridization assays categorize Her2 status as either negative/non-amplified or positive/amplified (Wolff et al. 2018).

The importance of an accurate Her2 status is critical for the patient to receive optimal treatment. A patient with either Her2 gene amplification and/or protein overexpression is a candidate for targeted monoclonal antibody treatment with Herceptin (Wilbur et al. 2015; Koopman et al. 2019). Equivocal cases with Her2 score 2+ need reflex ISH testing to determine their Her2 status. Digital image analysis has emerged as an objective technique to score Her2 IHC staining and may reduce the number of equivocal cases currently seen (Koopman et al. 2019). Some facilities currently employ DIA on routine FFPE IHC techniques developed with DAB chromogen and counterstained with haematoxylin to solve Her2 equivocal cases (Hall et al. 2008; Koopman et al. 2019).

Digital image analysis relies on AI through the extensive development of algorithms and deep learning of morphological patterns (Qaiser et al. 2018; Dimitriou et al. 2019; De Logu et al. 2020). After the development of complex algorithms, the system needs extensive training and validation to learn the patterns. Part of the process is the need to teach the program to recognize certain cells or cell patterns and to develop algorithms to detect these. For Her2 studies, an algorithm needs to be developed to isolate the membrane staining pattern and to detect the quality of membrane staining (Hall et al. 2008). The deep learning is generally performed on ROIs selected by the pathologist or operator to focus on the pattern specific to that area (Dimitriou et al. 2019; De Logu et al. 2020).

To start the learning process, an ROI is selected and scanned and measurements are taken of the analyte. For instance, the DAB staining of linear structures on the cell membrane would be targeted for Her2 scoring (Koopman et al. 2018). To train the platform a large amount of data are required, and many images of ROIs are scanned so as to improve the accuracy of the algorithm (De Logu et al. 2020). Some commercially available systems provide algorithms based on morphology of cancer cells for Her2 overexpression and they provide a universal cut-off for positivity (Hall et al. 2008; Qaiser et al. 2018). There is a difference between the various available algorithm platforms, but the key concept of optimal system calibration is universal (Loughrey et al. 2018). The American Society of Clinical Oncology/College of American Pathologists (ASCO/CAP) guidelines have acknowledged DIA as a valid diagnostic scoring method for Her2 assessment (Koopman et al. 2019).

Although the concept of DIA with the assistance of AI has potential for scoring IHC slides, there are also many obstacles to overcome before it can be introduced into a clinically diagnostic pathology laboratory. Other things to consider are the intra- and inter-laboratory variability in staining intensity as well as the time needed to perform the digital scanning and analysis (Qaiser et al. 2018). Each of these scanned images and analysis create large files of data which need to be stored appropriately, an issue common to all digital pathology platforms. Another generic requirement is for slides to be of high quality and specimens need to undergo optimal pre-analytical conditions. Artefacts found on the stained images can generally be ignored by a trained pathologist along with staining variability. It is difficult for AI to replicate this type of 'fuzzy logic'. Extra attention needs to be paid to these details to either use a filter to remove the artefacts or to train the algorithm to detect them, which requires more extensive deep learning (Dimitriou et al. 2019).

There is considerable training and validation to be done and the time to analyse the samples is extensive and may not be practical in a diagnostic laboratory at the moment (Qaiser et al. 2018; Dimitriou et al. 2019; De Logu et al. 2020). Various studies have used AI and machine learning to distinguish between cell types. The algorithm used to analyse the difference in cell morphology must distinguish between the *in situ* and invasive carcinoma as well as stromal and tumour cell staining, just to highlight two possible scenarios (Loughrey et al. 2018).

Tissue Microarrays

Tissue microarrays (TMA) are paraffin blocks containing multiple cores of tissue from multiple sources (Dixon et al. 2015). They are made by taking representative tissue cores from FFPE tissue 'donor' blocks and inserting them into an empty paraffin 'recipient block' (Jawhar 2009; Glinsmann-Gibson et al. 2020). This technology has been available for a while now, especially in the research field. With advances in testing techniques and the need for more information to be extracted from less tissue, TMAs may hold the key to maximizing the use from available patient tissue (Jawhar, 2009; Dixon et al. 2015).

Large amounts of information can be obtained using this high throughput technique. Tissue microarrays can be used to analyse protein, DNA or RNA via IHC, fluorescence *in situ* hybridization (FISH) or RNA *in situ* hybridization (ISH), as well as routine histology haematoxylin and eosin (H&E) and histochemical stains – for instance, if a particular assay is prohibitively expensive to perform on one patient at a time. Constructing a TMA encompassing 30 patient cores and performing the expensive assay would be more feasible and a better use of laboratory resources. It is for these situations that there may be scope for its routine use on patient samples in routine diagnostic pathology.

When constructing a TMA there needs to be careful planning and preparation so each core can be identified in the block. A map is required with a marker embedded in the block for orientation so each core can be traceable on the X and Y-axis (Jawhar 2009). If each individual core cannot be identified within the TMA, then they cannot be scored and the block is of no significant use. Cores can vary in size from 0.6 mm to 2.0 mm in diameter and should be selected depending on the information required. Figure 9.3 highlights the basic steps necessary to construct a TMA.

Tissue microarray blocks have many different uses. They can be made from a series of different tissue types or the same tissue type from multiple patient blocks. Small TMAs are commonly used in a diagnostic histology laboratory as a control block for IHC staining (Jawhar 2009). The steps to making

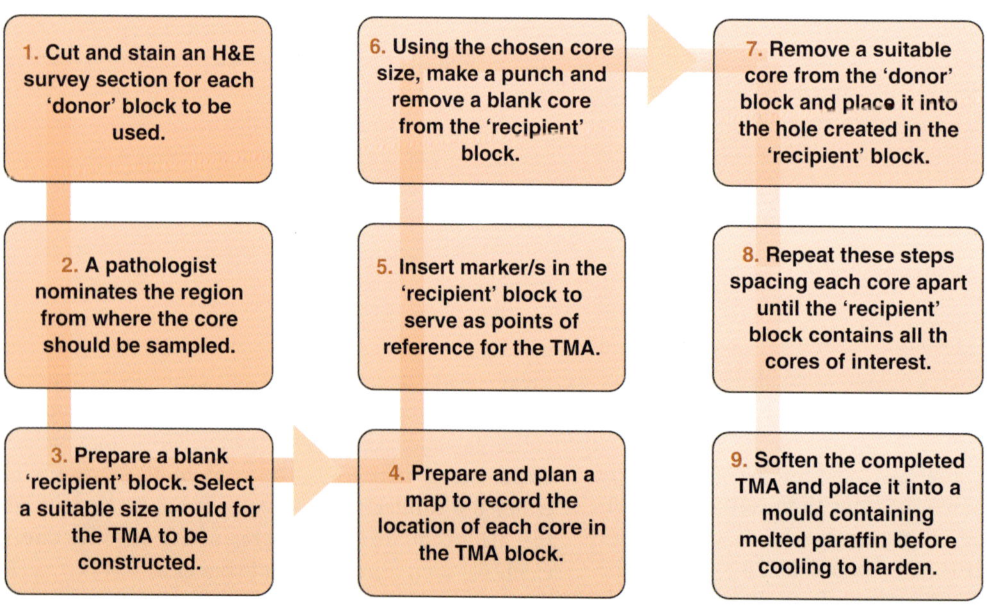

Figure 9.3 Tissue microarray construction

a TMA are relatively simple, but require attention to detail to ensure the planning and construction is robust. A TMA is usually constructed manually using a tissue microarray instrument which makes the holes in the 'recipient' block and takes the tissue cores from the 'donor' block, providing uniformity (Jawhar, 2009). The biggest challenge, however, is core length consistency. For example, take a TMA containing 50 cores. Each core diameter can be consistently achieved to be 0.5 mm because of the 'needle' size used. Conversely, it can be technically difficult to achieve the same length for each of the 50 cores. Some may be short whilst other may be long. When these cores are embedded into a 'recipient' paraffin block and sections are obtained, naturally the shorter cores will be exhausted first. Another hurdle holding the use of TMAs back from routine diagnostics is the time-consuming and costly nature of constructing the TMA block. It is currently not efficient for routine diagnosis due to the construction time.

Tissue microarrays are commonly used in a research setting with the initial construction of the TMA block being very laborious (Dixon et al. 2015; Glinsmann-Gibson et al. 2020). Studies have shown just using two cores per case in 95% of cases is equivalent to analysing the whole slide (Jawhar 2009). Once a TMA has been constructed it can be used to obtain a large amount of information while using fewer antibodies and reagents. Being able to test 50 patients at once for an important biomarker will save time and be cost-effective (Glinsmann-Gibson et al. 2020). Tissue microarrays are also a good tool for validating or screening novel antibodies (Jawhar 2009).

Conclusion

What the future holds for diagnostic IHC is unknown, but having seen how IHC has evolved with advances in molecular biology techniques, it seems there will be a place for IHC in some capacity in the future. Looking forward to new technologies on the horizon, the continual evolution of IHC will be exciting nonetheless. New techniques have the potential to radicalize the way IHC is performed. With emerging technologies such as MSIHC continually maturing, the equipment currently used to perform these assays may be expensive, but as technology progresses and these techniques become more commonly used, the costs may come down.

A raft of new challenges will accompany these new technologies. The largest new frontier of diagnostic pathology currently lies with digitalization of some aspects of pathology. Issues which need to be addressed in the present and future include data management and storage capacity. Digital pathology and the 'next-generation' IHC techniques create excessive amounts of data, and this can be complex to analyse. A new requirement of expertise in data analysis employing statisticians or biostatisticians may soon be commonplace in a routine histology laboratory. There is also the practicality of novel techniques being performed in a diagnostic laboratory alongside new levels of instrumentation. The skill set required to work in an IHC laboratory may change as these new forms of technology progresses. All of these issues need to be contemplated and addressed together as the discipline of IHC expands into the latter half of the 21st century.

References

Ahmed M, Broeckx G, Baggerman G, Schildermans K, Pauwels P, Van Craenenbroeck AH, Dendooven A 2020. Next-generation protein analysis in the pathology department. *J Clin Pathol* **73**(1):1–6.

Aljakna A, Lauer E, Lenglet S, Grabherr S, Fracasso T, Augsburger M, Sabatasso S, Thomas A 2018. Multiplex quantitative imaging of human myocardial infarction by mass spectrometry-immunohistochemistry. *Int J Legal Med* **132**(6):1675–84.

Angelo M, Bendall SC, Finck R, Hale MB, Hitzman C, Borowsky AD, Levenson RM, Lowe JB, Liu SD, Zhoa S, Natkunam Y, Nolan GP 2014. Multiplexed ion beam imaging of human breast tumors. *Nat Med* **20**(4):436–42.

Baharlou H, Canete NP, Cunningham AL, Harman AN, Patrick E 2019. Mass cytometry imaging for the study of human diseases: Applications and data analysis strategies. *Front immuno* **10**:2657.

Bendall SC, Nolan GP, Roederer M, Chattopadhyay PK 2012. A deep profiler's guide to cytometry. *Trends Immunol* **33**(7):323–32.

Borowsky AD, Glassy EF, Wallace WD, Kallichanda NS, Behling CA, Miller DV, Oswal HN, Feddersen RM, Bakhtar OR, Mendoza AE, Molden DP, Saffer HL, Wixom CR, Albro JE, Cessna MH, Hall BJ, Lloyd IE, Bishop JW, Darrow MA, Gui D, Jen KY, Walby JAS, Bauer SM, Cortez DA, Gandhi P, Rodgers MM, Rodriguez RA, Martin DR, McConnell TG, Reynolds SJ, Spigel JH, Stepenaskie SA, Viktorova E, Magari R, Wharton KA, Qiu J, Bauter TW 2020. Digital whole slide imaging compared with light microscopy for primary diagnosis in surgical pathology. *Arch Pathol Lab Med* **144**(10):1245–53.

Carvajal-Hausdorf DE, Schalper KA, Neumeister VM, Rimm DL 2015. Quantitative measurement of cancer tissue biomarkers in the lab and in the clinic. *Lab Invest* **95** (4):385–96.

Davidson TM, Rendi MH, Frederick PD, Onega T, Allison KH, Mercan E, Bunyé TT, Shapiro LG, Weaver DL, Elmore JG 2019. Breast cancer prognostic factors in the digital era: Comparison of Nottingham grade using whole slide images and glass slides. *J Pathol Inform* **10**:11.

De Logu F, Ugolini F, Maio V, Simi S, Cossu A, Massi D, Nassini R, Lourino M 2020. Recognition of cutaneous melanoma on digitized histopathological slides via artificial intelligence algorithm. *Front Oncol* **10**:1559.

Dimitriou N, Arandjelović O, Caie PD 2019. Deep learning for whole slide image analysis: An overview. *Front Med (Lausanne)* **6**:264.

Dixon AR, Bathany C, Tsuei M, White J, Barald KF, Takayama S 2015. Recent developments in multiplexing techniques for immunohistochemistry. *Expert Rev Mol Diagn* **15**(9):1171–86.

Fassler DJ, Abousamra S, Gupta R, Chen C, Zhao M, Paredes D, Batool SA, Knudsen BS, Escobar-Hoyos L, Shroyer KR, Samaras D, Kurc T, Saltz J 2020. Deep learning-based image analysis methods for brightfield-acquired multiplex immunohistochemistry images. *Diagn Pathol* **15**(1):100.

Giesen C, Wang HAO, Schapiro D, Zivanovic N, Jacobs A, Hattendorf B, Schüffler PJ, Grolimund D, Buhmann JM, Brandt S, Varga Z, Wild PJ, Günther D, Bodenmiller B 2014. Highly multiplexed imaging of tumor tissues with subcellular resolution by mass cytometry. *Nat Methods* **11**(4):417–22.

Glinsmann-Gibson B, Wisner L, Stanton M, Larsen B, Rimsza L, Maguire A 2020. Recommendations for tissue microarray construction and quality assurance. *Appl Immunohistochem Mol Morphol* **28**(4):325–30.

Goltsev Y, Samusik N, Kennedy-Darling J, Bhate S, Hale M, Vasquez G, Black S, Nolan GP 2018. Deep profiling of mouse splenic architecture with CODEX multiplexed imaging. *Cell* **174**(4):968–81.

Gorris MAJ, Halilovic A, Rabold K, Van Duffelen A, Wickramasinghe IN, Verweij D, Wortel IMN, Textor JC, De Vries IJM, Figdor CG 2018. Eight-color multiplex immunohistochemistry for simultaneous detection of multiple immune checkpoint molecules within the tumor microenvironment. *J Immunol* **200**(1):347–54.

Hall BH, Ianosi-Irime M, Javidian P, Chen W, Ganesan S, Foran DJ 2008. Computer-assisted assessment of the human epidermal growth factor receptor 2 immunohistochemical assay in imaged histologic sections using a membrane isolation algorithm and quantitative analysis of positive controls. *BMC Med Imaging* **8**:11.

Han G, Spitzer MH, Bendall SC, Fantil WJ, Nolan GP 2018. Metal-isotope-tagged monoclonal antibodies for high-dimensional mass cytometry. *Nat Protoc* **13**(10):2121–48.

Hanna MG, Reuter VE, Ardon O, Kim D, Sirintrapun SJ, Schüffler PJ, Busam KJ, Sauter JL, Brogi E., Tan LK, Xu B, Bale T, Agaram NP, Tang LH, Ellenson LH, Philip J, Corsale L, Stamelos E, Friedlander MA, Ntiamoah P, Labasin M, England C, Klimstra DS, Hameed M 2020. Validation of a digital pathology system including remote review during the COVID-19 pandemic. *Mod Pathol* **33** (11):2115–27.

Hanna MG, Reuter VE, Hameed MR, Tan LK, Chiang S, Sigel C, Hollmann T, Giri D, Samboy J, Moradel C, Rosado A, Otilano JR, England C, Corsale L, Stamelos E, Yagi Y, Schüffler PJ, Fuchs T, Klimstra DS, Sirintrapun SJ 2019. Whole slide imaging equivalency and efficiency study: Experience at a large academic center. *Mod Pathol* **32**(7):916–28.

Hoffmann F, Umbreit C, Krüger T, Pelzel D, Ernst G, Kniemeyer O, Guntinas-Luchius O, Berndt A, Von Eggeling F 2019. Identification of proteomic markers in head and neck cancer using MALDI-MS imaging, LC-MS/MS, and immunohistochemistry. *Proteomics Clin Appl* **13** (1):e1700173.

Hofman P, Badoual C, Henderson F, Berland L, Hamila M, Long-Mira E, Lassalle S, Roussel H, Hofman V, Tartour E, Ilié M 2019. Multiplexed immunohistochemistry for molecular and immune profiling in lung cancer: Just about ready for prime-time? *Cancers (Basel)*, **11**(3):283.

Jawhar NMT. 2009. Tissue microarray: A rapidly evolving diagnostic and research tool. *Ann Saudi Med* **29**(2):123–7.

Koopman T, Buikema HJ, Hollema H, De Bock GH, Van Der Vegt B 2019. What is the added value of digital image analysis of Her2 immunohistochemistry in breast cancer in clinical practice? A study with multiple platforms. *Histopathology* **74**(6):917–24.

Koopman T, De Brock GH, Buikema HJ, Smits MM, Louwen M, Hage M, Imholz ALT, Van Der Vegt B 2018. Digital image analysis of Her2 immunohistochemistry in gastric- and oesophageal adenocarcinoma: A validation study on biopsies and surgical specimens. *Histopathology* **72** (2):191–200.

Lee CW, Ren YJ, Marella M, Wang M, Hartke J, Couto SS 2020. Multiplex immunofluorescence staining and image analysis assay for diffuse large B cell lymphoma. *J Immunol Methods* **478**:112714.

Levenson RM, Borowsky AD, Angelo M 2015. Immunohistochemistry and mass spectrometry for highly multiplexed cellular molecular imaging. *Lab Invest* **95** (4):397–405.

Loughrey MB, Bankhead P, Coleman HG, Hagan RS, Craig S, McCorry AMB, Gray RT, McQuaid S, Dunne PD, Hamilton PW, James JA, Salto-Tellez M 2018. Validation of the systematic scoring of immunohistochemically stained tumour tissue microarrays using QuPath digital image analysis. *Histopathology* **73**(2):327–38.

Matea CT, Mocan T, Tabaran F, Pop T, Mosteanu O, Puia C, Iancu C, Mocan L 2017. Quantum dots in imaging, drug delivery and sensor applications. *Int J Nanomedicine*, **12**: 5421–31.

Parra ER, Francisco-Cruz A, Wistuba II 2019. State-of-the-art of profiling immune contexture in the era of multiplexed staining and digital analysis to study paraffin tumor tissues. *Cancers (Basel)* **11**(2):247.

Parra ER, Jaing M, Solis L, Mino B, Laberiano C, Hernandez S, Gite S, Verma A, Tetzalff M, Haymaker C, Tamegnon A, Rodriguez-Canales J, Hoyd C, Bernachez C, Wistuba I 2020. Procedural requirements and recommendations for multiplex immunofluorescence tyramide signal amplification assays to support translational oncology studies. *Cancers (Basel)* **12**(2):255.

Parra ER, Uraoka N, Jiang M, Cook P, Gibbons D, Forget MA, Bernatchez C, Haymaker C, Wistuba II, Rodriguez-Canales J 2017. Validation of multiplex immunofluorescence panels using multispectral microscopy for immune-profiling of formalin-fixed and paraffin-embedded human tumor tissues. *Sci Rep* **7** (1):13380.

Phillips D, Schürch CM, Khodadoust MS, Kim YH, Nolan GP, Jiang S 2021. Highly multiplexed phenotyping of immunoregulatory proteins in the tumor microenvironment by CODEX tissue imaging. *Front Immunol* **12**:687673.

Qaiser T, Mukherjee A, Reddy PB C, Munugoti SD, Tallam V, Pitäaho T, Lehtimäki T, Naughton T, Berseth M, Pedraza A, Mukundan R, Smith M, Bhalerao A, Rodner E, Simon M, Denzeler J, Huang CH, Bueno G, Snead D, Ellis IO, Ilyas M, Rajpoot N 2018. Her2 challenge contest: A detailed assessment of automated Her2 scoring algorithms in whole slide images of breast cancer tissues. *Histopathology* **72**(2):227–38.

Rost S, Giltnane J, Bordeaux JM, Hitzman C, Koeppen H, Liu SD 2017. Multiplexed ion beam imaging analysis for quantitation of protein expression in cancer tissue sections. *Lab Invest* **97**(8):992–1003.

Shakya R, Nguyen TH, Waterhouse N, Khanna R 2020. Immune contexture analysis in immuno-oncology: Applications and challenges of multiplex fluorescent immunohistochemistry. *Clin Transl Immunology* **9**(10): e1183.

Shamai G, Binenbaum Y, Slossberg R, Duek I, Gil Z, Kimmel R 2019. Artificial intelligence algorithms to assess hormonal status from tissue microarrays in patients with breast cancer. *JAMA Netw Open* **2**(7):e197700.

Spitzer MH, Nolan GP 2016. Mass cytometry: Single cells, many features. *Cell* **165**(4):780–91.

Sun Z, Nyberg R, Wu Y, Bernard B, Redmond WL 2021. Developing an enhanced 7-color multiplex IHC protocol to dissect immune infiltration in human cancers. *PLoS One* **16** (2):e0247238.

Tan WCC, Nierurkar SN, Cai HY, Ng HHM, Wu D, Wee YTF, Lim JCT, Yeong J, Lim TKH 2020. Overview of multiplex immunohistochemistry/immunofluorescence techniques in the era of cancer immunotherapy. *Cancer Commun (Lond)* **40**(4):135–53.

Taube JM, Akturk G, Angelo M, Engle EL, Gnjatic S, Greenbaum S, Greenwald NF, Hedvat CV, Hollmann TJ, Juco J, Parra ER, Rebelatto MC, Rimm DL, Rodriguez-Canales J, Schalper KA, Stack EC, Ferreira CS, Korski K, Lako A, Rodig SJ, Schenck E, Steele KE, Surace MJ, Tetzlaff MT, Von Loga K, Wistuba II, Bifulco CB 2020. The Society for Immunotherapy of Cancer statement on best practices for multiplex immunohistochemistry (IHC) and immunofluorescence (IF) staining and validation. *J Immunother Cancer* **8**(1):e000155.

Viratham Pulsawatdi A, Craig SG, Bingham V, McCombe K, Humphries MP, Senevirathne S, Richman SD, QuirkeP, Campo L, Domingo E, Maughan TS, James JA, Salto-Tellez M 2020. A robust multiplex immunofluorescence and digital pathology workflow for the characterisation of the tumour immune microenvironment. *Mol Oncol* **14**(10):2384–2402.

Wilbur DC, Brachtel EF, Gilbertson JR, Jones NC, Vallone JG, Krishnamurthy S 2015. Whole slide imaging for human epidermal growth factor receptor 2 immunohistochemistry interpretation: Accuracy, precision, and reproducibility studies for digital manual and paired glass slide manual interpretation. *J Pathol Inform* **6**:22.

Willemsen M, Krebbers G, Bekkenk MW, Teunissen MBM, Luiten RM 2021. Improvement of opal multiplex immunofluorescence workflow for human tissue sections. *J Histochem Cytochem* **69**(5):339–46.

Wolff AC, Hammond MEH, Allison KH, Harvey BE, Mangu PB, Bartlett JMS, Bilous M, Ellis IO, Fitzgibbons P, Hanna W, Jenkins RB, Press MF, Spears PA, Vance GH, Viale G, McShane LM, Dowsett M 2018. Human epidermal growth factor receptor 2 testing in breast cancer: American Society of Clinical Oncology/College of American Pathologists Clinical Practice Guideline Focused Update. *J Clin Oncol* **36**(20):2105–22.

Zhang W, Hubbard A, Jones T, Racolta A, Bhaumik S, Cummins N, Zhang L, Garsha K, Ventura F, Lefever MR, Lu Z, Hurley JK, Day WA, Pestic-Dragovich L, Morrisonn LE, Tang L 2017. Fully automated 5-plex fluorescent immunohistochemistry with tyramide signal amplification and same species antibodies. *Lab Invest* **97**(7):873–85.

Zrazhevskiy P, Gao X 2013. Quantum dot imaging platform for single-cell molecular profiling. *Nat Commun* **4**:1619.

Index

accuracy, concept in terms of IHC, 212
adrenocorticotropin, 12
Agilent Dako Omnis, 120
  components, 121–33
    bulk reagents, 130
    hood and touch screen tablet, 122–5
    mixing station, 129
    PC and peripherals, 131–3
    pre-treatment modules, 127
    reagent storage, 129
    slide load drawers, 125–7
    unloading station, 127
    waste containers, 130–1
  detection kits, 136–7
  dimensions, 120
  dynamic gap technology, 133–4
  green credentials, 157
  IHC assay optimization, 151–3
  initial validation protocol, 150–1
  localization antibodies, 134–6
  maintenance tasks, 156–7
    dynamic gap lid clean, 156
    liquid system clean, 156
    minor maintenance tasks, 156–7
  overview, 120–1, 158–9
  principle, 121
  quality assurance programs, 155
  quality control, 150, 153–5
  record logs, 155
  staining protocols, 138–45
    double staining/labelling, 145–6
    immunofluorescence protocol, 140–1
    research protocols, 145
    in situ hybridization (ISH), 142–5
    standard protocol, 138–40
  suggestions for improvement, 157–8
  workflow management, 146–50
alkaline phosphatase (AP), 8
  chromogens capable of development with, 9
analytical processes
  quality management, 34–8, 39–47
  research applications, 164–6
  troubleshooting, 190–9
aniline dyes, 3
antibodies
  antibody cocktails, 232–3
  anti-peroxidase antibodies, 10
  concentrates vs RTUs, 20, 44, 98, 231–2
    BenchMark ULTRA, 97–9
    BOND III, 73
    Omnis, 134–6, 151–3
  conjugation fundamentals, 9–10
  current status of IHC, 230–4
  definition and function, 3
  discovery of serum antibodies, 1
  expired antibodies, avoiding use of, 45
  incorrect, 44, 211
  localization antibodies
    BenchMark ULTRA, 97–9
    BOND III, 73–5
    Omnis, 134–6
  manual titration, BenchMark ULTRA, 96–7
  monoclonal vs polyclonal antibodies, 20, 232
  optimizing for IHC, 168
  performance monitoring, 45
  primary antibody
    selection, 19, 20
    troubleshooting, 193–4
  quality assurance, 233–4
  regulatory framework, 58
  research applications, 164–5, 171–6
  selection process, 44
  standardization of nomenclature, 226
  stock level management, 45
  storage considerations, 44
  validation and verification, 42–4
antibody selection, quality management, 42–5
antibody validation
  NATA recommendations, 43
  parameters, 43
antigen, definition, 3
antigen retrieval
  BenchMark ULTRA, 97
  BOND III, 72–3
  common buffers, 41, 170
  comparison of strategies, 170–1
  heat induced, 40–1
  main methods, 39
  most common technique, 67
  Omnis, *see under* epitope retrieval.
  see also epitope retrieval.
antigen unmasking, 14–15, 41, 187
antigen–antibody interactions, research history, 3–4
artificial intelligence (AI), digital image analysis using, 261–2
Aschoff nodules, 7
auditing, importance of, 27
autofluorescence, 7, 177
automation, 17–19
  advantages of a fully automated system, 85
  benefits and drawbacks, 18–19
  comparison with manual methods, 96–7, 201–2
  definition of IHC automation, 120
  equipment controls, 54–5
  machine selection, 214
  overview, 67–8, 85
  quality management, 42
  see also Agilent Dako Omnis; Leica BOND III IHC system; Roche Ventana BenchMark ULTRA.
avidin, definition, 21
avidin-biotin-peroxidase complex (ABC), 13, 45

basic principles of IHC
  chemistry influences, 6
  histology concepts, 4–6
  immunology concepts, 3–4
BenchMark ULTRA, *see* Roche Ventana BenchMark ULTRA.
beta-galactosidase (β-gal), 9
biotin, definition, 22
block and slide storage, quality management, 38
blocking and quenching
  current status, 228
  research applications, 171
BOND III, *see* Leica BOND III IHC system.
Bouin's solution, 33
bowel cancer, current status of IHC, 243–6
breast cancer, current status of IHC, 246–8
bubble artefact, 33, 69, 189
bulk reagents

BenchMark ULTRA, 92–3
BOND III, 71–2
Omnis, 130

calcium elimination, *see* decalcification.
cauterization, troubleshooting, 185–6
cell block creation, to make the most of a small specimen, 204
chemistry, role in IHC, 6
chromogenic detection, benefits, 45
chromogenic multiplex staining, future applications, 254
chromogenic staining protocol, BenchMark ULTRA, 103–4
chromogens
definition, 22
troubleshooting, 196
clinicians/surgeons, tissue procurement role, 31
CO detection by indEXing (CODEX), future applications, 256–7
coeliac disease, 17
cold/prolonged ischaemic time, 44, 161, 216
definition, 185, 224
measuring, 224, 225
recommendations, 185
troubleshooting, 184, 185, 186
colloidal gold immunolabelling, 9, 12
companion diagnostics staining protocol, BenchMark ULTRA, 108–9
components, Omnis, 121–33
conjugation of antibodies, fundamentals, 9–10
counterstain, troubleshooting, 197
COVID-19 pandemic, 260
current status of IHC, 210, 248–9
antibodies, 230–4
bowel cancer, 243–6
breast cancer, 246–8
lung pathology, 236–40
melanoma, 240–3
protocol for diagnostic histopathology, 227–30
cytology specimens
BenchMark ULTRA staining protocol, 109–10
immunostaining with BOND III, 77–80
quality control, 53

DAB chromogen
antibody cocktails and, 232
avidin-biotin-peroxidase complex and, 13
biotin blocking and, 195–6
BOND III preparation routine, 69
default choice for routine FFPE sections, 227
detection kits
BenchMark ULTRA, 100–2
BOND III, 75, 79
Omnis, 137
double staining, 80, 206
BenchMark ULTRA, 110–11, 117
Omnis, 145–6
enhancement
BenchMark ULTRA, 102–3
Omnis, 139
false positives, 102, 211
haematoxylin and, 47
horseradish peroxidase and, 8–9
mixing strategy, 177
Omnis, 138
most common usage status, 45, 254
pigments and, 198, 227
polymer based detection systems and, 15
post-analytical considerations, 166
reagent selection and, 215
removing residue, 156
research protocols, Omnis, 145
safe disposal requirements, 94, 112, 131
SATB2 IHC staining protocol, 116
special stains and, 221
staining tone, Omnis, 151, 155
standard preparation practice, 129
typical IHC protocol using polymer detection for, 21
waste disposal and, 157
Dako Omnis, *see* Agilent Dako Omnis.
decalcification
available strategies, 34–5
definition, 34
gentler alternatives to hydrochloric acid, 187, 221
IHC assays deployed after, 220–1
quality management, 34–5
troubleshooting, 187
detection systems
BenchMark ULTRA, 102–3
BOND III, 74–5
Omnis, 136–7
polymer based, 15–17, 74–5
quality management, 45–7
research applications, 176–7
standardization, 226–7
troubleshooting, 194–6
dewaxing
temperature considerations, 70–1
troubleshooting, 191
diagnosis, role of IHC assays, 219–20
diagnostic applications for IHC, comparison with research applications, 160–1
diagnostic histopathology, current status of IHC protocol, 227–30
blocking and quenching, 228
epitope retrieval, 227–8
interpretation of IHC assays, 229
personal preferences, 228–9
diagnostic pathology, IHC facility, *see also* IHC facility requirements, 213–18
diaminobenzidine (DAB), *see also* DAB chromogen, 8, 45
digital image analysis, future applications, 261–2
digital pathology, future applications of IHC, 260, 263
diphtheria, 1, 4
direct immunofluorescence (DIF), BOND III, 76–7
direct immunohistochemistry, definition, 22
dispensers, BenchMark ULTRA, 87–9
double staining/labelling
BenchMark ULTRA, 110–11
BOND III, 78–80
concept of, 10
making the most of a small specimen through, 206–7
Omnis, 145–6
sequential, 79–80, 110–11
simultaneous, 78–9
troubleshooting
analytical problems, 197
post-analytical problems, 206–7
drying of slides, recommendations, 108, 190
dynamic gap technology, Omnis, 133–4
dynamic range controls, 51
example of, 52

environmental policies, Agilent, 157
enzyme immunoassay (EIA), 9
enzyme-immunolabelling techniques
comparison with IF methodologies, 10
problem-solving, 10–12
enzyme-linked immunosorbent assay (ELISA), 9
enzymes, visualization fundamentals, 7–9
epitope retrieval
ball of thread analogy, 41
Bond ULTRA, 72
combination approach, 41
current status, 210, 214, 227–8
methods for FFPE blocks, 170
Omnis, 127, 138, 146

epitope retrieval (cont.)
PIER vs HIER, 39–41
see also antigen retrieval; heat-induced epitope retrieval (HIER); proteolytic induced epitope retrieval (PIER).
epitope unmasking, 39, 149, 191
epitopes
definition, 22
immunology role, 3
Epstein Barr, 17, 105, 145
equipment, quality control, 54–5
external quality assurance (EQA) and proficiency programs, 56

facility requirements for IHC, 213–18
equipment and space, 214–15
less invasive techniques, 217–18
reagents and consumables, 215
staffing, 215
standardization of histological processes, 215–17
false negatives, concept in terms of IHC, 211
false positives
concept in terms of IHC, 211
troubleshooting, 102, 211
fixation of tissue
general recommendations, 184
importance of optimal fixation, 32–4
role in IHC success, 5
standardization, 224–6
troubleshooting, 184–5, 186–7
zonal, 36
Flippin protocol, BOND III staining protocol, 76
fluorescein isothiocyanate (FITC)
BenchMark ULTRA protocol, 103, 104
colour, 7, 140
conjugating antibodies, 9
DIF procedure, 219
Omnis protocol, 140–1
optimum dilution, 77
fluorescence, visualization fundamentals, 6–7
fluorescence microscopy, comparison with conventional light microscopy, 7
fluorescence techniques, future applications, 254
fluorochrome, definition, 22
fluorochromes, definition, 6
fluorophores, definition, 6, 22
formaldehyde
dilution rate for tissue fixation purposes, 14, 32, 224
see also formalin fixation.
historical use, 164
problem pigments derived from, 198
superiority as a tissue fixative, 14
formalin, tissue penetration rate, 186
formalin fixation
artefactual sequence alteration problems, 33
mode of action, 14
formalin fixed paraffin embedded (FFPE) blocks
antibody selection, 193
BenchMark ULTRA and, 86
blocking and quenching, 228
comparison with fresh/frozen tissue, 163
default chromogen, 227
dewaxing procedure, 191
diagnostic settings, 160, 213
digital image analysis, 261
double and triple staining, 233
elimination of calcium, 187
see also decalcification.
epitope retrieval methods, 170
front line diagnostic technique, 219
general staining protocol, 20
HIER and, 39–41
ion beam imaging, 259
mass spectrometry preparation requirements, 259
most important factors for IHC success, 5
multiple samples, 217–18
multiplex staining, 253
TSA, 254
Omnis staining protocol, 141
pre-treatment, 191–3
research settings, 168–70
special stains, 221–2
stages of IHC procedure, 20–1
standard protocol, 215
standardization for referral to different facilities for IHC staining, 215–16
tissue fixation and processing, 5, 224–6
tissue selection considerations, 34
typical IHC protocol using polymer detection for DAB, 21
fundamentals of IHC
antibody conjugation, 9–10
basic principles, 3–6
elements of the discipline, 1
modern era, 13–14
origins, 1–3
staining technique, 19–21
theory, 1
visualization via enzymes, 7–9
visualization via fluorescence, 6–7
future applications of IHC, 263
digital image analysis using AI, 261–2
digital pathology, 260, 263
multiplex staining, 253–4
chromogenic, 254
CO detection by indEXing (CODEX), 256–7
fluorescence techniques, 254
tyramide signal amplification, 254–6
nanocrystal quantum dots (QDs), 257
next generation, 253–63
see also next generation techniques.
quality management, 61–2
tissue microarrays, 262–3

glass slides, quality management, 38
glucose oxidase, 8
glutaraldehyde, 9, 33
gold, colloidal, 9, 12
green credentials, Omnis, 157
guidelines/technical advice, 178–9

haematoxylin and eosin (H&E), *see also* H&E staining, 5
H&E staining, 202
bowel cancer use, 243
breast cancer use, 247–8
complementary role of IHC assays, 218–19
decalcification and, 221
economic perspective, 37
formalin fixation and, 14
front line diagnostic technique, 219–20
gold standard of histology status, 228
importance of high quality tissue morphology, 187
limitations in cancer use, 248
lung pathology use, 237
melanoma use, 241
objective, 5
process, 5
re-staining, 205
tissue fixation and processing, 224
zonal fixation and, 36
heat induced epitope retrieval (HIER), quality management, 39–41
heat-induced epitope retrieval (HIER)
common buffers, 215
comparison with PIER, 39–41, 170
current status, 227–8
heating methods utilized for, 15
introduction, 67
microwave irradiation method, 67

hiding sections, to make the most of a small specimen, 202
histology, role in IHC, 4–6
hood
  BenchMark ULTRA, 87–9
  Omnis, 122–5
horseradish peroxidase (HRP), 8, 45, 101, 255
  chromogens capable of development with, 8
humidity control, Omnis, 127

IHC assay
  classification as medical device, 58–61, 63, 210
  comparison with IHS assay, 211
  interpretation
    current status, 229
    staff training requirements, 47–8
  in-vitro diagnostic (IVD) status, 210
  optimization with Omnis, 151–3
  quality management, 39–47, 48
    see also under quality management.
  report generation, 48
  roles served by, 218–23
    see also roles served by IHC assays.
immunochemistry, 4
immunofluorescence (IF)
  BenchMark ULTRA protocol, 104–5
  BOND III protocol, 76–7
  comparison with enzyme-immunolabelling techniques, 10
  definition, 22
  development history, 6–7
  faults, 7
  Omnis protocol, 140–1
  technique development, 67
immunoglobulin G (IgG) molecules, 9
immunoglobulin-enzyme bridge method, 10
immunohistochemical critical assay performance controls (ICAPCs), 45
immunohistochemistry (IHC), 13–14
  aim, 3
  current status, 210, 248–9
  definition, 22, 210
  early work, 253
  elements of the discipline, 1
  origins, 1–3
  overview, 1, 85
  practical limitations, 12
  staining technique, 19–21
    see also staining protocols.
  summary of steps in the process, 227
  theoretical basis, 1
  traditional model, 253
immunolabelling
  concept of, 6
  direct approach, 10
immunolabelling techniques, problem-solving, 10–12, 13
immunology, role in IHC, 3–4
indirect immunohistochemistry, definition, 22
indirect immunolabelling, layer-based technique, 10
in-situ hybridization (ISH)
  antigen retrieval for pre-treatment, 80
  automation and, 42
  BenchMark ULTRA, 85, 103, 105–8, 114
  BOND III and, 82
  combining IHC with, 16, 18
  concept in terms of IHC, 210
  definition, 22, 210
  double staining and, 206
  fluorescence microscopy and, 220
  molecular analysis, 234, 235
  Omnis, 120, 142–5
  referral to different facilities for, 216
  staining protocols, 75
  tissue microarrays (TMAs), 262
  tray allocation and, 71
International Quality Network for Pathology (IQNPAth), 57
inventory controls, 54
in-vitro diagnostics (IVD), 60
  classification of IHC assay as, 210
  classifications, 211
  and in-house IVD tests, 59–60
  medical devices, regulatory framework, 58–61
ion beam imaging, 259
ischaemia/ischaemic effect, 33, 111
ischaemic time, cold/prolonged, *see* cold/prolonged ischaemic time.

labelled streptavidin-biotin-enzyme conjugate (LSAB), 13
laboratory requirements, *see* facility requirements for IHC.
Leica BOND III IHC system
  antigen retrieval, 72–3
  bulk reagent storage, 69–70
  covertiles, 69
  dimensions, 68
  immunostaining cytology specimens, 77–80
    cell blocks, 78
    double staining technique, 78–80
    sequential double staining, 79–80
    simultaneous double staining, 78–9
    smears, 77–8
  localization antibodies, 73–5
    optimum titration, 73–4
    polymer detection kits, 74–5
  maintenance, 81–2
  pre-staining processes, 70–1
  principle, 68–73
  proprietary bulk solutions, 71–2
  quality control, 80–1
  reagent drawer, 69
  robotic systems, 68
  slide drawers, 68
  staining protocols, 75–7
    Flippin protocol, 76
    immunofluorescence protocol, 76–7
  suggested enhancements for future models, 82
  tray allocation, 71
less invasive techniques, *see also* small specimen samples, 217–18, 253
lifting sections, to make the most of a small specimen, 204–6
liquid coverslip technology, BenchMark ULTRA, 85, 95–6
localization antibodies
  BenchMark ULTRA, 97–9
  BOND III, 73–5
  Omnis, 134–6
LSAB technique, 13, 15
lung pathology, current status of IHC, 236–40
lymphoma queries, tissue procurement requirements, 32

macro cut-up, selection of tissue at, 34
maintenance
  BenchMark ULTRA, 112–14
  BOND III, 81–2
  Omnis, 156–7
mass spectrometry immunohistochemistry (MSIHC), 258–9
  advantages and disadvantages, 260
medical device, classification of IHC assays as, 58–61, 63, 210
melanoma, current status of IHC, 240–3
microarrays, *see* tissue microarrays (TMAs).
microwave burn pattern, 72, 97
mixed-antibody method, 10
mixing station, Omnis, 129
molecular technologies
  IHC and, 234–6
  limitations, 235
monoclonal antibodies, vs polyclonal, 20, 232
morphology, definition, 22

mouse on mouse studies, 161
multiplex ion beam imaging, 259
multiplex staining, 10
  future applications, 253–4
multiplexing, 45
  research applications, 161

nanocrystal quantum dots (QDs), future applications, 257
negative controls, 51–2
next generation techniques, 253–63
  mass spectrometry immunohistochemistry (MSIHC), 258–9
  multiplex ion beam imaging, 259
  scanning mass cytometry, 260
nomenclature of antibodies, standardization, 226
Nordic immunohistochemical quality control (NordiQC), 57

Omnis, *see* Agilent Dako Omnis.
on-line resources, quality control, 58
optimum titration of localization antibodies, BOND III, 73–4
overheating of tissue sections, as source of poor immunostaining, 70

packaging, environmental perspective, 157
PC and peripherals, Omnis, 131–3
periodic acid Schiff (PAS) reaction, 17
peroxidase anti-peroxidase (PAP) technique, 11–12, 67
pigments, troubleshooting, 198–9
poka-yoke, Japanese principle, 121
polyclonal antibodies, vs monoclonal, 20, 232
polymer based detection systems, 15–17
  BOND III, 74–5
polysaccharides, 4
post-analytical processes
  quality management, 48
  research applications, 166–7
  troubleshooting, 199–207
pre-analytical processes
  quality management, 31–4, 38–9
  research applications, 161–4
  troubleshooting, 184–90
precision, concept in terms of IHC, 212
pre-cut controls, quality management, 39
predictive markers, concept in terms of IHC, 211
pre-treatment, quality management, 39–41
pre-treatment modules, Omnis, 127
pre-treatment process, troubleshooting, 191–3
primary antibodies, definition, 22
processing of tissue
  quality management, 35–7
  role in IHC success, 5
  standardization, 224–6
procurement of tissue
  considerations for clinicians/surgeons, 31–2
  importance of avoiding ischaemic effects in tissues, 33
  importance of optimal fixation, 32–4
  thickness considerations, 34
prognostic markers, concept in terms of IHC, 212
proteolytic induced epitope retrieval (PIER), 15, 41
  common digestion enzymes, 42
  comparison with HIER, 39–41, 170
  quality management, 41

quality assurance, 25–7
  antibodies, 233–4
  definition, 25
  examples of activities, 25–6
quality assurance programs, Omnis, 155
quality control
  BenchMark ULTRA, 111–12
  BOND III, 80–1
  definition, 25
  external, 56–8
  internal, 50–6
  Omnis, 150, 153–5
  research applications, 167–8
quality improvement
  concept of, 27–8
  definition, 27
quality management
  analytical processes
    block and slide storage, 38
    decalcification, 34–5
    general histology, 34–8
    IHC assay, 39–47
      antibody selection, 42–5
        performance monitoring, 45
        selection process, 44
        storage considerations, 44
        validation and verification, 42–4
      automation, 42
      detection system, 45–7
    processing of tissue, 35–7
    sectioning of tissue, 37–8
    selection of tissue at macro cut-up, 34
  external quality control, 56–8
    EQA and proficiency programs, 56
    IQNPAth, 57
    NordiQC program, 57
    on-line resources, 58
    RCPA QAP, 57–8
  future of quality management in IHC, 61–2
  IHC controls, 48
  IHC staining, influencing factors, 28–30
  internal quality control, 50–6
    cytology specimens, 53
    dynamic range controls, 51
    equipment controls, 54–5
    IHC system control, 56
    internal tissue controls, 55–6
    inventory controls, 54
    negative controls, 51–2
    renal IHC controls, 53
    specific controls for specific situations, 52
    staffing controls, 54
    tissue control banks, 53
  key elements, 24
  overview, 24, 62, 183
  post-analytical processes, IHC assay, 48
    IHC interpretation, 47, 48
    report generation, 48
  pre-analytical processes, 31–4
    fixation of tissue, 32–4
    general histology, 38
    IHC assay, 38–9
      glass slides, 38
      pre-cut controls, 39
      pre-treatment, 39–41
        combination approach to epitope retrieval, 41
        heat induced epitope retrieval (HIER), 39–41
        proteolytic enzymes, 41
    tissue procurement, 31–2
  quality assurance, 25–7
    definition, 25
  quality control, 25
  quality improvement, 27–8
  regulatory framework, 58
  therapeutic goods administration, 58–61
    IVD and in-house IVD tests, 59–60
    medical device terminology, 59
    TGA standards application, 60–1
  troubleshooting IHC issues, 63
quantitative/qualitative analysis, role of IHC assays, 223

reagent application, troubleshooting, 191

reagent storage, Omnis, 129
reagents
  access points, BenchMark ULTRA, 96
  accidental loading, 121
  bulk, *see* bulk reagents.
reagents and consumables, IHC facility requirements, 215
record logs, Omnis, 155
renal biopsies, limitations, 53
report generation, IHC assays, 48
research applications for IHC
  analysis of the staining assay, 177–8
  analytical stage, 164–6
    aliquot contents, 165
    antibody host species, 165
    antibody name, 164
    antibody source, 164
    clonality and Ig class, 165
    enrichment/purification process, 166
    lot/serial number, 165
    manufacture and expiry dates, 165
    protein concentration, 165
    storage, 165
    visualization, 166
  antibody optimization, 168
  antigen retrieval, 170–1
    common buffers, 41, 170
  blocking and quenching, 171
  comparison with diagnostic applications, 160–1
  detection system, 176–7
  guidelines/technical advice, 178–9
  overview, 160, 179
  post-analytical stage, 166–7
    localization, 166
    morphology requirements, 166
    staining pattern, 166
  pre-analytical stage, 161–4
    background information, 163
    fixation, 163–4
    nature of test tissue, 163–4
    section thickness, 163
    tissue origin, 163
    tissue source, 163
  quality control, 167–8
    control tissue, 167
      nature and fixation, 167
      source, 167
    stereological analysis, 167–8
    Western blot optimization, 167
  test material selection, 168–70
  test/primary antibody, 171–6
  visualization, 177
research protocols, Omnis, 145
resolution, concept in terms of IHC, 212
resolving power, concept in terms of IHC, 212
re-staining slides, to make the most of a small specimen, 202
retrieval solution, common examples, 41
rheumatic fever, 7
Roche Ventana BenchMark ULTRA, 85
  antigen retrieval, 97
  components, 86–95
    bulk reagents, 92–3
    PC and peripherals, 94–5
    reagent hood and dispensers, 87–9
    slide drawers, 89–92
    waste containers, 93–4
  detection kits, 99–103
    amplification kits, 102–3
    OptiView DAB, 101–2
    UltraView DAB, 100–1
    UltraView Fast Red, 102
  dimensions, 87
  general buffers with corresponding histology nomenclature, 115
  IHC reagents with corresponding histology nomenclature, 115
  ISH reagents with corresponding histology nomenclature, 116
  liquid coverslip technology, 85, 95–6
  localization antibodies, 97–9
  maintenance, 112–14
  manual antibody titration, 96–7
  maximization of enzyme labels, 15
  overview, 85, 114
  principle, 85–6
  quality control, 111–12
  reagent access points, 96
  research applications, 86
  staining protocols, 103–11
    chromogenic protocol, 103–4
    companion diagnostics, 108–9
    cytology preparations, 109–10
    double labelling, 110–11
      sequential, 110–11
    immunofluorescence protocol, 104–5
    PIN4 protocol, 118
    SATB2 IHC staining protocol, 117
    in situ hybridization, 85, 103, 105–8
  tray allocation of commonly used reagents, 88
  unique technology, 114
roles served by IHC assays, 218–23
  complementing the H&E stain, 218–19
  deployed after tissue decalcification, 220–1
  front line diagnostic technique, 219–20
  quantitative and qualitative analyses, 223
  special stains and IHC, 221–3
Royal College of Pathologists of Australasia Quality Assurance Program (RCPA QAP), 57–8

scanning mass cytometry (SCM), 260
secondary antibodies, definition, 22
sectioning of tissue
  good practice, 37–8
  troubleshooting, 188–90
sensitivity, concept in terms of IHC, 211
Serotherapeutic Institute, Vienna, 3
serum antibodies, discovery of, 1
slide load drawers, Omnis, 125–7
slide storage, quality management, 38
slides, glass slides, 38
small specimen samples
  benefits of using, 217–18
  multiple testing options, 202–7
    lifting section technique, 208
smears, 77–8
special stains, relationship with IHC, 221–3
specificity, concept in terms of IHC, 211
staff training, requirements for IHC interpretation, 47–8
staffing
  controls, 54
  IHC facility requirements, 215
staining assay analysis, requirements, 177–8
staining modules, Omnis, 127
staining protocols
  BenchMark ULTRA, 103–10
  BOND III, 75–7
  controls selection, 20
  influencing factors, 28–30
  Omnis, 138–45
  primary antibody selection, 19, 20
  procedure, 20–1
  validation requirements, 25
standardization, 223–7
  detection system and chromogen choice, 226–7
  IHC facility requirements, 215–17
  nomenclature of antibodies, 226
  for referral to other facilities, 215–16
  tissue fixation and processing, 224–6
stock level management, 54
Stoke's shift, 7
surgeons, tissue procurement role, 31

temperature control, Omnis, 127

terminology, key concepts, 210–13
accuracy, 212
false negative, 211
false positive, 211
IHC and ISH, 210
precision, 212
predictive markers, 211
prognostic markers, 212
resolution, 212
resolving power, 212
sensitivity, 211
specificity, 211
verification/validation, 212–13
tetanus, 2
Therapeutic Goods Administration (TGA), 24
application of standards, 60–1
therapeutic goods administration, quality management, 58–61
tissue controls
banking, 53
cytology specimens, 53
dynamic range, 51
internal, 55–6
negative, 51–2
positive and negative, 25
renal IHC controls, 53
for specific situations, 52
troubleshooting, 190–1
tissue fixation, *see* fixation of tissue.
tissue microarrays (TMAs), future applications, 262–3
tissue processing, *see* processing of tissue.
tissue procurement, *see* procurement of tissue.
tissue specimens
decalcification considerations, 34–5, 220–1
examples of poor tissue processing, 36–7
good sectioning practice, 37–8
processing considerations, 35–7
see also small specimen samples.
touch screen tablet, Omnis, 122–5
transurethral resection of prostate (TURPs), 185
trichrome stain technique, 5
troubleshooting
accidental loading of reagent vial, 121
analytical problems, 190–9
chromogens, 196
counterstain, 197
detection systems, 194–6
dewaxing, 191
double staining, 197
pigments, 198–9
pre-treatment process, 191–3
primary antibody, 193–4
reagent application, 191
tissue controls, 190–1
expired antibodies, 45
false negatives, 211
false positives, 102, 211
immunolabelling techniques, 10–12, 13
making the most of a specimen, 202–7
creating cell blocks, 204
double staining, 206–7
hiding sections, 202
lifting sections, 204–6
re-staining, 202
manual vs automated methods, 96–7, 201–2
overheating of tissue sections, 70
overview, 183
post-analytical problems, 199–207
hints for troubleshooting, 199–201
pre-analytical problems, 184–90
cauterization, 185–6
cold ischaemic time, 185
decalcification, 187
sectioning, 188–90
tissue fixation, 184–5, 186–7
tissue processing, 186–7
tracking possible causes of sub-optimal IHC results, 25
troubleshooting IHC issues, 63
unreliable protocols, 12–13
use of incorrect antibody, 44, 211
tubulitis, 17
tyramide signal amplification, future applications, 254–6

unlabelled antibody method, 10
unloading station, Omnis, 127

validation protocol, Omnis, 150–1
verification/validation, concept in terms of IHC, 212–13
Vimentin, 'canary in the mine' role, 56
visualization
research applications, 177
via enzymes, 7–9
via fluorescence, 6–7

waste handling
BenchMark ULTRA, 93–4
DAB chromogen, 157
Omnis, 130–1
water quality, importance of, 35, 227
Western blots, 3, 161, 167, 179, 216